Clinical Nephrogeriatrics

Carlos Guido Musso • José Ricardo Jauregui
Juan Florencio Macías-Núñez • Adrian Covic
Editors

Clinical Nephrogeriatrics

An Evidence-Based Guide

Springer

Editors
Carlos Guido Musso
Nephrology Division
Hospital Italiano de Buenos Aires
Buenos Aires
Argentina

José Ricardo Jauregui
Hospital Italiano de Buenos Aires
Buenos Aires
Argentina

Juan Florencio Macías-Núñez
Departamento de Medicina
Salamanca
Spain

Adrian Covic
University of Medicine "Grigore T. Popa"
and University Hospital "C. I. Parhon"
Iasi
Romania

ISBN 978-3-030-18713-2 ISBN 978-3-030-18711-8 (eBook)
https://doi.org/10.1007/978-3-030-18711-8

This Springer imprint is published by the registered company Springer Nature Switzerland AG
The registered company address is: Gewerbestrasse 11, 6330 Cham, Switzerland

"To Professors Dr. Stewart Cameron,
Dr. Dimitios G. Oreopoulos, Dr. Isidoro Fainstein,
Dr. David Galinsky. Dr. Roberto Kaplan,
and Dr. Hugo A. Schifis"

Foreword

The population of the world is growing older at an unprecedented rate. In 2015, about 620 million persons were over age 65 years, and this number is expected to grow to 1.6 billion by 2050. Wide disparities exist among the regions of the world concerning the fraction of elders in the population. For example, in Europe in 2018, about 1 of every 6 individuals was over 65 years of age, whereas the comparable statistic for Africa is 1 out of every 33 individuals. The frequency of the "oldest old" (over 80 years of age) is expected to increase globally from 125 million currently to about 450 million by 2050. Global life expectancy (at birth) is now 69 years and is projected to grow to 76 years by 2050. The origin of this changing population dynamics is complex but entails lower birth rates, control of communicable diseases affecting the young, and more effective control of noncommunicable disease afflicting the older adults, most dramatically cardiovascular disease. These sobering statistics make geriatric and gerontology disciplines of great and growing interest broadly and specifically for nephrology. Kidney diseases, both acute and chronic, are quite common in the older and elder adult and therefore are expected to increase as the world ages. Thus, a comprehensive monograph on clinical nephrogeriatrics is both needed and timely. Dr. Musso and his editorial colleagues have assembled a distinguished group of international authors to bring forth a detailed examination of the physiology, anatomy, pathology, and clinical expression of diseases of the kidney in aging. The topics covered are broad in scope and practical in orientation, so as to make the volume of high value to practitioners dealing with older patients with kidney diseases, including those that eventuate in the need for renal replacement therapy. Disorders of fluid, electrolyte, and acid-base, blood pressure regulation, infection, nutrition, and urolithiasis in older subjects receive appropriate attention. The important topic of medication prescribing in the elderly patients is given a thorough review. Finally, palliative and conservative care for those unfortunate elderly patients with end-stage kidney disease and limited life expectancy is covered in a compassionate way.

All in all, this monograph fills an important gap in the literature of nephrology. I predict that it will be widely read. As this tome addresses an ever-changing topic of high and growing interest, I expect that it will undergo an evolution through multiple editions, especially as our knowledge of the fundamental biology of the aging kidney expands in future years. Congratulations to the editors and authors for such a successful start to a long-term enterprise.

Richard J. Glassock, MD, MACP
Department of Medicine
David Geffen School of Medicine at UCLA
Los Angeles, CA
USA

Contents

Contributors

Ahmed H. Abdelhafiz, MBChB, MSc, MD, FRCP (UK) Department of Geriatric Medicine, Rotherham General Hospital, Rotherham, UK

Department of Elderly Medicine, Rotherham General Hospital, Rotherham, UK

Nneoma Agbasi, RMN, MSc, PGDip NELFT Quality Improvement Programme, NELFT NHS Foundation Trust, Basildon, Essex, UK

Filippo Aucella, MD Department of Nephrology and Dialysis, Scientific Institute for Research and Health Care "Casa Sollievo della Sofferenza" IRCCS, San Giovanni Rotondo, Italy

Joanne M. Bargman, MD, FRCPC University Health Network and University of Toronto, Toronto, ON, Canada

Vincenzo Bellizzi, MD, PhD Division of Nephrology, Dialysis and Transplantation, Nephrology Unit, University Hospital "San Giovanni di Dio e Ruggi d'Aragona", Salerno, Italy

European Renal Nutrition (ERN) Working Group at the European Renal Association – European Dialysis Transplant Association (ERA-EDTA), London, UK

Waldo H. Belloso, MD Clinical Pharmacology Section, Internal Medicine Service, Hospital Italiano de Buenos Aires, Buenos Aires, Argentina

Angela Benjumea, MD Internal Medicine and Geriatrics, Universidad de Caldas, Manizales, Colombia

Patrizia Calella, RD, PhD Department of Movement Sciences and Wellbeing, Parthenope University, Naples, Italy

Maria Mercedes Capotondo, MD Nephrology Division, Hospital Italiano de Buenos Aires, Buenos Aires, Argentina

Philippe Chauveau, MD European Renal Nutrition (ERN) Working Group at the European Renal Association – European Dialysis Transplant Association (ERA-EDTA), London, UK

Aurad Aquitaine et Service de Néphrologie CHU de Bordeaux, Bordeaux, France

Ricardo Correa-Rotter, MD Nephrology Department, National Institute of Medical Sciences "Salvador Zubiran", Mexico City, Mexico

Adrian Covic, PhD, FERA, FRCP, FESC University of Medicine "Grigore T. Popa" and University Hospital "C. I. Parhon", AOSR, Iasi, Romania

Neera K. Dahl, MD, PhD Section of Nephrology, Yale School of Medicine, New Haven, CT, USA

Nada Dimkovic, MD, PhD Clinical Department for Renal Diseases, Zvezdara University Medical Center, Belgrade, Serbia

Meguid El Nahas, MD, PhD, FRCP Global Kidney Academy, Sheffield, UK

Theodoros Eleftheriadis, MD, PhD Division of Nephrology and Hypertension, 1st Department of Internal Medicine, AHEPA Hospital, Medical School, Aristotle University of Thessaloniki, Thessaloniki, Greece

Myrto Giannopoulou, MD, PhD Division of Nephrology and Hypertension, 1st Department of Internal Medicine, AHEPA Hospital, Medical School, Aristotle University of Thessaloniki, Thessaloniki, Greece

David S. Goldfarb, MD Nephrology Section, New York Harbor VA Healthcare System and NYU Langone Health, New York, NY, USA

Eirini Grapsa, MD, PhD Nephrology Department Aretaieio University Hospital, National and Kapodistrian University of Athens, Athens, Greece

Kristian Heldal, MD, PhD, MHA Clinic of Internal Medicine, Telemark Hospital Trust, Skien, Norway

Institute of Clinical Medicine, Faculty of Medicine, University of Oslo, Oslo, Norway

Department of Transplantation Medicine, Section of Nephrology, Oslo University Hospital, Oslo, Norway

José Ricardo Jauregui, MD, PhD Ageing Biology Unit, Hospital Italiano de Buenos Aires, Buenos Aires, Argentina

Lina Johansson, RD, PhD European Renal Nutrition (ERN) Working Group at the European Renal Association – European Dialysis Transplant Association (ERA-EDTA), London, UK

Department of Nutrition and Dietetics, Imperial College Healthcare NHS Trust, London, UK

Clare B. Jones, MB, ChB University Health Network and University of Toronto, Toronto, ON, Canada

Joseph Kavanagh, MBChB, MRCP (UK) Department of Geriatric Medicine, Rotherham General Hospital, Rotherham, UK

Vassilios Liakopoulos, MD, PhD Division of Nephrology and Hypertension, 1st Department of Internal Medicine, AHEPA Hospital, Medical School, Aristotle University of Thessaloniki, Thessaloniki, Greece

Juan Florencio Macías-Núñez, MD, PhD Departamento de Medicina, University of Salamanca, Salamanca, Spain

Rachel Marshall, MBChB, MRes, MRCP (UK) Department of Geriatric Medicine, Rotherham General Hospital, Rotherham, UK

Carlos Guido Musso, MD, PhD Nephrology Division, Hospital Italiano de Buenos Aires, Buenos Aires, Argentina

Physiology Department, Instituto Universitario del Hospital Italiano de Buenos Aires, Buenos Aires, Argentina

Ageing Biology Unit, Hospital Italiano de Buenos Aires, Buenos Aires, Argentina

Arunraj Navaratnarajah, MA BMBCh (Oxon) MRCP West London Renal and Transplant Centre, Hammersmith Hospital, Imperial NHS Healthcare Trust, London, UK

Macaulay Amechi Chukwukadibia Onuigbo, MD MSc, FWACP, FASN, MBA The Robert Larner, M.D. College of Medicine, University of Vermont, Burlington, VT, USA

College of Business, University of Wisconsin MBA Consortium, Eau Claire, WI, USA

Lucas Petraglia, MD Internal Medicine Department, Hospital Italiano de Buenos Aires, Buenos Aires, Argentina

Chrysoula Pipili, MD, PhD Nephrology Department Aretaieio University Hospital, National and Kapodistrian University of Athens, Athens, Greece

Luis Miguel Gutiérrez Robledo, MD, PhD National Institute of Geriatrics, Mexico City, Mexico

Stefanos Roumeliotis, MD, PhD Division of Nephrology and Hypertension, 1st Department of Internal Medicine, AHEPA Hospital, Medical School, Aristotle University of Thessaloniki, Thessaloniki, Greece

Paula Scibona, MD Clinical Pharmacology Section, Internal Medicine Service, Hospital Italiano de Buenos Aires, Buenos Aires, Argentina

Daniel Teta, MD, PhD European Renal Nutrition (ERN) Working Group at the European Renal Association – European Dialysis Transplant Association (ERA-EDTA), London, UK

Service of Nephrology, Hospital of Sion and University of Lausanne, Lausanne, Switzerland

Manuel F. Vilas, MD Nephrology Division, Hospital italiano de Buenos Aires, Buenos Aires, Argentina

Luminita Voroneanu, MD, PhD University of Medicine "Grigore T. Popa" and University Hospital "C. I. Parhon", Iasi, Romania

Michelle Willicombe, MA, MBBS, MRCP, MD West London Renal and Transplant Centre, Hammersmith Hospital, Imperial NHS Healthcare Trust, London, UK

Structural and Functional Renal Changes Secondary to Aging

1

Nada Dimkovic

A complex process involves all organs along the time, which is reflected in structural and functional changes that delineate the process of "organ aging." The basis of this process are numerous, known and less known mechanisms that vary not only by age but also by genetic factors, gender, ethnicity, and comorbidities. Although the aging process is controlled by signaling pathways very similar to disease processes, age-related alterations are different to those induced by diseases. Sometimes, these two processes cannot be easily distinguished, and this diagnostic problem is much more common in older than in younger patients.

Interest in the aging kidney has gained significance from the time when the limit for the diagnosis of chronic kidney disease (CKD) was established. Namely, the threshold for defining CKD based on estimated glomerular filtration rate (eGFR) was value less than 60 ml/min/1.73 m^2. Accepted limit led to the diagnosis of a large number of elderly with CKD. Although this limit is not necessarily true for a group of elderly, a reduced kidney function along with a normal aging process has an important role in daily clinical practice to drug dosing, kidney donor selection, and the definition of the risk of acute kidney damage due to a reduced renal reserve. Therefore, most of the papers were related to renal function and determination of glomerular filtration rate (GFR) in the elderly.

Changes in the kidneys during the aging process can be detected by the imaging procedure (IP) [1–5], kidney biopsy [6–8], and by functional testing [9, 10] (Table 1.1).

The first molecular biology of aging at the cellular level was proposed by Dr. Harman who suggested oxidative stress and free radicals as a major cause of aging [9]. Additionally, accumulation of pro-fibrogenic mediators, mitochondrial damage, and loss of telomeres correlate with the process of kidney aging [11]. The process

N. Dimkovic (✉)
Clinical Department for Renal Diseases, Zvezdara University Medical Center, Belgrade, Serbia
e-mail: dim@eunet.rs

C. G. Musso et al. (eds.), *Clinical Nephrogeriatrics*,
https://doi.org/10.1007/978-3-030-18711-8_1

Table 1.1 Basic structural and functional changes in the kidney during the aging process

IP finding	Biopsy finding	Functional changes
More and larger kidney cysts Focal scars Increased surface roughness Decreased cortical volume Atherosclerosis of kidney artery	Global glomerulosclerosis Thickening of GBM Increase in mesangial matrix Tubular atrophy Tubular diverticula Interstitial fibrosis Arteriosclerosis Arteriolar hyalinosis Nephron hypertrophy	GFR decline Increased glomerular capillary permeability Reduced tubular reabsorptive capacity (sodium, urea, magnesium) Reduced secretory capacity (potassium, creatinine) Reduced urine concentration-dilution capacity Production of kidney hormones: preserved (erythropoietin, parathyroid hormone) and reduced (renin)

of kidney aging involves Klotho gene which is expressed in the distal convoluted tubules. Downregulation of Klotho gene increases the susceptibility to oxidative stress via stimulation of IGF-1 pathway [12]. Increased oxidative stress acts at the three levels [12, 13]:

1. Activate angiotensin II pathway and transcription of transforming growth factor B1 (TGF-B1),
2. Leads to shortening of telomeres via inhibition of telomerase.
3. Activate rapamycin target (TOR) leading to accumulation of malignant mitochondria in cells.

Structural Changes

The first findings of changes in the kidney structure as part of the aging process are based on postmortem studies. It has been established that aging increases the number of sclerotic glomeruli and the frequency of changes in tubules and blood vessels [14]. Precious data was obtained in the era of transplantation by analysis of kidney from healthy donors from six decades. The advantage of these analyses over autopsy was that structural changes in the kidneys obtained by pre-implantation biopsy could be compared with a clinical finding, results in urine and blood (including functional tests) and finding on the computed tomography (CT) angiogram. For a better understanding, changes in the kidneys during aging can be classified into micro- and macroanatomical changes.

Microanatomical Changes

These changes involve three basic components of the kidney: glomeruli, tubules, and vasculature. Changes in glomeruli during the aging process can be characterized as senile glomerulosclerosis with the glomeruli being replaced by fibrous tissue. Simultaneously with the increase in the number of sclerotic glomeruli, the remaining functional glomeruli can be increased. With time, they show progressive folding and thickening of glomerular basal membrane, increasing the volume of the mesangial matrix due to the imbalance between formation and decomposition and finally glomerular tuft collapse: globally sclerotic glomeruli (GSG) [15, 16]. Glomerulosclerosis is a non-specific process, can be due to several factors including ischemia and changes in the light microscope reminiscent of ischemic changes. Prevalence of GSG begins about 30 years of life (25%) and reaches as much as 82% in the eighth decade of life [17]. The number of glomeruli per area of cortex (glomerular density) inversely correlates with glomerular size. Glomerular density is lower in biopsies where less than 10% of glomeruli are sclerotic suggesting that the nephron hypertrophy with age can be detected in regions without significant nephrosclerosis. If the number of sclerotic glomeruli is more than 10%, the density increases due to a large number of small, sclerotic glomeruli and atrophic tubules in the region of significant nephrosclerosis. The described changes lead to discrepancies between weight and size of the kidney in old age. Although the renal weight decreases from 400 g (in the fourth decade) to 300 g (in the ninth decade), the volume of the kidney determined by computerized tomography is not necessarily changed.

Mesangial cells and endothelial cells have been shown to increase in number until the age of 50 years and number progressively decline thereafter. The ratio of the number of mesangial cells to enlarged glomerular volume is therefore initially maintained. Podocytes do not increase in number, and there are some reports that their number decreases over time along with the decreased capacity for their regeneration and repair. Also, podocytes can undergo hypertrophy together with glomerulus hypertrophy. Such changes affect kidney glomerular filtration rate and albumin permeability [18, 19].

Tubulointerstitial changes during the aging process include infarction, scarring, and fibrosis. Fibrosis is an active process that begins with interstitial inflammation and activation of fibroblasts as well as increased expression of adhesive proteins osteopontin and intercellular adhesion molecules 1. Additionally, accumulated collagen contributes to tubulointerstitial changes. Experimental model showed increased collagen deposits and increased expression of genes for fibronectin and TGF-B [20]. In distal tubules, the number of diverticula increases, which can eventually be transformed into simple cysts. Namely, it is well known that the number of simple cysts increases with the aging process [21]. Changes in tubular morphology have also been observed including a decrease in tubule volume and length and increased tubular atrophy [22]. The previously described changes in glomeruli, together with tubulointerstitial changes and changes in blood vessels, constitute the basis of nephrosclerosis. Its prevalence among living donors is 2.7% in the young and up to 73% in the oldest living donors [17].

Blood vessels of the kidney are most usually atheromatous and, if present, can lead to renovascular hypertension, ischemic nephropathy, and/or intrarenal atheroembolic events with consequent chronic renal failure [23]. Pre-arteriolar subendothelial accumulation of hyaline and collagen deposits lead to intimal thickening which can compromise blood vessel lumen and lead to sclerosis of the glomeruli, most often in the area of the kidney cortex. This so-called vascular aging of the kidneys results in the formation of aglomerular circulation in the juxtamedullary glomeruli, which is the communication between the afferent and the efferent arterioles and the redistribution of blood into the medulla [24]. At the same time, intima of small arteries is thickened due to the proliferation of elastic tissue and atrophy of the media. The arcuate arteries become more angulated, and the interlobular arteries become more tortuous and spiral [25, 26]. Data support that there are changes in vascular responsiveness and autoregulation. While vasoconstrictive response to angiotensin was not altered with aging, vasodilatatory response to acetylcholine or to acute sodium load was impaired with aging [27].

Macroanatomical Changes

These changes include modifications in kidney volume, presence of cysts and tumors, often benign. There are many controversies about the kidney volume in the elderly and they come from different measurement methods (CT scan, ultrasound, histology). Also, kidney volume is an unspecific finding since it does not reflect true changes in kidney disease. Earlier data obtained from ultrasound examinations of over 600 volunteers showed that the volume of the kidney correlates with the younger age, weight, heights, and total body surface area [28]. Subsequent data obtained by an examination of individuals without kidney disease showed that the thickness of the kidney parenchyma decreased by 10% with each decade of age [29], data confirmed by the more recent study [30]. More precious data are obtained from the potential kidney donors of a wide range of age. It has been shown that the volume of the kidney is stable up to 50 years of age when it begins to decline [5]. Namely, for up to 50 years, the decrease in cortical volume is compensated by an increase in the volume of the medulla which maintains the dimension of the kidney. After 50 years, the volume of the medulla decreases in women and remains stable in men. Reduction of the cortical volume is the result of an increasing number of globally sclerotic glomeruli (GSG) with atrophy of corresponding tubules (nephrosclerosis). Hypertrophy of non-sclerotic glomeruli and tubules helps to maintain the volume of kidney parenchyma. However, after 50 years, this hypertrophy cannot compensate for the loss of volume due to nephrosclerosis [5, 31].

It has already been noted that changes in the tubules in the form of diverticula can predispose to renal cysts that become more frequent and larger with older age [2]. These cortical and medullar cysts correlate with larger body size, male gender, hypertension, and proteinuria. Parapelvic cysts and angiomyolipomas are also more frequent in older age. Since parapelvic cysts are of lymphatic origin, they are not associated with hypertension and albuminuria [32].

Other structural changes in kidney related to aging include cortical scars, parenchymal calcifications, fibromuscular dysplasia, and kidney artery atherosclerosis with the prevalence of 25% for patients between 65 and 75 years as compared with 0.4% for those younger than 30 years [3].

Functional Changes

Glomerular Functional Changes

Since the early 1950s, it has been known that the urea clearance and GFR decrease with aging process [33, 34]. At present, it is not possible to establish single-nephron GFR, and therefore, there can be considerable heterogeneity of single-nephron GFR between subjects with the same GFR. The GFR remains constant until the fourth decade when it is reduced by an average of 46% from that in young people until the age of 90 [34]. It is worth mentioning that there is reduction in mean creatinine clearance despite no difference in serum creatinine and this can be explained by the so-called senile sarcopenia and by reduced protein intake. At the same time, functional reserve of the kidney (increase of basal GFR by 20% after amino acid load) is decreased in healthy elderly persons and reach its maximum of 50% for 60 min which is less and slower than in younger persons (80% for period of 30 min) [35, 36]. The decline in GFR is associated with a decrease in the effective renal plasma flow (ERPF), from 600 ml/min/1.73 m^2 at youth to 300 ml/min/1.73 m^2 in 80 years old healthy persons. This is followed by an increase in the filtration fraction as the EFRF was disproportionately lower than the GFR [37].

The GFR decline during the aging process can be calculated by Keller's equation that shows eGFR in aged with no signs of kidney weakness [38]:

$$\text{GFR} = 130 - \text{age}\left(\text{in years}\right)$$

Additionally, BIS equation (based on serum creatinine or cystatin C) is currently considered the reliable equations for estimating GFR in the elderly [39, 40]:

$$\text{BIS1 equation} : \text{GFR} = 3736 \times \text{creatinine}^{-0.87} \times \text{age}^{-0.95} \times 0.82\left(\text{if female}\right)$$

$$\text{BIS2 equation} : \text{GFR} = 767 \times \text{cystatin C}^{-0.61} \times \text{creatinine}^{-0.40} \times \text{age}^{-0.57} \times 0.87\left(\text{if female}\right)$$

The causes of decreased glomerular filtration were debated, and it was postulated that reduced GFR was probably associated with existing nephrosclerosis in old age. However, in multivariable models (adjusting for age and gender), biopsy-revealed nephrosclerosis was associated with urinary albumin excretion, nocturnal blood pressure and hypertension but not with GFR [17]. In living donor biopsy series, GFR declined with age independently of nephrosclerosis raising the question of the other pathological changes in the kidney and extrarenal factors contributing to the decline in GFR [41]. The opinion that cortical atrophy and GFR fall under the same mechanism(s) is not always justified given that the GFR decrease is possible regardless of the reduction in cortical volume [5].

Finally, about three decades ago, Lindeman et al. described that about one-third of 254 healthy individuals had an increase in creatinine clearance with aging. Apart from possible imprecision of calculation of the slope of GFR over time, it is possible that transient comorbidities that are associated with aging such as obesity, diabetes, and subclinical cardiovascular disease may lead to transient hyperfiltration and preserved or even increased GFR [42].

Tubulointerstitial Functional Changes

Tubular-interstitial changes related to aging include changes in water, sodium, potassium, urea, creatinine, and divalent cation handling. These are usually interpreted as three "nephrogeriatric giants," which means frequent structural and physiological renal changes in the elderly, which influence the course of the disease and the therapeutic strategies in the elderly [23]:

- Tubular dysfunction
- Medullary hypotonicity
- Tubular frailty

Tubular dysfunction includes changes in water and electrolyte handling which, unrecognized, can cause serious problems in the elderly, particularly in special clinical conditions. Compared to younger persons, reabsorption of sodium in proximal tubules is not different in elderly but it is reduced in the thick ascending loop of Henle (Table 1.2). Therefore, the amount of urinary loss of sodium is increased and the free water clearance is reduced. These changes lead to reduced osmolality of the interstitium and reduced ability of the medulla to concentrate urine. Sodium urinary loss is also potentiated by reduced plasma renin and aldosterone levels. According to some reports, serum and urinary natriuretic peptides are elevated which in turn may increase natriuresis [43]. Elderly individuals also seem to have more sodium excretion at the night suggesting an impaired circadian variation. Knowing about these specificities in sodium handling is very important to avoid hyponatremia and hypovolemia and to adjust fluid intake and therapy in the aged.

Table 1.2 The tubulointerstitial changes in electrolyte handling during the aging process

	Functional change	Consequence
Sodium	Reduced reabsorption in the thick ascending loop of Henle Reduced plasma renin and aldosterone level Elevated serum/urinary natriuretic peptides	Urinary loss Hyponatremia (trend) Dehydration (trend)
Potassium	Reduced muscle mass Low-potassium diet Hyporeninemic hypoaldosteronism	Hyperkalemia (trend)
Magnesium	Increased excretion in volume overload Poor intestinal absorption Decreased intake	Hypomagnesemia (trend)

There are several reasons for the change in potassium handling in the aged. Apart from reduced muscle mass and low potassium diet [44], the elderly have significantly lower renal excretion of potassium compared with the young. Impaired potassium secretion is directly associated with disorders in sodium reabsorption and tubular atrophy and interstitial scarring. Additionally, hyporeninemic hypoaldosteronism and suppression of water and sodium delivery into the distal nephron are associated with potassium secretion disorders in the aging kidney [45]. An increase in H+K+ATPasa pump at collecting tubules leads to increased potassium reabsorption [46].

Magnesium excretion is increased in the scenario of volume overload lowering its serum level. Hypomagnesemia in the elderly may also be explained by decreased intake and poor intestinal absorption that lead to hypomagnesemia. Since in healthy old people sodium reabsorption is reduced in the thick ascending loop of Henle and magnesium reabsorption occurs chiefly at this tubular segment, it has been hypothesized that a urinary magnesium loss could explain this increased Mg excretion [47]. There is no data on altered calcium handling in the elderly with normal renal function, adequate diet, and sunlight exposure.

Experimental data revealed that distal urea reabsorption is decreased in old rats due to the reduction of urea channels (UT1) in the collecting tubules. Urea excretion contributes to osmotic diuresis and together with medullary hypotonicity makes the elderly prone to dehydration [48]. With regard to creatinine, there are data on decreased tubular secretion and even tubular reabsorption in dehydrated elderly [49].

During the aging process, no physiological changes were observed in the level of serum vitamin D, parathormone, or erythropoietin. Therefore, hyperphosphatemia, hyper- and hypocalcemia, and anemia cannot be explained by the process of aging, and one should look for other possible causes.

Elderly people are capable of secreting an acid load and maintain normal serum bicarbonate level and urine pH on a 70 g protein diet [50]. However, following an acid load, senescent kidneys do not increase acid excretion and lower urinary pH to the degree that younger kidneys do. Also, the maximal value of ammonia and titratable acid excretion were reached in 6–8 hours as compared to 4 hours in the young. Therefore, elderly have difficulties to cope acidosis particularly in acute setting [47].

Medullary Hypotonicity

Elderly individuals are not capable to dilute or concentrate urine as well as younger ones and they are more prone to water disorders and volume depletion. The ability to generate free water depends on several factors including sufficient GFR, functional intact distal diluting site, and suppression of antidiuretic hormone to avoid water reabsorption in the collecting duct. According to experimental data from aged rats, there is downregulation of V2 receptors in renal tubules and also lower abundance of aquaporins 2 and 3 [51]. Knowing the changes in kidney function with aging (defect in sodium reabsorption, reduced distal urea reabsorption), the maximal urinary concentration capacity decreases by 30 mOsm/kg per decade after the age of 30. Decreased effect of antidiuretic hormone and water reabsorption capability may cause severe dehydration in elderly who have increased threshold for the thirst [52].

At the same time, there is a decrease in capacity to dilute urine in the aged; maximum free water clearance is reduced from 12.2 to 5.9 ml/min, and minimum urine concentration is 90 mOsm/kg in the elderly as compared with 50 mOsm/kg in the young [43].

Tubular Frailty

Renal tubular cells are more vulnerable to ischemic and toxic injury and also they recover more slowly from acute tubular necrosis [23]. Consequently, aged are predisposed for developing acute kidney injury and chronic kidney disease [53].

Age-Related Changes and Definition of Chronic Kidney Disease

According to the Kidney Disease Improving Global Outcomes (KDIGO) guidelines [54], CKD is present if the patient has a GFR <60 ml/min/1.73 m^2 that persists for 3 months even in the absence of the finding of kidney damage (increased albuminuria). The most commonly used formulas for the calculation of glomerular filtration rate are based on serum creatinine: The Modification of Diet in Renal Disease (MDRD) study equation and Chronic Kidney Disease Epidemiology (CKD-EPI) equation. However, both formulas underestimate measured GFR in healthy adults since they have higher muscle mass as compared to CKD patients.

Namely, in healthy patients with an eGFR between 45 and 59 ml/min/1.73 m^2 CKD-EPI equation underestimate GFR by 16% and the MDRD study equation by 25% [55]. Age-related decline in GFR and underestimation of GFR in healthy older patients are the reasons for overdiagnosis of CKD in the elderly. Therefore, KDIGO 2012 guidelines suggest eGFR measurement based on serum cystatin C, particularly in those with eGFR 45–59 ml/min/1.73 m^2 (according to creatinine-based formulas) and without albuminuria. Still, precaution is needed in case of obesity, inflammation, and atherosclerosis [56].

The importance of determining glomerular filtration in the old ones is reflected in the prediction of the outcome, i.e., the prognosis of the elderly. It has been confirmed that an increase in cardiovascular mortality in individuals over 65 years starts when eGFR is less than 45 ml/min/1.73 m^2 [57]. By analyzing 46 cohorts with more than 2 million individuals, CKD Prognosis Consortium concluded that eGFR less than 60 ml/min/1.73 m^2 is a threshold for CKD in all age groups [58]. However, elderly individuals with eGFR of 45–59 ml/min/1.73 m^2 rather have a reduced kidney reserve than CKD.

Another contribution to more adequate presumptive diagnosis of CKD in the elderly is the HUGE formula based on hematocrit, urea, and gender [59]:

$$\begin{aligned}\text{HUGE} = 2.303458 - (0.264418 \times \text{Hematocrit}) \\ + (0.118100 \times \text{Serum Urea}) [+1.383960 \text{ if male}]\end{aligned}$$

Values less than zero exclude CKD while values equal or higher than zero point to CKD. Although this equation has sensitivity of 92.8%, specificity of 93.2%, and positive predictive value of 95.8%, it is screening method that has to be confirmed by appropriate medical evaluation. However, a prospective study recently conducted in the population of Buenos Aires (Argentina) documented a lower performance of the HUGE formula for detecting CKD, even in the elderly population (sensitivity, 40.0%), also verifying that the performance of the HUGE formula improved when combined with the calculated GFR (MDRD-4) and urinary sediment (sensitivity, 95.8%) [60].

Conclusion

Knowledge about which are the renal aging changes is crucial to differentiate renal aging from chronic kidney disease and understand the trend to the internal milieu alterations and kidney disorders in the elderly.

References

1. Al-Said J, Brumback MA, Moghazi S, Baugarten DA, O'Neill WC. Reduced renal function in patients with simple renal cysts. Kidney Int. 2004;65(6):2303–8.
2. Rule AD, Sasiwimonphan K, Lieske JC, Keddis MT, Torres VE, Vrtiska TJ. Characteristics of renal cystic and solid lesions based on contrast-enhanced computed tomography of potential kidney donors. Am J Kidney Dis. 2012;59(6):611–8.
3. Lorenz EC, Vrtiska TJ, Lieske JC, et al. Prevalence of renal artery and kidney abnormalities by computed tomography among healthy adults. Clin J Am Soc Nephrol. 2010;5(3):431–8.
4. Duan X, Rule AD, Elsherbiny H, et al. Automated assessment of renal cortical surface roughness from computerized tomography images and its association with age. Acad Radiol. 2014;21(11):1441–5.
5. Wang X, Vrtiska TJ, Avula RT, et al. Age, kidney function, and risk factor associate differently with cortical and medullary volumes of the kidney. Kidney Int. 2014;85(3):677–85.
6. Kubo M, Kiyohara Y, Kato I, et al. Risk factors for renal glomerular and vascular changes in an autopsy –based population survey: the Hisayama study. Kidney Int. 2003;63(4):1508–15.
7. Baert L, Steg A. Is the diverticulum of the distal and collecting tubules a preliminary stage of the simple cist in the adult? J Urol. 1977;118(5):707–10.
8. Elsherbiny HE, Alexander MP, Kremers WK, et al. Nephron hypertrophy and glomerulosclerosis and their association with kidney function and risk factors among living kidney donors. Clin J Am Soc Nephrol. 2014;9(11):1892–902.
9. Harman D. Aging: a theory based on free radical and radiation chemistry. J Gerontol. 1956;11(3):298–300.
10. Dai DF, Chiao YA, Marcinek DJ, Szeto HH, Rabinovitch PS. Mitochondrial oxidative stress in aging and health span. Longev Healthspan. 2014;3:6.
11. Perico N, Remuzzi G, Benigni A. Aging and the kidney. Curr Opin Nephrol Hypertens. 2011;20:312–27.
12. Yang H, Fogo A. Cell senescence in the aging kidney. J Am Soc Nephrol. 2010;21:1436–9.
13. Zhou X, Saxena R, Liu Z, et al. Renal senescence in 2008: progress and challenges. Int Urol Nephrol. 2008;40:823–39.
14. Darmady EM, Offer J, Woodhouse MA. The parameters of the ageing kidney. J Pathol. 1973;109(3):195–207.
15. Martin JE, Sheaff MT. Renal ageing. J Pathol. 2007;211(2):198–205.
16. Hoy WE, Douglas-Denton RN, Highson MD, Cass A, Johnson K, Bertram JF. A stereological study of glomerular number and volume: preliminary findings in a multiracial study of kidneys at autopsy. Kidney Int Suppl. 2003;63(83):S31–7.

17. Rule AD, Amer H, Cornell LD, et al. The association between age and nephrosclerosis on renal biopsy among healthy adults. Ann Intern Med. 2010;152(9):561–7.
18. Huber TB, Edelstein CL, Hartleben B, et al. Emerging role of autophagy in kidney function, diseases and aging. Autophagy. 2012;8(7):1009–31.
19. Wiggins JE. Aging in the glomerulus. J Gerontol A Biol Sci Med Sci. 2012;67(12):1358–64.
20. Gagliano N, Arioso B, Santanbrogio B, et al. Age-dependent expression of fibrosis-related genes and collagen deposition in rat kidney cortex. J Gerontol A Biol Sci Med Sci. 2000;55(8):365–72.
21. Lauks SP Jr, McClachlan MS. Aging and simple cysts of the kidney. Br J Radiol. 1981;54(637):12–4.
22. Lindeman RD, Goldman R. Anatomic and physiologic age changes in the kidney. Exp Gerontol. 1986;21(4–5):379–406.
23. Musso CG. Geriatric nephrology and the "nephrogeriatric giants". Int Urol Nephrol. 2002;34:255–6.
24. Takazakura E, Sawabu N, Handa A, et al. Intrarenal vascular changes with age and disease. Kidney Int. 1972;2:224–30.
25. Silva FG. The ageing kidney: a review – part I. Int Urol Nephrol. 2005;37:185–205.
26. Silva FG. The ageing kidney: a review – part II. Int Urol Nephrol. 2005;37:419–32.
27. Hollenberg NK, Adams DF, Solomon HS, et al. Senescence and the renal vasculature in normal man. Circ Res. 1974;34:309–16.
28. Emamiam SA, Nielsen MB, Pedersen JF, Ytte L. Kidney dimensions at sonography: correlation with age, sex, and habitus in 665 adult volunteers. AJR Am J Roenthenol. 1993;160(1):83–6.
29. Gourtsoyiannis N, Prassopoulos P, Cavouras D, Pantelidis N. The thickness of the renal parenchyma decreases with age: a CT study of 360 patients. AJR Am J Roentgenol. 1990;155(3):541–4.
30. Glodny B, Unterholzner V, Taferner B, et al. Normal kidney size and its influencing factors – a 64-slice MDCT study of 1040 asymptomatic patients. BMC Urol. 2009;9:19.
31. McLachlan M, Wasserman P. Changes in sizes and distensibility of the aging kidney. Br J Radiol. 1981;54(642):488–91.
32. Schwarz A, Lenz T, Klaen R, Offermann G, Fiedler U, Nussberger J. Hygroma renale: pararenal lymphatic cysts associated with renin-dependent hypertension (page kidney). Case report on bilateral cysts and successful therapy by marsupialization. J Urol. 1993;150(3):953–7.
33. Smith HW. The kidney: the structure and function in health and disease. New York: Oxford University Press; 1951.
34. Davies DF, Shock NW. Age changes in glomerular filtration rate, effective renal plasma flow, and tubular excretory capacity in adult males. J Clin Invest. 1950;29(5):496–507.
35. Musso CG. Renal reserve test: its methodology and significance. Saudi J Kidney Dis Transpl. 2011;22(5):990–3.
36. Musso CG, Reynaldi J, Martinez B, Pierángelo A, Vilas M, Algranati L. Renal reserve in the oldest old. Int Urol Nephrol. 2011;43(1):253–6.
37. Alvarez Gregori J, Musso C, Macias Núñez JF. Renal ageing. In: Sastre J, Pamolona R, Ramón J, editors. Medical biogerontology. Madrid: Ergon; 2009. p. 111–23.
38. Keller F. Kidney function and age. Nephrol Dial Transplant. 1987;2(5):382.
39. Swedish Council on Health Technology Assessment. Methods to estimate and measure renal function (glomerular filtration rate): a systematic review, SBU Yellow Report No. 214. Stockholm: Swedish Council on Health Technology Assessment (SBU); 2011.
40. Musso CG, Álvarez-Gregori J, Jauregui J, MacíasNúñez JF. Glomerular filtration rate equations: a comprehensive review. Int Urol Nephrol. 2016;48(7):1105–10.
41. Rule AD, Cornell LD, Poggio ED. Senile nephrosclerosis-does it explain the decline in glomerular filtration rate with aging? Nephron Physiol. 2011;119(Suppl):6–11.

42. Eriksen BO, Lochen ML, Arntzen KA, et al. Subclinical cardiovascular disease is associated with high glomerular filtration rate in the nondiabetic general population. Kidney Int. 2014;86(1):146–53.
43. Musso CG, Macías-Núñez JF. Dysfunction of the thick loop of Henle and senescence: from molecular biology to clinical geriatrics. Int Urol Nephrol. 2011;43(1):249–52.
44. Lye M. Distribution of body potassium in healthy elderly subjects. Gerontologie. 1981;27:286–92.
45. Phelps KR, Lieberman RL, Oh MS, et al. Pathophysiology of the syndrome of hyporeninemic hypoaldosteronism. Metabolism. 1980;29:186–99.
46. Musso CG, Miguel RD, Algranati L, Farias Edos R. Renal potassium excretion: comparison between chronic renal disease patients and old people. Int Urol Nephrol. 2005;37(1):167–70.
47. Musso CG, Juarez R, Vilas M, Navarro M, Rivera H, Jauregui R. Renal calcium, phosphorus, magnesium and uric acid handling: comparison between stage III chronic kidney disease patients and healthy oldest old. Int Urol Nephrol. 2012;44(5):1559–62.
48. Musso CG, Alvarez Gregori J, Jauregui JR, Macías Núñez JF. Creatinine, urea, uric acid, water and electrolytes renal handling in the healthy oldest old. World J Nephrol. 2012;1(5):123–6.
49. Musso CG, Michelángelo H, Vilas M, Reynaldi J, Martinez B, Algranati L, Macías Núñez JF. Creatinine reabsorption by the aged kidney. Int Urol Nephrol. 2009;41(3):727–31.
50. Wagner EA, Falciglia GA, Amlal H, et al. Short-term exposure to high-protein diet differentially affect glomerular filtration rate but not acid-base balance in older compared to younger adults. J Am Diet Assoc. 2007;107:1404–8.
51. Preisser L, Teillet L, Aliotti S, et al. Downregulation of aquaporin-2 and -3 in aging kidney is independent of V(2) vasopressin receptor. Am J Phyiol Renal Physiol. 2000;279:F144–52.
52. Musso CG, Macías Núñez JF. Renal handling of water and electrolytes in the old and old-old healthy aged. In: Núñez M, Cameron S, Oreopoulos D, editors. Renal ageing: health and disease. New York: Springer; 2008. p. 141–54.
53. Musso CG, Liakopoulos V, Ioannidis I, Eleftheriadis T, Stefanidis I. Acute renal failure in the elderly: particular characteristics. Int Urol Nephrol. 2006;38(3–4):787–93.
54. Stevens PE, Levin A. Evaluation and management of chronic kidney disease: synopsis of the kidney disease improving global outcomes 2012 clinical practise guideline. Ann Intern Med. 2013;158(11):825–30.
55. Murata K, Bauman NA, Saenger AK, Larson TS, Rule AD, Lieske JC. Relative performance of the MDRD and CKD-EPI equations for estimating glomerular filtration rate among patients with varied clinical presentations. Clin J Am Soc Nephrol. 2011;6(8):1863–972.
56. Rule AD, Glassock RJ. GFR estimating equations: getting closer to the truth? Clin J Am Soc Nephrol. 2013;8(8):1414–20.
57. Stengel B, Metzger M, Froissart M, et al. Epidemiology and prognostic significance of chronic kidney disease in the elderly –the Three-City prospective cohort study. Nephrol Dial Transplant. 2011;26(10):3286–95.
58. Hallan SI, Matsushita K, Sang Y, et al. Age and association of kidney measures with mortality and end-stage renal disease. JAMA. 2012;308(22):2349–60.
59. Robles NR, Felix FJ, Lozano L, Miranda I, Fernandez-Berges D, Macías JF. The H.U.G.E. formula (Hematocrit, Urea, Sex) for screening chronic kidney disease (CKD) in an age-stratified general population. J Nutr Health Aging. 2015;19(6):688–92.
60. Musso CG, Maytin S, Conti P, Terrasa S, Primerano A, Reynaga A, Vilas M, Jauregui J. HUGE equation accuracy for screening chronic kidney disease: a prospective study. J Aging Res Clin Pract. 2017;6:158–62.

Renal Aging and Chronic Kidney Disease in the Elderly: Which Are the Differences?

2

Carlos Guido Musso and Juan Florencio Macías-Núñez

Introduction

First of all, the difference among the concepts of *aging, senescence, and chronic disease* should be clarified: *Aging* is not synonymous of illness but part of the normal vital cycle. Aging is a universal asynchronic and heterogeneous process which induces a series of changes in the organisms through time, characterized by the attenuation of functional performance compared to the maximal functional strength reached around the second decade of life (25–30 years of age). Aging is universal since it is part of everybody's vital cycle, asynchronic since it has its particular rate in each individual, and heterogeneous since it has its particular rate in each individual's organ. However, aging becomes *senescence* when its changes significantly reduce the body homeostatic capability making the organism vulnerable and frail [1–3]. Regarding the concept of *disease,* it is an abnormal process that deteriorates the functionality of any organ or system of organs. When this functional alteration installs abruptly in a previously normal organ, it is considered an *acute disease,* while when it installs slowly and progressively it is considered a *chronic disease* [3–5]. Finally, when senescence combined with a chronic condition, the evolution and prognosis of this condition worsens, and it requires adjusting the conventional therapeutic targets to the patient's frailty status. Because of that, it has been proposed

C. G. Musso
Nephrology Division, Hospital Italiano de Buenos Aires, Buenos Aires, Argentina

Physiology Department, Instituto Universitario del Hospital Italiano de Buenos Aires, Buenos Aires, Argentina

Ageing Biology Unit, Hospital Italiano de Buenos Aires, Buenos Aires, Argentina

J. F. Macías-Núñez (✉)
Departamento de Medicina, University of Salamanca, Salamanca, Spain
e-mail: jfmacias@usal.es

C. G. Musso et al. (eds.), *Clinical Nephrogeriatrics*,
https://doi.org/10.1007/978-3-030-18711-8_2

Table 2.1 Clinical guide for distinguishing an aged kidney from a chronic kidney disease (CKD) and senescent nephropathy

	Healthy oldest old	Stage III – CKD	Senescent nephropathy
GFR	Low (expected value for age)	Low (any value)	Low (any value)
Serum urea	Normal	High	High
Serum creatinine	Normal	High	High
Hematocrit	Normal	Normal/low	Normal/low
Parathyroid hormone	Normal	Elevated	Elevated
Urinalysis	Normal	Normal/altered	Normal/altered
Renal image	Normal	Abnormal	Abnormal
Frailty phenotype	No	No	Yes

GFR glomerular filtration rate

that when a chronic disease suffers from the influence of the senescence process, it should be considered a different condition known as a *senescent chronic disease,* for instance when chronic nephropathy is combined with senescence, it becomes a new condition called *senescent chronic nephropathy*) [6] (Table 2.1). This concept is deeply explained in the chapter dedicated to "nephroprevention in chronic kidney disease in elderly patients."

One of the main points in clinical nephrology is to clearly distinguish between normal renal aging (RA) and chronic kidney disease (CKD) in order to avoid unnecessary medicalization of what is a normal change associated with aging, the potential harmful consequences of such overdiagnosis, such as the exclusion of healthy elderly people from medical procedures due to an erroneous diagnosis of CKD. Besides, among the adverse effects of treating healthy old individuals as CKD patients is the prescription of a low protein diet which can induce malnutrition and sarcopenia, as well as the prescription of renin-angiotensin-aldosterone system inhibitors which can induce hyperkalemia, hyponatremia, hypotension, or/and acute kidney injury [1].

Although RA and CKD are different entities, they share some similarities and because of that they are frequently confused in clinical practice. However, they have important and clear differences which can easily help to distinguish both clinical settings [1].

Since the knowledge of these similarities and differences between RA and CKD are crucial in order not to confuse both entities, they are described in detail as follows.

Chronic Kidney Disease: Renal Aging Similarities

Reduced Glomerular Filtration Rate (GFR) [2, 7–9]

This similarity is the main reason why RA and CKD are usually confused when CKD diagnosis is erroneously based only on the GFR reduction, since healthy oldest old individuals (age ≥ 80 years) and stage III – CKD patients usually have the same low GFR value, around 50 ml/min/1.73 m^2.

This aged induced GFR reduction is caused by renal and systemic mechanisms, such as the senile glomerulosclerosis process, capillary obliteration, arteriosclerosis, tubular atrophy and interstitial fibrosis among the former, and the characteristically reduced basal metabolism in the elderly among the latter. As a consequence there is a progressive renal mass reduction and GFR decline at a rate of 1 ml/year since the fourth decade on. Moreover, the renal reserve (RR) which is the kidney's ability to increase its basal GFR in response to an oral protein overload is usually reduced in both settings (RR, 40%) compared to healthy young people (RR, 80%), although it can be even negative in advanced CKD patients (RR, 0%). This characteristic predisposes RA and CKD people to develop acute kidney injury.

Keller et al. described a simple equation to estimate creatinine clearance (CrCl) in people between 25 and 100 years old with normal serum creatinine value. Thus, Keller equation (CrCl = 130 − age (in years)) is currently the most useful one to determine the expected GFR reduction secondary to aging in healthy elderly people.

This reduction in GFR predisposes both, healthy elderly and CKD patients, to require adjusting the dose of those drugs (or their metabolites) which are excreted by glomerular filtration [2].

Reduced Urine Dilution: Concentration Capability [10, 11]

Maximal urine dilution and concentration capability are significantly reduced in healthy old individuals and chronic nephropathy patients compared to healthy young individuals. This change predisposes both, healthy old individuals and chronic nephropathy patients, to develop over hydration status (due to reduced urine dilution capability), as well as dehydration status (due to reduced urine concentration capability) on particular clinical settings, such as water overload and water deprivation, respectively.

Reduced Sodium and Urea Reabsorption [5, 12]

Maximal sodium and urea reabsorption capability is significantly reduced in healthy old individuals and chronic nephropathy patients compared to healthy young individuals. This characteristic of the aged kidney has been attributed to a reduced number of sodium carriers (thick ascending limb of the loop of Henle) and urea channels (distal tubule), as well as to a sort of aldosterone resistance in the collecting ducts. In the case of CKD, this phenomenon has been attributed to the renal parenchyma (tubular) damage induced by the renal disease.

Regarding the reduced sodium and urea reabsorption capability, this phenomenon leads healthy old individuals and CKD patients to present an increased basal fractional excretion of these substances, and consequently to develop hypovolemia, and even low extracellular volume hyponatremia if they are submitted to an excessive negative sodium balance, as well as not to lower fractional excretion of sodium and urea during low renal perfusion status in both groups compared to healthy young people.

Chronic Kidney Disease: Renal Aging Differences

Despite the above-described renal functional similarities that the healthy old individuals and chronic nephropathy patients have, they have many and important structural and functional differences which allow physicians to distinguish them. These differences are the following ones.

Glomerular Filtration Rate Value According to Age [5, 8, 9]

The glomerular filtration rate reduction secondary to aging has a particular rate, 1 ml/min per year since the age of 40, but this is not necessarily the declination rate in chronic nephropathy. As it was mentioned above, the expected lower limit of GFR which accompanies the normal aging can be calculated by applying the Keller equation. Thus, since healthy elderly (old and very old) usually have a GFR between 70 and 40 ml/min/1.73 m^2, the only stage of CKD which can be confused with RA is the stage III – CKD (GFR between 60 and 30 ml/min/1.73 m^2).

Another important difference between the reduced GFR in RA and moderate CKD (stage III – CKD) is that the former has normal serum creatinine and urea levels, while the latter usually has abnormal elevated serum creatinine and urea values. Normal serum creatinine levels in the elderly can be explained by the muscle mass reduction (sarcopenia), which leads to low creatinine production. Additionally, normal serum urea in old individuals can be explained by the low protein diet that they usually have, which leads to low urea production, and their habitual increased fractional excretion of urea compared to healthy young individuals.

Erythropoietin and Parathyroid Hormone [5, 9, 13]

Erythropoietin synthesis is preserved in healthy elderly people, while it is usually reduced in moderate CKD (stage III – CKD) patients. Thus, RA has no anemia while moderate CKD usually has. Serum parathyroid hormone levels are normal in healthy old individuals who are well-nourished and have adequate sunlight exposition. Conversely, moderate CKD (stage III – CKD) patients usually present secondary hyperparathyroidism.

Calcium, Phosphorus, and Magnesium [13, 14]

Serum calcium, phosphorus, and magnesium values are usually normal in RA, while they are usually altered (low calcemia and high magnesemia and phosphatemia) in moderate CKD (stage III – CKD) patients. On the other hand, fractional excretion of calcium, magnesium, and phosphorus values are usually similar between healthy old individuals and young people, while they are characteristically elevated in moderate CKD (stage III – CKD) patients compared to those documented in RA.

Tubular Potassium Handling [5, 15–17]

Fractional excretion of potassium is lower in healthy old people compared to the one in chronic nephropathy patients. This phenomenon is attributed to a low aldosterone level and aldosterone distal tubules resistance induced by aging. These differences in the renal handling of potassium between healthy elderly and moderate CKD (stage III – CKD) patients explains why the former develop more frequently hyperkalemia compared to the latter, when they are on a high potassium diet or on sparing potassium drugs.

Tubular Creatinine Handling [5, 18]

Proximal tubular creatinine secretion is reduced in the elderly compared to healthy young people, and it is even much more reduced compared to chronic nephropathy patients. It has been proposed that this phenomenon could be explained by the creatinine back-filtration (reabsorption) at the proximal tubules observed in healthy aged individuals.

Urinary Acidification [5, 19]

Even though the maximal values of ammonia and titratable acid excretion were reached after an acid load in 4 hours in the young and in 6–8 hours in the healthy old, there are no differences in titratable acid, ammonia, or net acid excretion in response to an acute acid load in the healthy elderly people compared to healthy young individuals. Consequently, it takes longer to reach peak proton (acid) excretion in elderly individuals, and they experience a greater difficulty in handling acidosis. Conversely, distal tubular acidification is frequently altered in moderate CKD (stage III – CKD) patients, and because of that they usually suffer from hyperchloremic metabolic acidosis (normal GAP anion metabolic acidosis).

Kidney Imaging [1, 5]

Despite finding a slightly reduced kidney size and few simple cysts, kidney imaging is usually normal in healthy elderly people. On the contrary, kidney imaging is usually altered in most of the CKD patients.

Urinalyses [1, 5]

Despite finding a mild proteinuria (≤0.3 g/day), urinalyses is normal in healthy elderly. Conversely, urinalysis is usually altered (proteinuria and/or hematuria) in CKD patients.

Based on all the above-exposed reasons, it is clear that a mere reduced GFR at a level expected for age, in absence of elevated creatininemia, elevated uremia, anemia, hyperparathyroidism, abnormal urinalysis, and/or altered kidney imaging, should not be interpreted and diagnosed as CKD (Table 2.1). It is worth mentioning that there are borderline clinical cases, for instance when a hypertensive elderly patient with a GFR value according to age has no alteration in his/her renal complementary studies, in this situation the follow up is crucial since would surely clarify in the future if he/she is a healthy elderly or an elderly person suffering from CKD: If the previously mentioned patient starts suffering from proteinuria, he/she will be clearly defined as a CKD patient. Thus, follow- up and clinical and complementary study re-evaluation is also part of the differential diagnosis strategy, and this will be always much better than over diagnosing CKD, with its negative consequences [1].

HUGE Equation

Chronically reduced GFR in an old individual does not always mean that he/she suffers from CKD. Besides, not every CKD presents GFR reduction, as is the case of stage I – CKD patients, who have an altered urinalysis and/or an abnormal renal image but with a normal GFR value [1, 5].

Because of the above-exposed reasons, Alvarez-Gregori et al. originally described a new equation (HUGE) for detecting CKD, which precisely does not take into account patients' GFR value but their hematocrit, serum urea, and gender (HUGE is an acronym that comes from these three words) [20].

HUGE equation is as follows:

$$\text{HUGE} = 2.505458 - (0.264418 \times \text{Hematocrit}) + (0.118100 \times \text{Serum urea}) [+1.383960 \text{ if male}]$$

However, later studies documented that HUGE equation showed a better performance for screening CKD when it was combined with MDRD equation and urinalysis [6, 21, 22].

What a "Normal GFR" Rate Means in the Elderly?

Since there is a classical report that documented no GFR reduction in one-third of the elderly studied individuals, and even we have documented in the clinical practice these individuals (personal communication), some authors have stated that this finding is enough to consider age-related GFR decline as an abnormality [9]. However, this is a wrong point of view because of the following reasons:

- Firstly, the concept of abnormality in nature refers to a value which is not far from the arithmetic average of the observed values, therefore if the majority of the healthy very old people (aged 80 years of age and over) have a GFR ranging 60–40 ml/min/1.73 m^2, should be interpreted as normal GFR according to age [5, 23].

- Secondly, CKD patients have an increased overall mortality rate compared to the general population, but it has been documented that there is an increased overall mortality rate in the elderly only when their GFR value was below 45 ml/min/1.73 m^2. A very low GFR level like this is usually not explained by normal aging but by chronic nephropathy [1].
- Thirdly, some reports showed that the healthy old people who had a "normal" GFR value, which means a GFR value higher than the expected to age, had no renal reserve. This phenomenon could be interpreted as they were suffering from hyperfiltration [24].
- Fourthly, as it was previously mentioned aging is a heterogenous process, which means that it does not affect all individuals at the same rate. Thus, the fact that a number of people age successfully, at a slower rate, does not invalidate the way in which such process develops in most of the people (normality) [25]. Even, it has recently proposed a classification for the successful renal aging, which is based on three levels, in elderly subjects with normal creatininemia, uremia, urinalysis, renal imaging, and a preserved renal reserve (RR ≥20%):
  - Level I: elderly individual (age > 65 years old) with a GFR >65 ml/min/1.72 m^2
  - Level II: old individual (age 65–79 years old) with a GFR higher than 65–50 ml/min/1.72 m^2
  - Level III: a very old individual (age > 80 years old) with a GFR higher than 49–30 ml/min/1.72 m^2

  Thus, a relative high GFR in the elderly can be attributed to an early chronic nephropathy status (hyperfiltration) or to a successful renal aging process.

Conclusion

A glomerular filtration rate reduction according to age, in a setting of normal creatininemia, uremia, hemoglobin, parathyroid hormone level, urinalysis, and kidney imaging, should be interpreted as normal renal aging instead of chronic kidney disease.

References

1. Musso CG, Jauregui JR. How to differentiate renal senescence from chronic kidney disease in clinical practice. Postgrad Med. 2016;128(7):716–21. https://doi.org/10.1080/00325481.2016.1209963.
2. Musso CG. Geriatric nephrology and the 'nephrogeriatric giants'. Int Urol Nephrol. 2002;34(2):255–6.
3. Musso CG, Núñez JF. Feed-back between geriatric syndromes: general system theory in geriatrics. Int Urol Nephrol. 2006;38(3–4):785–6.
4. Forciea M, Lavizzo-Mourey R, Schwab E. Geriatric secrets. Philadelphia: Hanley & Belfus; 2000.
5. Rennke H, Denker B. Renal pathophysiology. Philadelphia: Lippincott Williams & Wilkins; 1994. p. 267–90.

6. Aiello F, Dueñas EP, Musso CG. Senescent nephropathy: the new renal syndrome. Healthcare (Basel). 2017;5(4):E81. https://doi.org/10.3390/healthcare5040081.
7. Musso CG, Macías Nuñez JF, Oreopoulos DG. Physiological similarities and differences between renal aging and chronic renal disease. J Nephrol. 2007;20(5):586–7.
8. Keller F. Kidney function and age. Nephrol Dial Transplant. 1987;2(5):382.
9. Musso CG, Oreopoulos DG. Aging and physiological changes of the kidneys including changes in glomerular filtration rate. Nephron Physiol. 2011;119(Suppl 1):p1–5. https://doi.org/10.1159/000328010.
10. Musso CG, Oreopoulos D. Renal changes in the elderly. In: Katlic, editor. Cardiothoracic surgery. London: Springer; 2011. p. 293–9.
11. Musso CG, Macías-Núñez JF. Dysfunction of the thick loop of Henle and senescence: from molecular biology to clinical geriatrics. Int Urol Nephrol. 2011;43(1):249–52.
12. Musso CG, Alvarez Gregori J, Jauregui JR, Macías Núñez JF. Creatinine, urea, uric acid, water and electrolytes renal handling in the healthy oldest old. World J Nephrol. 2012;1(5):123–6.
13. Musso CG, Musso CAF, Joseph H, De Miguel R, Rendo P, Gonzalez E, Algranati L, dos Ramos Farias E. Plasma erythropoietin levels in the oldest old. Int Urol Nephrol. 2004;36(2):259–62.
14. Musso CG, Juarez R, Vilas M, Navarro M, Rivera H, Jauregui R. Renal calcium, phosphorus, magnesium and uric acid handling: comparison between stage III- chronic kidney disease and healthy oldest old. Int Urol Nephrol. 2012;44(5):1559–62.
15. Musso CG. Potassium metabolism in patients with chronic kidney disease (CKD). Part I: patients not on dialysis (stages 3–4). Int Urol Nephrol. 2004;36(3):465–8.
16. Musso CG, de Miguel R, Algranati L, Farias E. Renal potassium excretion: comparison between chronic renal disease patients and old people. Int Nephrol and Urol. 2005;37:167–70.
17. Musso C, Liakopoulos V, De Miguel R, Imperiali N, Algranati L. Transtubular potassium concentration gradient: comparison between healthy old people and chronic renal failure patients. Int Urol Nephrol. 2006;38(2):387–90.
18. Musso CG, Michelángelo H, Vilas M, Martinez B, Bonetto A, Jauregui R, Algranati L. Renal creatinine handling in very old patients with chronic renal disease. Int Urol Nephrol. 2011;43(3):899–902.
19. Musso CG, Alvarez-Gregori J, Macias-Nuñez JF. Renal handling of uric acid, magnesium, phosphorus, calcium, and acid-base in the elderly. In: Macias-Nuñez J, Cameron S, Oreopoulos D, editors. The ageing kidney in health and disease. New York: Springer; 2008. p. 155–71.
20. Álvarez-Grégori J, Robles N, Mena C, Ardanuy R, Jauregui J, Macías Nçuñez JF. The value of a formula including haematocrit, blood urea and gender (HUGE) as a screening test for chronic renal insufficiency. J Nutr Health Aging. 2011;15(6).2011):1–5.
21. Musso CG, Maytin S, Conti P, Terrasa S, Primerano A, Reynaga A, Vilas M, Jauregui J. HUGE equation accuracy for screening chronic kidney disease: a prospective study. J Aging Res Clin Pract. 2017;6:158–62.
22. Musso CG, de Los Rios E, Vilas M, Terrasa S, Bratti G, Varela F, Diez GR, Jauregui J, Luna D. The HUGE formula (hematocrit, urea, gender) for screening for chronic kidney disease in elderly patients: a study of diagnostic accuracy. Int Urol Nephrol. 2016. https://doi.org/10.1007/s11255-016-1486-6.
23. Dawson-Saunders B, Trapp R. Medical biostatistics. Mexico. Manual Moderno. 1993. p. 51–2.
24. Musso CG. Renal reserve test: its methodology and significance. S J Kidney Dis Transpl. 2011;22(5):990–3.
25. Musso CG, Jauregui J. The ageing kidney: a proposal for its classification. Electron J Biomed. 2016;1:3–6.

Frailty in Chronic Kidney Disease Elderly Patients

3

Angela Benjumea and José Ricardo Jauregui

Introduction

Frailty is a construct originally coined by gerontologists to describe cumulative declines across multiple physiological systems that occur with aging and lead individuals to a state of diminished physiological reserve and increased vulnerability to stressors [1–3]. Fried et al. provided a standardized definition for frailty and created the concept of frailty phenotype which incorporates disturbances across interrelated domains (shrinking, weakness, poor endurance and energy, slowness, and low physical activity level) to identify old people who are at risk of disability, falls, institutionalization, hospitalization, and premature death [4].

Older adults (aged ≥ 65 years) comprise the largest segment of the chronic kidney disease (CKD) population, and impaired kidney function is linked with unsuccessful aging. It is worth mentioning that young adult CKD patients can also have frailty phenotype clinical features, suggesting that frailty is not confined to old age people. This phenomenon manifests as a high prevalence of impaired physical performance, emergent geriatric syndromes, disability, and risk of death. Considering the multiple system involvement underlying the symptoms and deficits seen in CKD, especially in its severe stages, the concept of frailty is a highly useful tool to identify older adults with kidney disease who are frail, and consequently in high risk of death [1–3].

Frailty treatment can be based on different strategies, such as exercise, nutritional interventions, drugs, vitamins, and antioxidant agents. Finally, conservative and palliative cares are very important alternative treatments for very frail and sick patients [1–4]. Since the diagnosis and treatment of frailty and sarcopenia is crucial

A. Benjumea (✉)
Internal Medicine and Geriatrics, Universidad de Caldas, Manizales, Colombia
e-mail: angela.benjumea@ucaldas.edu.co

J. R. Jauregui
Ageing Biology Unit, Hospital Italiano de Buenos Aires, Buenos Aires, Argentina

C. G. Musso et al. (eds.), *Clinical Nephrogeriatrics*,
https://doi.org/10.1007/978-3-030-18711-8_3

in geriatrics and all CKD patients, it would be very important to incorporate these evaluations in pre-dialysis, peritoneal dialysis, hemodialysis, and kidney transplant patients in order to detect and consequently treat the frailty phenotype in these groups.

Frailty as a Multicomponent in Geriatrics

Frailty is described in the geriatric literature as a multidimensional phenotype that reflects declining physical function and a global vulnerability to adverse outcomes in the setting of stress, such as illness or hospitalization [1–5]. Moreover, frailty phenotype is associated with increased risk of falls, hospitalization, disability, and death [4]. Multiple instruments to diagnose frailty have been created and validated [1]. One well-validated index, proposed by Fried and colleagues, defines frailty as the presence of three or more of five criteria, such as [4]:

- Shrinking: unintentional weight loss (≥10 lb or 4.5 kg of unintentionally weight loss in prior year)
- Exhaustion: self-report exhaustion
- Weakness: grip strength in the lowest 20% at baseline, adjusted to gender and body mass index
- Slow walking speed: walking time/15 f (4.5 m), slowest 20%, adjusting to gender and standing height
- Low physical activity level: kilocalories (Kcals) expended per week, lowest 20% (male <383 Kcals/week and female <270 Kcals/week)

Based on Fried et al.'s criteria, the estimated prevalence of frailty varies from 7% in old population (≥65 year) to 40% in very old population (≥80 years) [2–4].

Individual components of clinical frailty have been associated with some of the classical geriatric syndromes such as falls, depression, incontinence, and functional impairment. Frailty is likely the underlying process that leads to clinical manifestations that present as geriatric syndromes [5]. A geriatric syndrome is a multifactorial health condition that occurs when the accumulated effects of impairments in multiple systems render an elderly vulnerable to stressors [6]. Geriatric syndromes represent a final common pathway arrived at through multiple contributing causes. Most geriatric syndromes share common underlying risk factors [6]. It can exist a positive feedback relationship between shared risk factors, geriatric syndromes, and frailty, which increases the propensity to progress to poor outcomes [5, 7, 8]. Targeting shared risk factors (e.g., mobility impairment and poor physical performance) can be a useful way to intervene in the prevention of frailty, geriatric syndromes, and their associated sequelae [7, 8].

Even though there is frequently an overlap among frailty, comorbidity, and disability, they are in fact different concepts. Disability is defined as difficulty or dependency in carrying out activities essential to independent living, including essential roles, tasks needed for self-care and living independently at home, and desired activities important to one's quality of life [9, 10]. Comorbidity is the concurrent

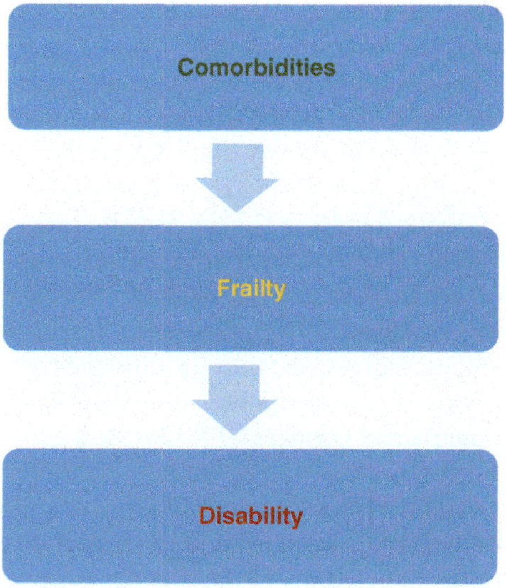

Fig. 3.1 Evolutionary relationship between comorbidities, frailty, and disability

presence of two or more chronic diseases. In addition, both frailty and comorbidity predict disability, adjusting for each other; disability may well exacerbate frailty and comorbidity can contribute to the development of frailty [9, 10] (Fig. 3.1). It has been suggested that the presence of disability or frailty could contribute to development or progression of chronic diseases, possibly through the lower activity levels associated with the former two conditions, or through other pathways affecting some basic biological mechanism essential to the maintenance of homeostasis, such as inflammation, or sympathetic–parasympathetic equilibrium [11, 12]. These causal relationships provide explanation for the frequent co-occurrence of these conditions, and suggest the clinical importance of differentiating them in order to choose the appropriate preventive intervention.

A systematic geriatric assessment (GA) is defined as a multidimensional, interdisciplinary diagnostic process focusing on determining an elderly individual's medical, psychosocial, and functional capabilities in order to develop a coordinated and integrated plan for his/her treatment and long–term follow-up [13]. This GA has been shown to successfully identify patients at risk of poor outcome in geriatric oncology [14]. Besides, the GA improves outcomes in older patients admitted to the emergency department and it is increasingly recommended for the treatment decision–making process in elderly patients [15, 16].

The Intersection of Geriatrics and Chronic Kidney Disease

Assessment and Prevalence of Geriatric Impairments

It is known that CKD, and particularly, end-stage renal disease is known to be associated with impaired health status and physical function. However, few studies have examined the association between CKD and frailty [17–21]. Shlipak et al.

found a strong association between CKD and frailty in elderly participants in the Cardiovascular Health Study [22]. Johansen et al. even documented a strong association between end-stage renal disease (ESRD) and frailty in younger patients [23]. Moreover, prevalence of frailty was approximately twofold higher in patients suffering from mild or early-stage CKD, compared with those without chronic nephropathy. Patients suffering from severe CKD were more likely to be frail. Frailty was also more common in persons with moderate to severe CKD than in those with other chronic illnesses, such as vascular disease, cancer, and other degenerative diseases of aging. Finally, frailty CKD were independently associated with an increased risk of death [23]. Emilee et al. found that the association was especially strong among individuals with an estimated glomerular filtration rate (eGFR) <45 mL/min/1.73 m^2, but was even also significant among those individuals with microalbuminuria and normal eGFR [24].

Studies were systematically identified which assessed the association between mortality risk or hospitalization with one or more geriatric impairments at the start of dialysis therapy, including impairment of cognitive function, mood, performance status or activities of daily living (instrumental), mobility (including falls), social environment, or nutritional status. Most studies focused on one or two geriatric domains only, whereas two studies assessed multiple impairments. The domain most frequently assessed was performance status, which was described in 12 of the 27 included studies, followed by depression (7 of 27), nutrition (5 of 27), and cognition (5 of 27) [25].

A systematic assessment aids to stage aging, thereby discriminating between fit and relatively vulnerable patients, and revealing deficits that are not routinely captured in standard history and examination. The GA has been proposed as a supportive instrument for treatment decision-making in oncologic patients and in ESRD patients as well. It provides the best available evidence on the patients' physiologic reserves and consequently a better estimation of residual life expectancy. Concrete information on impaired domains that could compromise dialysis treatment may facilitate shared decision-making with the patient and relatives. In addition, it may reveal treatable conditions that would otherwise be overlooked, thereby forming a starting point for preventive interventions to optimize quality of life, by improving patient's physical, activities of the daily living (ADL), and social problems. Finally, the information derived from a GA may help to estimate adverse outcomes of surgical interventions and other complex interventions [25]. In nephrology, a systematic approach to frail patients is currently lacking, but it is clear that geriatric impairment across multiple physical and mental domains at dialysis initiation is related to poor outcome. However, systematic assessment of impairment in relation to outcome is scarce, especially in the elderly. Whether systematic assessment of geriatric impairments could discriminate between fit and vulnerable patients in the context of treatment decisions concerning dialysis initiation should be assessed in more detail before the implementation in clinical practice.

Frailty in the CKD Population

The study of frailty among elderly CKD patients is a new and important area of investigation. Although studies are few, they highlight that kidney disease, even in the earlier stages, is associated with the clinical manifestations of frailty. This supports the concept that CKD itself might serve as a clinical phenotype of frailty; age-related physiologic changes may not be the only (or necessary) pathway to deficit accumulation in multiple systems. One published study reported the prevalence of chronic renal insufficiency, frailty, and disability among 5808 community dwelling participants aged ≥65 years in the Cardiovascular Health Study [4, 22, 26–28]. Shlipak et al. found that 11% of the studied population had creatinine values above the specified threshold for CKD, 1.3 mg/dL (female) and 1.5 mg/dL (male), 6% were frail, and 8% were disabled in one or more ADL [28]. Kidney disease was associated with double higher prevalence of frailty and disability, particularly among black women. The kidney disease associated with frailty remained significant after multivariable adjustment for comorbidity, anemia, inflammation (C-reactive peptide and fibrinogen), lipid status (low-density lipoprotein and high-density lipoprotein cholesterol), and subclinical cardiovascular disease [22, 28].

This cross-sectional study highlighted the strong association between kidney disease and frailty, even at milder stages of impairment. It was also found that factors such as anemia, inflammation, and lipid status were related to frailty and survival in non-CKD populations [29, 30]. Other authors have also found an association between CKD, frailty, and inflammatory markers [31]. If frailty is already detectable among older adults in the early stages of kidney disease, ESRD patients might be expected to have a higher burden of frailty and its consequences. Johansen et al. measured the prevalence and consequences of frailty in the ESRD adult patients ($n = 2275$), approximately half of whom were aged ≥65 years [23]. A remarkable two thirds of dialysis patients of all ages met criteria for frailty, as defined by the presence of low physical function scores and low vitality scores on the Medical Outcomes Survey Short Form-36 (SF-36), inactivity, and the presence of malnutrition [27]. Although older age was associated with a higher prevalence of each of the component factors and with frailty overall, a sizeable proportion of the younger age groups (age < 60) had deficits, reinforcing the notion that frailty is not confined to old age among vulnerable populations. This phenomenon was most marked for physical functioning and vitality where more than 50% of the youngest participants (age < 40) met criteria for poor status (SF-36 scores <75 for physical functioning and <55 for vitality). Moreover, the prevalence of poor physical function was as high as 90% among very old individual (≥80 years). Poor self-reported physical function was a major component of the frailty detected among this population, suggesting that this may be a key area for further investigation and intervention. These authors also documented that frailty correlated with variables such as older age, female sex, comorbidity (diabetes mellitus, stroke, and low albumin), and hemodialysis as a treatment modality, particularly among those without permanent vascular

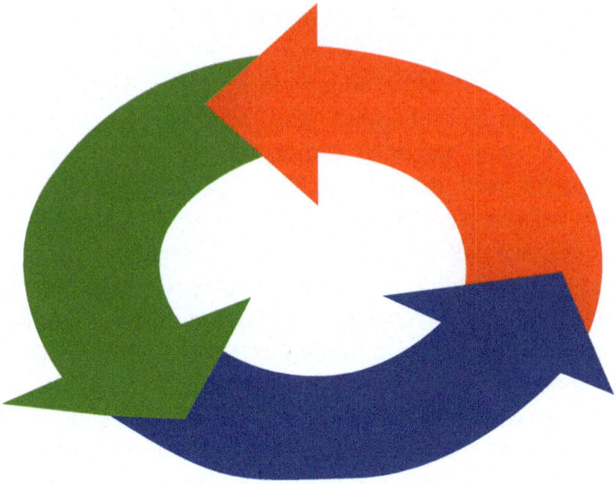

Fig. 3.2 Feedback among frailty (red arrow), nephropathy (green arrow), and senescence nephropathy (blue arrow)

access. Although the documentation of these factors represents an important start characterizing frailty phenotype among the ESRD people. Regardless of their age, frail dialysis patients have approximately double risk of hospitalization and death within 1 year, compared with nonfrail patients [23].

Each of the variables used to identify the frailty phenotype was independently associated with subsequent mortality, supporting the validity of their use in the ESRD individuals.

In addition, it has recently been considered the coexistence and mutual enhancement of frailty and chronic nephropathy in elderly patients, as a new condition, the *senescence nephropathy*, which leads the patients to a spiral of deterioration which makes their clinical status and therapeutic targets different from the ones in nonfrail CKD patients [26, 32] (Fig. 3.2).

Disability in Older Adults with Kidney Disease

Frailty can be diagnosed before the onset of disability, raising the possibility of targeting interventions to prevent functional decline. Disability is defined as difficulty or dependency in performing activities essential to independent living. These tasks include self-care (basic activities of daily living) and household management (instrumental activities) as well as those related to social roles or activities that maintain quality of life. Individuals are considered functionally dependent when they lose independence in basic ADL such as bathing, grooming, dressing, toileting, ambulating, and transferring [33–35]. The high burden of disability among ESRD adult patients has been recognized for some time, and has been linked with increased mortality [38, 39]. Increasing age has been associated with poorer functional status among patients on dialysis [36, 37, 40]. Among studies limited to elderly on dialysis, functional status is confined to activities at home, representing a decline in comparison with their predialysis functional status [41].

The ability to perform mobility-related ADL (bathing, stairs, walking blocks, and heavy housework) was significantly lower in older adults on dialysis compared to age, race, and sex-matched peers without CKD [38]. About one of three dialysis patients needs help with at least one self-care ADL [42]. Very few (5%) older adults on dialysis are fully independent in both basic and instrumental activities [43]. Dependence in instrumental activities is most common, occurring in more than 90%, whereas 52% of older dialysis patients have additional dependence in personal ADL [43]. Among elderly (≥65 years) hemodialysis patients, disability in personal care was associated with polypharmacy, lower education level, and mainly with poor mobility performance on a timed *get up and go* test [43, 44]. This latter finding raises the possibility that impaired physical performance can be an important disability inducing factor in ESRD patients, which is also seen in elderly without kidney disease [34]. Physical performance evaluation can prove to be a sensitive screening tool for detecting disability risk in CKD elderly patients; even the individuals who were independent for self-care in this study had impaired physical performance [43].

Disability, particularly in mobility, is a dynamic state with individuals experiencing transitions in the severity and duration of their functional dependence [45, 46]. Changes can happen insidiously or acutely, as seen during hospitalization. One prospective study measured the change in disability among 35 elderly dialysis patients admitted to hospital and documented a pervasive decline in physical and functional performance. All the studied individuals had instrumental activity dependence, and 77% had basic activity dependence at baseline. The evaluation for all daily functions, except telephone use, showed a trend to worsening. The most common new complaint was difficulty to transfer in and out of bed (27%). Further evidence for an accelerated physical decline with acute hospitalization was the significant decrease in mobility documented by using the timed *get up and go* test [47]. The ability to walk is a simple but robust marker of disability and mortality risk. Ten percent of incident dialysis patients are unable to walk, and surprisingly 40% develop a new walking disability (abnormal gait, use of an assistive device, or falls) during the 1st year on dialysis [45, 46]. Even in earlier stages of CKD in elderly patients, it seems to be an association between kidney function with disability, although adjustment for comorbidity attenuates this relationship [22, 28]. Frailty has been associated with an increased likelihood of transitioning to or remaining at more severe levels of disability in non-ESRD populations but this has not yet been examined in ESRD elderly patients [45, 46].

Geriatric Syndromes in CKD

Falls

Mild to moderate kidney dysfunction is associated with incident hip fracture in community dwelling elderly people [48]. This relationship cannot be confined to its effects on bone metabolism. A decreased creatinine clearance ˂60 mL/min predicted incident falls among community-dwelling elderly women (65–77 years old) [49]. This effect was mitigated by vitamin D supplementation, which could have improved muscle strength, balance, and physical performance to reduce falls [49, 50]. A smaller study found a similar association with fall risk using a creatinine clearance ˂65 mL/min [51] among community-dwelling elderly individuals over 70 years of age. Among ESRD elderly patients, prospective studies have confirmed that fall incidence (1.2–1.6 falls/person-year) is higher than reported rates for seniors residing in nursing homes (1.0–1.4 falls/resident-year) [52–54]. Falls are independently associated with increased mortality in elderly dialysis patients [55]. Some of the falls' risk factors are similar to those associated with functional decline, such as age, comorbidity, systolic blood pressure, prior falls, diabetes mellitus, polypharmacy, and mobility dependence [52, 53]. More investigation is needed to characterize fall risk factors specific of the kidney disease population and to identify which ones are amenable to intervention.

Cognitive Impairment

Elderly CKD patients have an increased risk of cognitive impairment which can manifest acutely as delirium and chronically as dementia. An estimated glomerular filtration rate (GFR) ˂60 mL/min was associated with poorer neuropsychological test performance among 923 community-dwelling adults (aged > 40 years) without dementia compared with a GFR above this level [56, 57].

This phenomenon was also evident in a large national sample using a brief cognitive screening instrument, which highlighted that impairment is detectable very early in the course of kidney disease [58]. Among ESRD elderly patients, the prevalence of cognitive impairment is higher, with only 13% found to have normal function on detailed testing [59]. Dementia is associated with an increased risk of death and withdrawal from dialysis [20, 60]. Dementia, along with stroke, is associated with the highest frequency of walking difficulties in the adult dialysis population, highlighting the common co-occurrence of geriatric syndromes among vulnerable elderly individuals. These conditions are likely a manifestation of underlying frailty, and diminished homeostatic reserve in brain function, as would be expected in cognitive impairment, can increase an individual's vulnerability to acute stressors, leading to recurrent delirium or acute confusion. Delirium can often occur during dialysis, since the combination of the acute decline in cerebral perfusion that occurs during dialysis, together with large fluid and solute shifts and associated brain edema, can increase the risk of acute delirium during dialysis [61–64].

One study examined the magnitude of variation in global cognitive function over a 2-day dialysis cycle in 28 patients using a cognitive summary score from a 45-min cognitive battery. They found that cognitive function plummeted during dialysis, recovered almost to baseline at 1 hour after dialysis, and was best on the day after dialysis [65]. The possibility that these recurrent episodes of cerebral hypoperfusion and delirium might contribute to the high rates of cognitive impairment in hemodialysis patients needs further exploration.

Additionally, ESRD patients are prone to accelerated aging, since underlying mechanisms, such as inflammation and microvascular damage, contribute to both decline of kidney function and impairment of other physiologic domains. Thus, a high prevalence of impairment in physical and psychosocial domains, such as dependency in ADL, cognitive impairment, depression, and malnutrition, can be found in both young and elderly dialysis population.

Protein-Energy Wasting and Sarcopenia

Elderly patients represent an increasing proportion of people with stage 5 CKD pre-dialysis, chronic hemodialysis (CHD), or chronic peritoneal dialysis (CPD) [66–69]. Frailty and protein-energy wasting (PEW) are common complications in ESRD elderly patients on CHD or CPD [70]. This phenomenon is clinically relevant, because many manifestations of frailty and PEW are strong risk factors for low quality of life, morbidity, and mortality. Frailty and PEW may be caused by aging, advanced kidney failure, or both combined conditions. PEW is defined as the loss of somatic and circulating body protein and energy reserves. The term PEW is used rather than protein-energy malnutrition, because some causes of PEW are unrelated to inadequate nutrient intake. Causes of PEW in ESRD patients include inadequate nutrient intake, losses of nutrients during dialysis, superimposed catabolic illnesses, nonspecific inflammation, acidemia, catabolic stress from the dialysis procedure, low levels of resistance to such anabolic hormones (insulin, growth hormone, and IGF-1), increased levels of catabolic hormones (parathyroid hormone and glucagon), blood losses (blood drawing, gastrointestinal bleeding), and possibly, oxidative and carbonyl stress [70].

In addition, two related concepts are sarcopenia and dynapenia. Sarcopenia is derived from the Greek words sarx (flesh) and penia (loss) [71]. Two common definitions for sarcopenia are progressive muscle mass decline caused by aging, which results in decreased functional capacity of muscles. Dynapenia, derived from the Greek words dyn (power) and penia (loss), is defined as loss of strength with aging. These definitions may not be optimal, because reduced muscle mass and strength are not always present in elderly people, and morbidity, malnutrition, or just physical inactivity can even reduce muscle mass and strength in younger people. Skeletal muscle mass size seems to be the most important predictor of muscle strength or physical performance and in chronic dialysis patients' survival. However, skeletal muscle mass and strength can be disassociated. As normal people age, the rate of decline in muscle strength is greater than the rate of loss of muscle mass, and strength can diminish even while muscle mass is maintained or increases. Physical performance is defined as the capability to conduct normal daily physical activities. Physical performance is often measured by such activities as the time required to climb a defined number of stairs or the distance walked or number of rises from a chair during a given time period. Physical performance and mortality may be associated more with muscle strength than muscle mass. Another age-related change in body composition, sarcopenic obesity, refers to low muscle mass (sarcopenia) combined with increased body fat (obesity). Sarcopenic obesity may develop without weight changes if the decrease in muscle mass is similar to the gained body fat [72].

Increased Prevalence of Frailty and PEW in Elderly ESRD Patients

Frailty and PEW are well described in ESRD adult patients independently of age. PEW is found in 18–75% of chronic dialysis patients in different reports [66–69]. There is less information concerning the prevalence and magnitude of these abnormalities in ESRD elderly patients. However, PEW, sarcopenia (reduced mid-arm muscle circumference [MAMC]), and dynapenia (decreased hand grip strength) seem to be more common in elderly (>65 years) than younger chronic dialysis patients [38] In CHD patients, decreased lean body mass and thigh muscle area are associated with aging. The prevalence of sarcopenia increases also with aging in non-ESRD patients. However, muscle wasting tends to be more severe in chronic dialysis patients than non-dialysis CKD patients [72]. Sarcopenic obesity is more pronounced in aged non-diabetic CHD patients than in aged controls. The volume of visceral fat, standardized by body mass index, is greater in nondiabetic CHD patients (mean age 57.5 years) compared to people with normal kidney function of similar age. Compared with the prevalence of frailty in community-dwelling elderly people (6.9–16.3%), frailty is substantially greater in elderly and near-elderly chronic dialysis patients (67.7%). Moreover, the prevalence of frailty increases with age in CHD patients, and elderly stage 3 CKD have greater prevalence of frailty than normal or mildly reduced kidney function in elderly patients (15% vs. 6%, respectively) [72].

Causes of Frailty and PEW in ESRD Elderly Patients

Some changes associated to aging which may potentially contribute to frailty can be categorized into genetic and environmental exposure, including epigenetic factors. Hundreds of genetic variations have been identified that are associated with longevity, and a number of these genetic variations involve the insulin pathways including insulin, IGF, their receptors, and the signal transduction system that they induce. Alterations that suppress activity of this pathway seem to be particularly associated with increased longevity. Since in many species calories intake increases longevity, this phenomenon could be related to the fact that carbohydrates and some amino acids stimulate the insulin, IGF-1, and IGF binding protein release. The IGF-1 exerts anabolic, anticatabolic, and antiapoptotic actions on skeletal muscle, helping to maintain its mass and enhance physical performance. There is an age-related decline in IGF-1 activity that stems from the growth hormone (GH) decline which can lead to muscle mass and strength loss, as well as reduced exercise capability [72]. Other environmental disorders which could contribute to aging are:

1. Mitochondrial dysfunction and oxidative stress. The accumulation of free radicals can participate in inducing age-related sarcopenia and DNA damage, protein crosslinking, nonenzymatic glycation or other carbonyl reactions with proteins, accumulation of partially or completely denatured proteins, and cellular inflammation, which is commonly present in the aged [28, 72]. In addition, the limits of cellular replication cycles because of telomere shortening as well as DNA damage and oncogene expression in aging lead to the accumulation of dysfunctional senescent cells, which may contribute to dysfunctional tissues and organ systems [72, 73].
2. Immune dysfunction secondary to aging predisposes elderly people to suffer from chronic inflammation. Inflammation not only stimulates protein degradation and skeletal muscle mass wasting but also suppresses appetite, stimulates resistance to insulin and GH, and enhances energy expenditure. A higher inflammatory state is associated with parenchymal fibrosis, less muscle mass and strength, and lower physical performance and functionality in the elderly [73].
3. Hormonal dysfunction secondary to aging leads to resistance to several hormones, such as testosterone, insulin, IGF-1, and thyroid hormone, as well as to 25-hydroxy vitamin D deficiency, particularly in industrialized societies. This phenomenon can be attributed to their reduced time to sunlight exposure and frequent use of sunscreen or clothing that covers the skin. Despite older age does not alter vitamin D intestinal absorption, decreased vitamin D intake and its reduced cutaneous synthesis of vitamin D (decreased skin thickness secondary to aging) can contribute to lower serum vitamin D levels in the elderly. Moreover, healthy elderly with low serum vitamin D levels are at higher risk of sarcopenia and dynapenia compared to elderly persons with high serum vitamin D levels. Even more, vitamin D supplementation in the elderly can improve lower extremity muscle performance and increases the number and diameter of type II muscle fibers [28, 72, 74].

On the other hand, some changes associated to CKD can also contribute to frailty. In this sense, severe neuropathy is often observed in CKD patients, which often presents clinically with impaired sensation, and could progress to hypoesthesia, reduced deep tendon reflexes, paresis, and ultimately, frank paralysis. Tendons in both, elderly individuals and ESRD patients have an increased risk of rupturing or separating from their bony insertion when subjected to increased contractile force. Skeletal muscle mass within the lower normal percentile is observed in up to 62% of dialysis patients, and physical activity is usually decreased in dialysis patients and tends to decrease with age in the general and dialysis population [28, 72–74]. Decline in physical activity with advancing age, measured by accelerometry, is much greater in CHD patients than in sedentary people without kidney disease. Dialysis patients are likely to describe a greater reduction in moderate or vigorous physical activity with aging. Physical inactivity in elderly dialysis patients is associated with lower serum albumin and serum creatinine levels, which are indicative of PEW and small skeletal muscle mass. Even more, in elderly dialysis patients, reduced frequency of daily physical activity is correlated with higher mortality risk [75, 76]. Reduced food intake in advanced CKD patients is often caused by anorexia, which may be caused by uremic toxins, inflammation, superimposed illnesses, as well as depression or other psychiatric disorders [76, 77]. Dietary protein intake is lower in healthy elderly people compared to healthy young people. Besides, dementia is frequent in elderly ESRD patients, and can reduce food intake. Edentulous state can impair the ability of ESRD patients to eat, and CHD is negatively associated with intake of energy and protein. Losses of amino acids, peptides, and water-soluble vitamins into dialysate may contribute to PEW and frailty [72–77].

Kidney failure intensifies many of the processes associated with aging. Kidney failure per se, like aging, engenders inflammation. In advanced CKD, there are impaired removal of proinflammatory cytokines (e.g., increased serum TNF-α and IL-6, etc.) and exposure to inflammatory stimulants (e.g., uremic toxins), including those toxins engendered by the dialysis procedure itself (dialysis catheters, tubing, dialyzer membranes, etc.) [26].

In CKD and aging, there is also an increased oxidant stress with enhanced generation of reactive oxygen species (ROS), elevated serum oxidants, and reduced levels of antioxidants. ROS induced mitochondrial injury. Oxidative stress caused by aging can cause atrophy and loss of muscle fibers, and oxidative stress can also be associated with muscle fiber atrophy in CHD patients. There are increased levels of protein carbonyls, such as advanced glycation end-products and advanced lipid end-products, which cause damage by reaction with endogenous proteins. Protein carbonyls, an indicator of oxidative proteins damage, are directly associated with grip strength and decline in walking speed in the elderly [78].

As with aging, CKD generates a cascade of changes in gene function, cell signaling, and metabolism that ultimately leads to expression of many of the phenotypic characteristics of the aged person. Serum levels of gluconeogenic hormones (glucagon and parathyroid hormone) are increased, and there is resistance to anabolic hormones (insulin, GH, and IGF-1) in advanced CKD. Vitamin D deficiency, obesity, metabolic acidosis, chronic inflammation, and accumulation of uremic toxins contribute to insulin resistance in ESRD patients. Insulin resistance in this population may activate caspase-3 and the ubiquitin–proteasome system, thereby enhancing muscle protein degradation [73, 78]. Since insulin also stimulates protein synthesis, in diabetic compared with nondiabetic CHD and CPD patients, insulin resistance may contribute to greater loss of skeletal muscle mass during the 1st year of dialysis treatment [78]. Type 2 diabetes mellitus elderly patients without ESRD also show greater declines in leg muscle mass compared with nondiabetics. A progressive decline in serum testosterone occurs with aging in normal men. In addition, low serum free testosterone is associated with frailty in elderly men. Treatment with supraphysiological doses of testosterone may increase muscle size and strength in otherwise normal men [79]. Metabolic acidosis, which is common in CKD patients, promotes frailty and PEW in many ways, such as causing bone loss, more rapid progression of kidney failure, other endocrine disorders, systemic inflammation with increased proinflammatory cytokines, enhanced β2-microglobulin formation, and hypertriglyceridemia, anorexia (reduced food intake), malaise, and hypotension [72].

Clinical Consequences of Frailty and PEW in ESRD Elderly Patients

Frailty and PEW are associated with impaired physical performance, poorer quality of life, and reduced survival in ESRD elderly patients. In CHD elderly patients, age-related decreases in skeletal muscle mass and increases in fat mass (intramuscular and intermuscular adipocytes) are associated with decreased isometric strength and impaired physical performance (6-min walk test and gait speed). Reduced anterior tibialis muscle mass, which is more common in CHD patients than in age- and sex-matched sedentary controls without ESRD, is significantly associated with reduced gait speed and isometric ankle dorsiflexor strength [80]. CHD adult patients with lower MAMC had worse mental health scores which were assessed by the Short Form 36-item health survey (SF-36) questionnaire and poorer survival. ESRD in adults of any age is associated with decreased physical performance. Scores of the Short Physical Performance Battery, an indicator of physical performance, are significantly lower in CHD patients compared with normal values for the elderly population.

The physical functioning subscale of the SF-36 questionnaire in these CHD patients was also reduced. In CHD elderly patient, both sit-to-stand scores and staircase climbing scores showed 50% and 54% fewer cycles, respectively, compared to age- and sex-matched control subjects without CKD [81].

In adult chronic dialysis patients, frailty compared with no frailty are usually associated with greater hospitalization risk and higher mortality [69, 75]. In the general population, decreased whole-leg extension strength exposes the elderly to more falls, while CHD elderly patients commonly fall. Fall rates in CHD elderly patients are higher than rates in community-dwelling elderly people without CKD (1.6 vs. 0.6–0.8 falls/person year). Impaired physical performance (10-m walking test) increases the risk of falls and fall-related fractures in CHD elderly patients; and falls are independently associated with increased mortality in this group. Impaired neuromuscular function (documented by increased time of *get up and go* test, reduced functional reach, and slower 6-min walk test) is associated with an increased risk of bone fracture in CHD elderly patients [72, 75].

It has been reported that chronic dialysis patients who suffered from a hip, vertebral, or pelvic fracture had a 2.7 times greater mortality than those patients who did not sustain such fractures. Regarding the body mass index (BMI), conversely to general population, the BMI is inversely related to mortality in chronic dialysis patients. This phenomenon has been attributed to the fact that obese CHD and CPD patients often have greater muscle mass than nonobese dialysis patients. Larger skeletal muscle mass, indicated by higher serum creatinine or MAMC, increased body fat mass; and gain in skeletal muscle mass or body fat are each independently associated to increased survival in chronic dialysis patients of any age. It is worth mentioning that is still unclear why skeletal muscle mass or obesity should promote longer lifespan, although muscle mass may be more important than fat mass for survival. Obesity combined with sarcopenia may be considered a form of PEW, which is associated with inflammation and increased mortality in chronic dialysis patients. Finally, the location of the increased fat mass influences mortality in CHD elderly patients since an abdominal fat excess seems to be associated, as in general population, with higher mortality rate [72].

Decision-Making

Dialysis Options

Dialysis for elderly frail individuals is a comparatively new treatment option. Proposing dialysis appears to be limited only by medical or social reasons as opposed to age alone. It is worth pointing out that the vast majority (94%) of octogenarians opt for treatment where dialysis was deemed appropriate by the renal team. Only 12.5% of those oldest old (≥80 years) patients would not recommend dialysis to patients of the same age. The declining independence levels seen in older people make HD an attractive option where dialysis can be managed by trained specialists. Patients incapable of self-care PD can be supported through assisted PD (aPD), where trained staff provided daily dialysis assistance either in nursing homes or in patients' homes. In this sense, there are several reports of successful PD for nursing home residents. In areas where aPD is available to support patients within their homes, 75% of those who chose PD received aPD compared to self-care PD [82].

Interventions

The construct of frailty would be without clinical utility unless it could be used to help guide interventions and stratify patients into those who will derive benefit, no benefit, or harm from any given intervention. To date, there are no simple one-step interventions that reverse frailty. Multidisciplinary care, nutritional supplementation, and exercise may attenuate the morbidity associated with frailty, particularly when applied early. In the renal population little work has been done to confirm the effectiveness, or clinical utility, of any of these interventions [28, 32].

The use of frailty indices to stratify patients into different treatment strategies is perhaps where its main advantage lies. This is widely accepted in several areas of medicine, particularly in oncology where treatment strategies incorporate physical performance tests and other markers of frailty. Recent data from the hypertension literature suggests that tight blood pressure control is less effective in those with frailty characteristics and suggests that targets be likewise adjusted [81–83].

Regarding ESRD patients, it is tempting to use frailty characteristics to determine if patients are best managed with non-dialysis renal care or with dialysis therapies. Although frailty is associated with adverse outcomes among incident dialysis patients, including higher risk of hospitalization and death, there is little data to support that frailty could improve after dialysis initiation and, rather on the contrary, there is a higher trend to increase dependence in ADLs. However, it remains to be evaluated if it is appropriate to restrict the use of dialysis in those who are deemed to be frail. Perhaps the main benefit of recognizing the frailty phenotype may lie in customized treatments that personalize targets and goals of care [84, 85].

Good Medical/Nephrology Care

Observational data indicate that, in general, the better the clinical status of the patient who starts dialysis, the better the prognosis of survival. PEW at the onset of dialysis is associated with poorer survival, and starting dialysis before patients develop PEW is associated with better long-term nutritional status and lower mortality. Dialysis initiation is often associated with the improvement in protein-energy status. Better control of uremia may lead to less frailty and PEW. Experience with CHD suggests that more than two times per week sessions and larger doses of dialysis may improve patients' appetite, nutritional status, and quality of life and reduce frailty and PEW. Thus, it would seem that ESRD patients who have inflammatory catabolic illnesses and are treated promptly covering their nutritional needs should have better clinical outcomes with less frailty and PEW. Moreover, given the high prevalence of inflammatory stress in ESRD patients, there should be a role for agents that correct these disorders. However, anti-inflammatory and antioxidant drugs have been used in many trials in dialysis patients, most without apparent success. Conversely, small-scale studies indicate that the antioxidants a-tocopherol and *N*-acetylcysteine may reduce adverse cardiovascular events in CHD patients [28, 73, 81].

Nutrient Intake

Frailty and PEW prevention and treatment always require adequate intake of nutrients. Multivitamin and trace element supplements are commonly needed. Most expert groups recommend similar amounts of dietary protein intake (DPI) for dialysis patients ranging from 1.0 to 1.3 g/kg per day with at least 50% of the DPI of high biologic value. It has been suggested that a safe protein intake that maximizes the probability of good protein nutrition for clinically stable CHD and CPD patients is 1.2 g/kg per day and 1.2–1.3 g/kg per day, respectively. The Kidney Disease Outcomes Quality Initiative (KDOQI) guidelines for energy intake in CHD and CPD patients recommend 35 kcal/kg per day for patients $<$60 years and 30 kcal/kg per day for CHD patients >60 years old. Energy prescription can be increased for patients who are underweight, have PEW, or engage in chronic heavy physical activity, and it can be reduced in patients who are very obese. Most people undergoing standard maintenance dialysis treatment will not be able to ingest these quantities of protein and energy, and their food intake may need to be augmented to meet these goals. In these circumstances, oral nutritional supplements can be used. Oral supplements of protein or primarily essential amino acids, usually including additional calories, may improve protein balance and PEW, promote protein accrual in skeletal muscle mass of people with ESRD, or prevent or retard the development of sarcopenia in elderly persons without CKD. Tube feeding, intradialytic parenteral nutrition, or total parenteral nutrition may be used for patients who are unable to take oral supplements. Tube feeding, intradialytic parenteral nutrition, and provision of amino acids through peritoneal dialysate may increase protein balance [86, 87].

Exercise

Although many benefits are ascribed to exercise training in CKD and dialysis patients, the most universally observed improvement is in endurance exercise capacity. Increased strength and physical performance are probably the most commonly reported improvement. Even though, exercise in young CKD patients is occasionally reported to reduce inflammatory cytokines, increased muscle mass with exercise training is less commonly described. This finding can be explained by less frequent or lower intensity strength training regimens for dialysis patients or their antianabolic status. Muscle intracellular protein remodeling without hypertrophy seems to be common with exercise training. It has been documented that 12 weeks of strength training of the thigh in CKD stage 4–5 elderly CKD patients significantly increased muscular strength and walking capacity to a similar extent as in elderly healthy individuals. Besides, CHD elderly patients who underwent low-intensity training of the leg and pelvic muscles, compared with nonexercising controls, displayed increased lower extremity strength and leg and whole-body lean mass, reduced body fat mass, and increased ADL scores [28, 85–87].

Conservative Care in CKD

ESRD elderly patients have increasing prevalence of co-morbidities and high mortality with a median 2.5 life years remaining for those over 75 years. Additionally, treatment withdrawal accounts for ~20% of overall deaths. Evidence is emerging that dialysis can be of little value, in terms of survival benefit and quality of life, to some frail patients with multiple co-morbid conditions and poor functional status. This has led to questioning of the suitability of renal replacement therapy for ESRD in this population and the impact on quality of life. ESRD is a life-limiting condition associated with substantially increased risks of morbidity and mortality. In a number of renal units in the UK, patients with ESRD are offered an alternative treatment to dialysis or transplantation known as conservative kidney management where supportive care is provided by the multidisciplinary team often in liaison with the community team and general practitioner [82, 88].

It is worth mentioning that despite conservative treatment and palliative care used neither dialysis nor renal prevention strategies (angiotensin-converting enzyme inhibitors and others), there are marked differences between them: The conservative treatment aim is to manage the ESRD complications without using dialysis, while the palliative treatment is applied to terminal patients, and its goal is to manage patient's symptoms secondary to advanced CKD. Deciding when to withhold dialysis in this population and provide conservative or palliative care as an alternative requires thorough ethical deliberation and complex decision-making process. Some patients may not benefit from dialysis, but there is limited evidence to guide patients, carers, and staff when making this important decision. Ideally, it should be able to accurately distinguish between a patient who will do well on dialysis and a patient who will do poorly; however, any attempt to define such a population has been largely unsuccessful. Some studies have explored age, functional status, and comorbidity burden as predictors of survival but the development of a criterion score to select people for dialysis has not been developed and individualized assessment is always necessary. The number of patients with advanced chronic kidney disease opting for conservative management rather than dialysis is unknown but likely to be growing [82].

Conclusion

Frailty, impaired physical performance, disability, and geriatric syndromes are common among older adults with kidney disease even at the early stages. Further work is necessary to characterize the mechanisms underlying the association of kidney disease with frailty and its consequences in order to guide approaches to prevent and mitigate multiple adverse outcomes. At present, recognition of the strong link between CKD and frailty, falls, cognitive impairment, disability, and mortality can be useful for informing prognosis and treatment plans.

References

1. Jones DM, Song X, Rockwood K. Operationalizing a frailty index from a standardized comprehensive geriatric assessment. J Am Geriatr Soc. 2004;52:1929–33.
2. Morley JE, Haren MT, Rolland Y, Kim MJ. Frailty. Med Clin N Am. 2006;90:837–47.
3. Slaets JP. Vulnerability in the elderly: frailty. Med Clin N Am. 2006;90:593–601.
4. Fried LP, Tangen CM, Walston J, Newman AB, Hirsch C, Gottdiener J, Seeman T, Tracy R, Kop WJ, Burke G, McBurnie MA, Cardiovascular Health Study Collaborative Research Group. Frailty in older adults: evidence for a phenotype. J Gerontol A Biol Sci Med Sci. 2001;56:M146–56.
5. Inouye SK, Studenski S, Tinetti ME, Kuchel GA. Geriatric syndromes: clinical, research, and policy implications of a core geriatric concept. J Am Geriatr Soc. 2007;55:780–91.
6. Tinetti ME, Inouye SK, Gill TM, Doucette JT. Shared risk factors for falls, incontinence, and functional dependence. Unifying the approach to geriatric syndromes. JAMA. 1995;273:1348–53.

7. Fried LF, Katz R, Cushman M, Sarnak M, Shlipak MG, Kuller L, Newman AB. Change in cardiovascular risk factors with progression of kidney disease. Am J Nephrol. 2009;29:334–41.
8. Manjunath G, Tighiouart H, Coresh J, Macleod B, Salem DN, Griffith JL, Levey AS, Sarnak MJ. Level of kidney function as a risk factor for cardiovascular outcomes in the elderly. Kidney Int. 2003;63:1121–9.
9. Pope A, Tarlov A. Disability in America: toward a national agenda for prevention. Institute of Medicine (U.S.) Committee on a National Agenda for the Prevention of Disabilities. Washington, DC: National Academy Press; 1991.
10. Adams PF, Hendershot GE, Marano MA. Current estimates from the national health interview survey, United States, 1996, Vital and Health Statistics, Series 10, No. 200. Hyattsville: National Center for Health Statistics; 1999.
11. Newman AB, Gottdiener JS, Mcburnie MA, Hirsch CH, Kop WJ, Tracy R, Walston JD, Fried LP. Associations of subclinical cardiovascular disease with frailty. J Gerontol Med Sci. 2001;56A:M158–66.
12. Walston J, McBurnie MA, Newman A, Tracy RP, Kop WJ, Hirsch CH, Gottdiener J, Fried LP, Cardiovascular Health Study. Frailty and activation of the inflammation and coagulation systems with and without clinical comorbidities: results from the Cardiovascular Health Study. Arch Intern Med. 2002;162(20):2333–41.
13. Ferrucci L, Guralnik JM, Studenski S, Fried LP, Cutler GB Jr, Walston JD. Designing randomized, controlled trials aimed at preventing or delaying functional decline and disability in frail, older persons: a consensus report. J Am Geriatr Soc. 2004;52:625–34.
14. Fried LP, Ferrucci L, Darer J, Williamson JD, Anderson G. Untangling the concepts of disability, frailty, and comorbidity: implications for improved targeting and care. J Gerontol A Biol Sci Med Sci. 2004;59:255–63.
15. Bortz WM. A conceptual framework of frailty: a review. J Gerontol A Biol Sci Med Sci. 2002;57:M283–8.
16. Anderson JE, Kraus J, Sturgeon D. Incidence, prevalence, and outcomes of end-stage renal disease patients placed in nursing homes. Am J Kidney Dis. 1993;21:619–27.
17. Brogan DJ, Haber M, Kutner NG. Functional decline among older adults: comparing a chronic disease cohort and controls when mortality rates are markedly different. J Clin Epidemiol. 2000;53:847–51.
18. Hailpern SM, Melamed ML, Cohen HW, Hostetter TH. Moderate chronic kidney disease and cognitive function in adults 20 to 59 years of age: Third National Health and Nutrition Examination Survey (NHANES III). J Am Soc Nephrol. 2007;18:2205–13.
19. Kurella M, Ireland C, Hlatky MA, Shlipak MG, Yaffe K, Hulley SB, Chertow GM. Physical and sexual function in women with chronic kidney disease. Am J Kidney Dis. 2004;43:868–76.
20. Kurella M, Mapes DL, Port FK, Chertow GM. Correlates and outcomes of dementia among dialysis patients: the Dialysis Outcomes and Practice Patterns Study. Nephrol Dial Transplant. 2006;21:2543–8.
21. Kurella M, Yaffe K, Shlipak MG, Wenger NK, Chertow GM. Chronic kidney disease and cognitive impairment in menopausal women. Am J Kidney Dis. 2005;45:66–76.
22. Shlipak MG, Stehman-Breen C, Fried LF, Song X, Siscovick D, Fried LP, Psaty BM, Newman AB. The presence of frailty in elderly persons with chronic renal insufficiency. Am J Kidney Dis. 2004;43(5):861–7.
23. Johansen KL, Chertow GM, Jin C, Kutner NG. Significance of frailty among dialysis patients. J Am Soc Nephrol. 2007;18:2960–7.
24. Wilhelm-Leen ER, Hall YN, Tamura MK, Chertow GM. Frailty and chronic kidney disease: the Third National Health and Nutrition Evaluation Survey. Am J Med. 2009;122(7):664–71. https://doi.org/10.1016/j.amjmed.2009.01.026.
25. Van Loon IN. The relevance of geriatric impairments in patients starting dialysis: a systematic review. Clin J Am Soc Nephrol. 2016;11:1245–59. https://doi.org/10.2215/CJN.06660615.
26. Aiello F, Dueñas EP, Musso CG. Senescent nephropathy: the new renal syndrome. Healthcare (Basel). 2017;5(4). pii: E81. doi:https://doi.org/10.3390/healthcare5040081.

27. Woods NF, LaCroix AZ, Gray SL, Aragaki A, Cochrane BB, Brunner RL, Masaki K, Murray A, Newman AB, Women's Health Initiative. Frailty: emergence and consequences in women aged 65 and older in the Women's Health Initiative Observational Study. J Am Geriatr Soc. 2005;53:1321–30.
28. Musso CG, Jauregui JR, Macías Núñez JF. Frailty phenotype and chronic kidney disease: a review of the literature. Int Urol Nephrol. 2015;47(11):1801–7. https://doi.org/10.1007/s11255-015-1112-z.
29. Arai Y, Takayama M, Gondo Y, Inagaki H, Yamamura K, Nakazawa S, Kojima T, Ebihara Y, Shimizu K, Masui Y, Kitagawa K, Takebayashi T, Hirose N. Adipose endocrine function, insulin-like growth factor-1 axis, and exceptional survival beyond 100 years of age. J Gerontol A Biol Sci Med Sci. 2008;63:1209–18.
30. Artz AS. Anemia and the frail elderly. Semin Hematol. 2008;45:261–6.
31. Swidler MA, Uribarri J, Siu AL. Characterization of frailty in older adults with chronic kidney disease (CKD): correlations with biomarkers of inflammation. J Am Soc Nephrol. 2005;16:514a.
32. Musso CG, Vilas M, de Quirós FG, Núñez JF. The importance of evaluating frailty and social-behavioral factors for managing drugs and dialysis prescription in elderly patients. Drug Res (Stuttg). 2016;66(4):223–4. https://doi.org/10.1055/s-0035-1565127.
33. Gill TM, Robison JT, Tinetti ME. Difficulty and dependence: two components of the disability continuum among community-living older persons. Ann Intern Med. 1998;128:96–101.
34. Gill TM, Williams CS, Tinetti ME. Assessing risk for the onset of functional dependence among older adults: the role of physical performance. J Am Geriatr Soc. 1995;43:603–9.
35. Delano BG, Suresh U, Feldman J, Schneider D, Friedman EA. Dismal rehabilitation in predominantly type II diabetics on dialysis in inner-city Brooklyn. Clin Nephrol. 2000;54:94–104.
36. Lowder GM, Perri NA, Friedman EA. Demographics, diabetes type, and degree of rehabilitation in diabetic patients on maintenance hemodialysis in Brooklyn. J Diabet Complicat. 1988;2:218–26.
37. Julius M, Hawthorne VM, Carpentier-Alting P, Kneisley J, Wolfe RA, Port FK. Independence in activities of daily living for endstage renal disease patients: biomedical and demographic correlates. Am J Kidney Dis. 1989;13:61–9.
38. Kutner NG, Brogan DJ. Assisted survival, aging, and rehabilitation needs: comparison of older dialysis patients and age-matched peers. Arch Phys Med Rehabil. 1992;73:309–15.
39. De Oreo PB. Hemodialysis patient-assessed functional health status predicts continued survival, hospitalization, and dialysis-attendance compliance. Am J Kidney Dis. 1997;30:204–12.
40. Ifudu O, Paul H, Mayers JD, Cohen LS, Brezsnyak WF, Herman AI, Avram MM, Friedman EA. Pervasive failed rehabilitation in center-based maintenance hemodialysis patients. Am J Kidney Dis. 1994;23:394–400.
41. Ifudu O, Mayers J, Matthew J, Tan CC, Cambridge A, Friedman EA. Dismal rehabilitation in geriatric inner-city hemodialysis patients. JAMA. 1994;271:29–33.
42. Leinau L, Murphy TE, Bradley E, Fried T. Relationship between conditions addressed by hemodialysis guidelines and non-ESRD-specific conditions affecting quality of life. Clin J Am Soc Nephrol. 2009;4:572–8.
43. Cook WL, Jassal SV. Functional dependencies among the elderly on hemodialysis. Kidney Int. 2008;73:1289–95.
44. Podsiadlo D, Richardson S. The timed "Up & Go": a test of basic functional mobility for frail elderly persons. J Am Geriatr Soc. 1991;39:142–8.
45. Gill TM, Allore HG, Hardy SE, Guo Z. The dynamic nature of mobility disability in older persons. J Am Geriatr Soc. 2006;54:248–54.
46. Hardy SE, Dubin JA, Holford TR, Gill TM. Transitions between states of disability and independence among older persons. Am J Epidemiol. 2005;161:575–84.
47. Lo D, Chiu E, Jassal SV. A prospective pilot study to measure changes in functional status associated with hospitalization in elderly dialysis-dependent patients. Am J Kidney Dis. 2008;52:956–61.

48. Fried LF, Biggs ML, Shlipak MG, Seliger S, Kestenbaum B, Stehman-Breen C, Sarnak M, Siscovick D, Harris T, Cauley J, Newman AB, Robbins J. Association of kidney function with incident hip fracture in older adults. J Am Soc Nephrol. 2007;18:282–6.
49. Gallagher JC, Rapuri PB, Smith LM. An age-related decrease in creatinine clearance is associated with an increase in number of falls in untreated women but not in women receiving calcitriol treatment. J Clin Endocrinol Metab. 2007;92:51–8.
50. Gallagher JC, Rapuri P, Smith L. Falls are associated with decreased renal function and insufficient calcitriol production by the kidney. J Steroid Biochem Mol Biol. 2007;103:610–3.
51. Dukas LC, Schacht E, Mazor Z, Stähelin HB. A new significant and independent risk factor for falls in elderly men and women: a low creatinine clearance of less than 65 ml/min. Osteoporos Int. 2005;16:332–8.
52. Cook WL, Tomlinson G, Donaldson M, Markowitz SN, Naglie G, Sobolev B, Jassal SV. Falls and fall-related injuries in older dialysis patients. Clin J Am Soc Nephrol. 2006;1:1191–6.
53. Desmet C, Beguin C, Swine C, Jadoul M, Université Catholique de Louvain Collaborative Group. Falls in hemodialysis patients: prospective study of incidence, risk factors, and complications. Am J Kidney Dis. 2005;45:148–53.
54. Ray WA, Taylor JA, Brown AK, Gideon P, Hall K, Arbogast P, Meredith S. Prevention of fall-related injuries in long-term care: a randomized controlled trial of staff education. Arch Intern Med. 2005;165:2293–8.
55. Li M, Tomlinson G, Naglie G, Cook WL, Jassal SV. Geriatric comorbidities, such as falls, confer an independent mortality risk to elderly dialysis patients. Nephrol Dial Transplant. 2008;23:1396–400.
56. Elias MF, Elias PK, Seliger SL, Narsipur SS, Dore GA, Robbins MA. Chronic kidney disease, creatinine and cognitive functioning. Nephrol Dial Transplant. 2009;24:2446–52.
57. Kurella M, Chertow GM, Fried LF, Cummings SR, Harris T, Simonsick E, Satterfield S, Ayonayon H, Yaffe KA. Chronic kidney disease and cognitive impairment in the elderly: the health, aging, and body composition study. J Am Soc Nephrol. 2005;16:2127–33.
58. Kurella Tamura M, Wadley V, Yaffe K, McClure LA, Howard G, Go R, Allman RM, Warnock DG, McClellan W. Kidney function and cognitive impairment in US adults: the Reasons for Geographic and Racial Differences in Stroke (REGARDS) Study. Am J Kidney Dis. 2008;52:227–34.
59. Murray AM, Tupper DE, Knopman DS, Gilbertson DT, Pederson SL, Li S, Smith GE, Hochhalter AK, Collins AJ, Kane RL. Cognitive impairment in hemodialysis patients is common. Neurology. 2006;67:216–23.
60. Rakowski DA, Caillard S, Agodoa LY, Abbott KC. Dementia as a predictor of mortality in dialysis patients. Clin J Am Soc Nephrol. 2006;1:1000–5.
61. Gottlieb D, Mildworf B, Rubinger D, Melamed E. The regional cerebral blood flow in patients under chronic hemodialytic treatment. J Cereb Blood Flow Metab. 1987;7:659–61.
62. Hata R, Matsumoto M, Handa N, Terakawa H, Sugitani Y, Kamada T. Effects of hemodialysis on cerebral circulation evaluated by transcranial Doppler ultrasonography. Stroke. 1994;25:408–12.
63. Ishida I, Hirakata H, Sugimori H, Omae T, Hirakata E, Ibayashi S, Kubo M, Fujishima M. Hemodialysis causes severe orthostatic reduction in cerebral blood flow velocity in diabetic patients. Am J Kidney Dis. 1999;34:1096–104.
64. Arieff A. Dialysis disequilibrium syndrome: current concepts on pathogenesis and prevention. Kidney Int. 1994;45:629–35.
65. Murray AM, Pederson SL, Tupper DE, Hochhalter AK, Miller WA, Li Q, Zaun D, Collins AJ, Kane R, Foley RN. Acute variation in cognitive function in hemodialysis patients: a cohort study with repeated measures. Am J Kidney Dis. 2007;50:270–8.
66. Oreopoulos DG, Dimkovic N. Geriatric nephrology is coming of age. J Am Soc Nephrol. 2003;14:1099–101.
67. Brown EA, Johansson L. Old age and frailty in the dialysis population. J Nephrol. 2010;23:502–7.

68. Cavalli A, Del Vecchio L, Locatelli F. Geriatric nephrology. J Nephrol. 2010;23(Suppl 15):S11–5.
69. US renal data system: USRDS 2010 annual data report: atlas of chronic kidney disease and end-stage renal disease in the United States. Bethesda, National Institute of Health, National Institute of Diabetes and Digestive And Kidney Disease; 2010.
70. Jassal SV, Chiu E, Li M. Geriatric hemodialysis rehabilitation care. Adv Chronic Kidney Dis. 2008;15:115–22.
71. Kim JC, Kalantar-Zadeh K, Kopple J. Frailty and protein-energy wasting in elderly patients with end stage kidney disease. J Am Soc Nephrol. 2013;24:337–5. https://doi.org/10.1681/ASN.2012010047.
72. Obi Y, Qader H, Kovesdy CP, Kalantar-Zadeh K. Latest consensus and update on protein energy-wasting in chronic kidney disease. Curr Opin Clin Nutr Metab Care. 2015;18(3):254–62. https://doi.org/10.1097/MCO.0000000000000171.
73. Musso CG, Giordani MC, Imperiali N. Aging kidney transplantation. Rev Investig Clin. 2016;68(2):68–74.
74. Musso CG, Jauregui JR. How to differentiate renal senescence from chronic kidney disease in clinical practice. Postgrad Med. 2016;128(7):716–21. https://doi.org/10.1080/00325481.2016.1209963.
75. Stack AG, Murthy B. Exercise and limitations in physical activity levels among new dialysis patients in the United States: an epidemiologic study. Ann Epidemiol. 2008;18:880–8.
76. Johansen KL, Chertow GM, Kutner NG, Dalrymple LS, Grimes BA, Kaysen GA. Low level of self-reported physical activity in ambulatory patients new to dialysis. Kidney Int. 2010;78:1164–70.
77. Pupim LB, Heimbürger O, Qureshi AR, Ikizler TA, Stenvinkel P. Accelerated lean body mass loss in incident chronic dialysis patients with diabetes mellitus. Kidney Int. 2005;68:2368–74.
78. Bhasin S, Storer TW, Berman N, Callegari C, Clevenger B, Phillips J, Bunnell TJ, Tricker R, Shirazi A, Casaburi R. The effects of supraphysiologic doses of testosterone on muscle size and strength in normal men. N Engl J Med. 1996;335:1–7.
79. Johansen KL, Shubert T, Doyle J, Soher B, Sakkas GK, Kent-Braun JA, Muscle atrophy in patients receiving hemodialysis. Effects on muscle strength, muscle quality, and physical function. Kidney Int. 2003;63:291–7.
80. Sterky E, Stegmayr BG. Elderly patients on haemodialysis have 50% less functional capacity than gender- and age-matched healthy subjects. Scand J Urol Nephrol. 2005;39:423–30.
81. Brown E, Johansson L. Dialysis options for end-stage renal disease in older people. Nephron Clin Pract. 2011;119(Suppl 1):c10–3. https://doi.org/10.1159/000328019.
82. Boaz M, Smetana S, Weinstein T, Matas Z, Gafter U, Iaina A, Knecht A, Weissgarten Y, Brunner D, Fainaru M, Green MS. Secondary prevention with antioxidants of cardiovascular disease in endstage renal disease (SPACE): randomised placebo controlled trial. Lancet. 2000;356:1213–8.
83. Noble HR, Agus A, Brazil K, Burns A, Goodfellow NA, Guiney M, McCourt F, McDowell C, Normand C, Roderick P, Thompson C, Maxwell AP, Yaqoob MM. Palliative Care in chronic Kidney diSease: the PACKS study—quality of life, decisión making, costs and impact on carers in people managed without dialysis. BMC Nephrol. 2015;16:104.
84. Tattersall J, Farrington K, Gentile G, Kooman J, Macias Núñez JF, Nistor I, Van Biesen W, Covic A, European Renal Best Practice Guidelines Group and the European Union of Geriatric Medicine Societies (EUGMS). Is Kt/V useful in elderly dialysis patients? Pro- and con arguments. Nephrol Dial Transplant. 2018;16:742–50. https://doi.org/10.1093/ndt/gfy042.
85. Musso CG, Schwartz P, Deira J, Macias Núñez JF. Is it correct to use a unique conventional dialysis prescription in the elderly? Four alternative schedules for dialyzing elderly patients. Int J Ren Dis Ther. in press.
86. Kidney Disease: Improving Global Outcomes (KDIGO) CKD Work Group. KDIGO 2012 clinical practice guideline for the evaluation and management of chronic kidney disease. Chapter 3: management of progression and complications of CKD. Kidney Int Suppl. 2013;3(1):73–90.

87. Guideline development group, Bilo H, Coentrão L, Couchoud C, Covic A, De Sutter J, Drechsler C, Gnudi L, Goldsmith D, Heaf J. Clinical Practice Guideline on management of patients with diabetes and chronic kidney disease stage 3b or higher (eGFR <45 mL/min). Nephrol Dial Transplant. 2015;30(Suppl 2);1:ii1–ii142.
88. Musso CG, Trigka K, Dousdampanis P, Jauregui J. Therapeutic alternatives and palliative care for advanced renal disease in the very elderly: a review of the literature. Int Urol Nephrol. 2015;47(4):647–54. https://doi.org/10.1007/s11255-014-0886-8.

Water, Electrolyte, and Acid-Base Disorders in the Elderly

4

Carlos Guido Musso and Manuel F. Vilas

Introduction

In healthy old and very old individuals, serum electrolyte levels are in the normal range, but they can be easily altered compared to the young individuals. This phenomenon can be attributed to a reduced homeostatic capability in the elderly, which is tightly related to the significant and prevalent structural and functional changes suffered by the aged kidney, known as the *nephrogeriatric giants*. Some of these renal aging changes have an important role in the development of the water and electrolyte disorders in aged individuals; therefore, they should always be taken into account before analyzing these conditions in this population. These *nephrogeriatric giants* are the following ones [1]:

- Age-related glomerular filtration rate (GFR) reduction (1 ml/year since 40 years of age), whose value can be calculated by applying Keller's equation (Creatinine clearance = 130 – age) [2]. This age-related reduced GFR contributes to the urine dilution capability reduction usually found in the elderly [3].
- Tubular dysfunction, which leads to reduced sodium, and reduced calcium and magnesium reabsorption (in particular circumstances), as well as reduced free

C. G. Musso (✉)
Nephrology Division, Hospital Italiano de Buenos Aires,
Buenos Aires, Argentina

Physiology Department, Instituto Universitario del Hospital Italiano de Buenos Aires,
Buenos Aires, Argentina

Ageing Biology Unit, Hospital Italiano de Buenos Aires,
Buenos Aires, Argentina
e-mail: carlos.musso@hospitalitaliano.org.ar

M. F. Vilas
Nephrology Division, Hospital italiano de Buenos Aires,
Buenos Aires, Argentina

C. G. Musso et al. (eds.), *Clinical Nephrogeriatrics*,
https://doi.org/10.1007/978-3-030-18711-8_4

water clearance, reduced potassium secretion, and slowed down distal proton secretion [3].

- Medulla hypotonicity, which contributes to the urine concentration capability reduction usually documented in the elderly [3]. Vasopressin release is not impaired with aging but this hormone level is relatively increased for any given plasma osmolality level compared to the young, indicating vasopressin kidney resistance [4]. This vasopressin kidney resistance can be explained by the aging-related medulla hypotonicity.

Dysnatremias

Dysnatremias are the most common electrolyte disturbances in aged individuals, and they are even considered an important risk factor for high morbidity and mortality since they can decrease brain function, compromise cardiac contractility, increase insulin resistance, induce bone disease and neuromuscular dysfunction. Salt and water imbalance can induce abnormalities in volemia and/or serum sodium depending on the nature of this alteration, magnitude, and how it alters the relative body sodium/water ratio [5–7].

Hypernatremia

Hypernatremia (serum sodium >145 mmol/L) is related to a clinical setting which induces significant salt and water depletion in excess of water [5]. Hypernatremia is present in about 1–3% of hospitalized patients, and it is associated with high mortality rate (40–60%), particularly in the oldest old [8–10]. Moreover, it has been reported that when serum sodium value is higher than 160 mmol/L, the patient's mortality rate increases to 75% [8]. Due to the fact that hypernatremia is usually associated to severe conditions with multi-organ failure in the setting of cardiac disease and sepsis, is not clear yet if hypernatremia associated high mortality rate is because of its deleterious effects (adverse metabolic and cardiac effects) or because it is just a marker of an exhausted organism; probably participate both of them [7, 11].

Factors that can cause hypernatremia include:

1. Low fluid supply: When old individuals are water restricted for 24 h, their thirst threshold is increased, and water intake is reduced compared to younger individuals [12]. Mouth dryness, taste decrease, malnutrition, altered mental capacity or cortical cerebral dysfunction (e.g., Alzheimer's disease), hypoangiotensinemia, and osmoreceptors and baroreceptors sensitivity reduction can contribute to this increased thirst threshold usually documented in the elderly [8, 9, 13, 14]. In addition, many elderly reduce intentionally their fluid intake to reduce incontinence or because they suffer from depression or dependency (reduced access to water) [14].
2. Loss of fluid: Dehydration secondary to water loss can be secondary to sweating (hot weather, febrile status), gastrointestinal losses (vomiting, diarrhea,

laxatives), respiratory losses (hyperventilation), urine losses (osmotic diuresis, diuretics, renin-angiotensin-aldosterone system (RAAS) blockers, diabetes insipidus). Regarding the abovementioned urine water loss hypernatremia-inducing mechanisms, it is worth mentioning that they are reinforced by the reduced urine concentration capability which is usually found in the elderly due to their medulla hypotonicity (nephrogeriatric giants) [1, 8, 9, 15].

3. Hypertonic saline gain:

   This is a very infrequent cause of hypernatremia which is the consequence of a hypertonic saline solution supply, such as sodium bicarbonate-containing solutions [4].

In addition, total body water is diminished with age, being 55% of total body weight (even lower in elderly women) compared to 65% in young. This decrease in total body water is due to a decrease in lean body mass and an increase in the percentage of body fat, and it seems to be due predominantly to a water decrease in the intracellular compartment [4, 5, 13, 14, 16].

Therefore, elderly people are more vulnerable to hypernatremia due to a combination of factors such as their reduced thirst threshold, diminished access to water, reduced water reabsorption capability, and their frequent exposure to dehydration inducing drugs (e.g., diuretics) and clinical conditions (e.g., sepsis) [10]. Thus, it is crucial to diagnose the particular hypernatremia-causing factor along with assessing their volume status, and clinical context in order to prescribe the appropriate fluid supply and rate of correction, and closely monitoring the patient's clinical status and laboratory values during his/her treatment [11].

Hyponatremia

Hyponatremia (serum sodium ˂135 mmol/L) appears in any clinical setting which leads to a significant reduced serum sodium/water ratio [5]. Hyponatremia is present in 10% of ambulatory elderly, 10–30% of hospitalized patients, and up to 53% of institutionalized elderly [7, 17]. Moreover, serum sodium levels lower with increasing age, being hyponatremia an independent predictor of mortality and rehospitalization [7, 17–20]. Most probably hyponatremia is both a marker of the severity of the underlying comorbidities and a direct contributor to prognosis [21].

Mild to moderate hyponatremia is usually asymptomatic, while severe hyponatremia (serum sodium ˂125 mmol/L) can be symptomatic, being the most common manifestation neurologic symptoms due to cerebral edema [4]. However, recent reports showed that asymptomatic chronic hyponatremia can induce cognitive disorders, gait instability, attention deficit, decreased reaction time, being an independent risk factor of falls and associated with the development of osteoporosis [6, 22–26]. Barsoney et al., based on their findings in hyponatremia animal models, have proposed that chronic hyponatremia could exacerbate (by increasing oxidative stress) multiple senescence manifestations such as osteoporosis, loss of adiposity, sarcopenia, and cardiomyopathy [27].

In acute hyponatremia sodium, potassium, and chloride leave the brain cell and water enters, inducing cerebral edema. Over time, the brain adapts to lower osmolality by shifting organic osmolytes (e.g., glutamate, etc.) from brain cells into the extracellular fluid. It has been hypothesized that this decrease in cellular organic osmolyte concentration could decrease cognitive function, mobility, and nerve conduction in chronic hyponatremia [28]. Thus, based on the above information, it can be proposed that the hyponatremia classically known as "asymptomatic hyponatremia" should be called in fact "paucisymptomatic hyponatremia" because a fine evaluation (tests) can find its symptoms.

Regarding hyponatremia pathophysiology, it is known that a significant salt and water depletion may generate real hypovolemia, and if this depletion involves a loss of salt and water in excess of salt, it can induce hyponatremia. Besides, a salt and water retention in excess of water can induce hyponatremia (with or without edema), which may present with hypervolemia (e.g., severe renal failure, etc.) or effective hypovolemia (cardiac failure, etc.) depending on its etiologic mechanism [5].

Additionally, another factor which can modify the sodium/water ratio is the body potassium content since its intracellular depletion induces hyponatremia by at least two mechanisms:

- Sodium shift to the intracellular compartment
- Inappropriate vasopressin release

Hyponatremia secondary to low potassium content can be documented in severe malnourished (severely sarcopenic) elderly patients [4, 16, 29].

Edelman summarized all these concepts in this equation [5]:

$$\begin{aligned}\text{Serum sodium} = {} & \text{body sodium content}\left(\text{exchangeable}\right)\\ & + \text{body potassium content}\left(\text{exchangeable}\right)\\ & /\text{total body water content}\end{aligned}$$

Based on these concepts, hyponatremia is usually classified depending on its inducing mechanism [5]:

Normotonic Hyponatremia

This is a pseudohyponatremia caused by an increase in the solid fraction of plasma which can be observed in severe dyslipidemia or paraproteinemia. This error can be avoided by using a direct ion-sensitive electrode potentiometry-based estimation for the blood analysis [30].

Hypertonic Hyponatremia

Hyperglycemia increases intravascular tonicity which extracts free water out of the intracellular compartment diluting the intravascular compartment, therefore inducing a hypertonic hyponatremia. This sort of hyponatremia is observed in a setting of hyperglycemia (diabetes mellitus decompensation) or intravenous treatments based on osmotic substances (e.g., manitol, etc.) [13].

Hypotonic Hyponatremia

This hyponatremia can be induced by different mechanisms [13, 31]:

- Excess of water supply (oral or intravenous)
- Impaired free water urine excretion due to a decreased circulatory delivery of fluid to the thick ascending limb of loop of Henle (TALH) (e.g., heart failure, severe renal failure), altered TALH function (e.g., tubular necrosis, inflammation), appropriate or inappropriate antidiuretic hormone release
- Deficit in salt supply
- Excess of sodium loss
- Combined mechanisms

Thus, through some of these pathophysiologic mechanisms, many diseases which compromise the lung (pneumonia, etc.), heart (cardiac failure), kidney (renal insufficiency), liver (cirrhosis), endocrine glands (hypothyroidism, adrenal insufficiency), or brain (psychiatric disorders, syndrome of inappropriate antidiuretic hormone release, cerebral salt wasting syndrome) can induce hypotonic hyponatremia [31].

Regarding the elderly people, there are two of the *nephrogeriatric giants* which predispose old individuals to develop hypotonic hyponatremia: the age-related reduced GFR and the tubular dysfunction. On one hand, aging-related GFR reduction and tubular dysfunction, particularly the reduced TALH function (diluting segment), induce a free water clearance reduction. On the other hand, the aging-related tubular dysfunction, particularly TALH and distal tubule reduced sodium reabsorption, induces an increased urine sodium loss [1] (Table 4.1).

Additionally, hypotonic hyponatremia is usually classified depending on its urine osmolality value, and extracellular fluid status, in [4, 21]:

- First, hyponatremia with adequate urine dilution (urine osmolality $<$100 mOsm/L). This condition occurs in particular clinical settings which can be found in the elderly, such as excessive water ingestion (psychiatric patients), or low filtered load of solutes (malnourished patients).
- Second, hyponatremia with inadequate urine dilution (urine osmolality $\geq$100 mOsm/L), which can be classified into three categories depending on the volume of extracellular fluid (ECF): normal, low, or high ECF.

Hyponatremia with Normal ECF

As it was mentioned above, two *nephrogeriatric giants* predispose the elderly to develop this sort of hyponatremia: the age-related GFR reduction and the tubular dysfunction, particularly the TALH dysfunction (diluting segment), since they reduce their free water excretion capability [1] (Table 4.1). However, despite these predisposing factors, one of the main causes of hyponatremia with normal ECF in this population is the syndrome of inappropriate antidiuretic hormone secretion (SIADH).

Table 4.1 Age-related body changes which predispose to internal milieu disorders in the elderly

Age-related changes	Internal milieu disorders
Age-related GFR reduction	Hyponatremia, hypermagnesemia, hypercalcemia, hyperphosphatemia
Sodium reabsorption reduction (tubular dysfunction)	Hyponatremia
Potassium secretion reduction (tubular dysfunction)	Hyperkalemia
Free water clearance reduction (tubular dysfunction)	Hyponatremia
Water reabsorption reduction (medulla hypotonicity)	Hypernatremia
Calcium reabsorption reduction (relative tubular dysfunction)	Hypocalcemia
Magnesium reabsorption reduction (relative tubular dysfunction)	Hypomagnesemia
Proton secretion reduced or slowdown (tubular dysfunction)	Hyperchloremic metabolic acidosis
Calcium intestinal absorption reduction	Hypocalcemia
Magnesium intestinal absorption reduction	Hypomagnesemia
Hypodipsia	Hypernatremia
Sarcopenia	Hyponatremia, hypokalemia (hypothesis)
Skin changes	Hypocalcemia
Taste decrease (hyporexia)	Hyponatremia, hypokalemia, hypomagnesemia, hypocalcemia, hypophosphatemia

SIADH induces free water retention, with little change in body sodium, due to an inappropriate (low serum osmolality) antidiuretic hormone release or an excessive response of its tubular receptor, in the context of normal GFR, normal thyroid, and adrenal function and in the absence of hyponatremia-inducing medication [4, 13]. SIADH is present in about 30% of hyponatremic elderly, which is described as a primary disorder or secondary to pulmonary or cerebral diseases [19, 29, 32].

Other causes of hyponatremia with normal ECF which should be taken into account in the elderly are hypothyroidism (central or peripheral) or glucocorticoid deficiency secondary to infectious, immunologic, or oncologic glucocorticoid axis damage [13, 29, 33].

The reset osmostat (RO) is considered a SIADH subtype (SIADH type C) which has a low plasma osmolality threshold (usually 280 mOsm/kg), that induces an elevation of antidiuretic hormone (ADH) at a lower plasma osmolarity with normal water load excretion and intact urine diluting ability while maintaining normal sodium balance. RO has been documented in many settings such as neurologic diseases, malignancy, alcoholism, malnutrition, and in general in patients suffering from debilitating diseases. Since it has already been described in the literature the concept of "sick cell syndrome," which consists of a membrane transport failure (sodium-potassium ATPase pump dysfunction), which leads to an increase in the intracellular sodium and a reduction in intracellular potassium, a phenomenon which can induce hyponatremia in severely ill patients, it has been recently proposed that the sick cell phenomenon could be responsible, not only of inducing hyponatremia in debilitated patients but also of a RO appearance in this group, leading osmostat cells to lower the body threshold for "normal" serum sodium value in order to adapt the whole organism to a new internal milieu order [34].

Hyponatremia with Low ECF

As it was mentioned above, one of the *nephrogeriatric giants* which predisposes the elderly to develop this sort of hyponatremia is the tubular dysfunction, particularly the reduced sodium reabsorption capability (TALH and distal tubule reduced sodium reabsorption) since it induces significant sodium loss [1] (Table 4.1).

Real hypovolemia may induce hyponatremia by stimulating the non-osmotic antidiuretic hormone release, in a setting of an adequate or excessive oral water (hypotonic solution) intake [13]. Sodium losses lead to hypovolemia and consequently induce adequate antidiuretic hormone secretion, thus hyponatremia is promoted in this case by a double mechanism: a reduction in body sodium content (sodium loss) and an increase in body water content (water retention).

Hyponatremia secondary to negative sodium balance is frequent in the elderly in the following clinical settings:

- Prolong low sodium intake (senile sodium leakage hyponatremia)
- Increased sodium loss (tubule damage, RAAS dysfunction)
- Salt and water loss in excess of sodium (potent diuretics or diarrhea with access to water intake) [35, 36]

Hyponatremia with High ECF

The nephrogeriatric giant that predisposes to high ECF hyponatremia is the age-related GFR reduction since it facilitates water retention [1] (Table 4.1). This sort of hyponatremia is typically observed in the elderly when they are suffering from severe edematous states secondary to heart, liver, or kidney failure or nephrotic syndrome. In these settings of effective hypovolemia, hypotonic hyponatremia appears as a consequence of an impaired circulatory delivery to diluting segments, in combination with vasopressin release induced by the effective hypovolemia [13]. Besides, in severe renal insufficiency, high ECF hypotonic hyponatremia appears as a consequence of an impaired capability of free water excretion due to a significantly decrease in GFR (GFR <5 ml/min/1.73 m^2) [13, 35]. Renal insufficiency is a frequent complication in the elderly patients, usually induced by different mechanisms: acute tubular necrosis (ischemic, drugs, etc.), intra-tubular obstruction (rhabdomyolysis, etc.), urological obstruction (prostatic hypertrophy, prostatic cancer, uterine prolapse, etc.), and/or tubule-interstitial damage (interstitial nephritis, etc.). In these clinical situations, a hypotonic solution load contributes to the appearance of hyponatremia [35].

It is worth mentioning that immobility syndrome (IS), one of the geriatric syndromes, consists of a reduction in the capability to perform daily activities due to a motor function deterioration that leads to characteristic body structural and physiological changes. Among these body physiology alterations are a decline cardiac output, ortostatism, and capillary leak. It has been hypothesized that a pre-renal state, which could be explained by the aforementioned functional changes, induces vasopressin release and free water retention (hyponatremia with increased ECF) in IS. In this sense, it has been documented that IS patients have a relatively higher vasopressin level regarding their serum osmolality value, enabling this hormonal excess to explain the free water retention status usually found in this group [37, 38].

Hyponatremia Secondary to Drugs

Drug-induced hyponatremia is the main cause of hyponatremia in the elderly (75% of hyponatremic elderly) [19, 23]. Moreover, there is an independent association between hyponatremia and polypharmacy in older people [19].

Drug-induced hyponatremia can be induced by water retention, sodium loss, and/or potassium loss mechanisms [4, 6, 39–41]:

1. Water retention
   - Severe renal insufficiency (e.g., aminoglycoside)
   - Cortisol deficiency (e.g., ketoconazol)
   - SIADH effect (e.g., antidepressants, antiepileptic, RAAS blockers, etc.)
2. Sodium loss
   - Reduced tubular salt reabsorption: RAAS blockers, potent diuretics
   - Tubular damage (drug-induced interstitial nephritis, non-steroidal anti-inflammatory toxicity, etc.)
3. Potassium loss
   - Loop diuretics
   - Cathartics

Therefore, it is very important to diagnose the particular hyponatremia-causing factor along with assessing patient's urine osmolality, volume status, and clinical context in order to indicate the adequate water and electrolyte prescription and rate of correction, as well as monitoring the patient's clinical status closely and laboratory values during his/her treatment [1].

Dyskalemia

Total body potassium content is lower in the old than in the young, and the correlation with age is linear [24]. As 85% of potassium is deposited in muscle, and muscular mass diminishes with age. This may largely account for the fall in total body potassium, with other factors such as poor intake also playing some role [42].

Hypokalemia

Prevalence of hypokalemia (serum potassium $<$3.5 mmol/L) is 12.8%, 11.4%, and 10.9% in the young, middle-age, and elderly people, respectively; being hypokalemia the second electrolyte disorder more prevalent in the elderly after hyponatremia [43, 44].

Under normal conditions, plasma potassium is normal in the elderly, but they have low body potassium stores due to the age-related muscle mass reduction (sarcopenia) which predispose them to develop hypokalemia, particularly in the context of malnutrition, enteric potassium losses (diarrhea, cathartics), and potent diuretics (loop diuretics or thiazide) [45, 46] (Table 4.1). In addition, the elderly develop hypokalemia more rapidly than do the young [45].

Even though patients with mild hypokalemia (3.0–3.4 mmol/L) are usually asymptomatic, they may present fatigue, lethargy, constipation, urinary retention, or polyuria. Lower serum potassium levels can induce limb paralysis, myonecrosis, or cardiac arrhythmias. Moreover, hypokalemia increases the risk of falls by 2.2-fold [44].

Another cause of hypokalemia in the elderly is the potassium redistribution from the intravascular compartment to the intracellular compartment induced by drugs, particularly found in those suffering from diabetes mellitus (e.g., insulin), and/or polypharmacy [5, 39].

Finally, adequate potassium supply with concomitant inactivation of the hypokalemia-inducing mechanism is the cornerstone of hypokalemia treatment [5].

Hyperkalemia

Prevalence of hyperkalemia (serum potassium >5.5 mmol/L) is 2.4%, 7.4, and 19.5% in the young, middle-age, and elderly people, respectively [43]. Older individuals usually have lower angiotensin-converting enzyme activity than younger individuals. Healthy elderly people have a lower plasma renin activity and aldosterone levels (in supine position and on normal sodium diet), than young healthy people. Under the stimuli of upright posture and sodium depletion, there are significant increases in serum renin and aldosterone in both age groups but their values are always lower in the elderly. The reduced plasma renin activity in the elderly may be related to the inhibitory effect of increased amounts of atrial natriuretic peptide on renin secretion. The lower serum aldosterone concentration with age appears to be a direct result of age-related decrease of plasma renin activity and not of aging changes in the adrenal gland, because aldosterone and cortisol responses to ACTH infusion are not altered in the elderly [47]. This reduced capability of the aging kidney to excrete potassium, which is one of the nephrogeriatric giants (tubular dysfunction), explains the vulnerability of the elderly to hyperkalemia [13, 48–50] (Table 4.1). This electrolyte disturbance is particularly frequent when elderly individuals are treated (either alone or in combination) with RAAS blockers: angiotensin-converting enzyme inhibitors (ACEI), angiotensin II receptor antagonists (ARA), as well as potassium-sparing diuretics, NSAIDs (hyporeninemic hypoaldosteronism secondary to prostaglandin E_2 and prostacyclin I_2 inhibition), and beta-blockers (decrease catecholamine-induced renin release) [20, 46, 51]. In addition, it has been documented that the use of hyperkalemia-inducing drugs is usually higher in the oldest patients, and in those who have comorbidities, and polypharmacy [46].

Other causes of hyperkalemia in the elderly are a severe GFR reduction (renal failure), obstructive nephropathy (renal tubule acidosis), adrenal insufficiency (type IV renal tubule acidosis), or potassium redistribution from the intracellular compartment to the intravascular compartment secondary to hyperkalemia-inducing drugs (e.g., digoxin) or gross cytolysis (e.g., rhabdomyolysis, tumor lysis) [5, 39].

Finally, an adequate serum potassium reduction initially by intracellular redistribution (beta 2 agonist, intravenous glucose, etc.), cardioprotection (intravenous calcium), and then potassium loss measures (e.g., loop diuretics, cationic exchange resins, dialysis, etc.), with concomitant inactivation of the hyperkalemia-inducing mechanism, are the cornerstones of hyperkalemia treatment [5].

Dysmagnesemia

Serum magnesium (Mg) normal range is 1.7–2.3 mg/dl, with no significant difference in serum magnesium or its urine fractional excretion value (3%) between healthy young and old individuals [52, 53]. However, in the setting of volume expansion old people present significantly higher urine magnesium loss compared to young people. Since most of the filtered Mg is normally reabsorbed in TALH, which is a segment functionally altered in the elderly, it has been proposed this aging-associated TALH dysfunction could explain the abovementioned phenomenon [52] (Table 4.1). Mg is mainly located in the intracellular compartment (99%), and 30–50% of the dietary magnesium is absorbed by the intestinal tract, being its absorption stimulated in part by vitamin D (1.25 cholecalciferol). Thus, hypovitaminosis D, which is frequently found in the elderly, could partially explain the reduced Mg absorption documented in old individuals [53, 54] (Table 4.1).

Regarding the nephrogeriatric giants' influence in dysmagnesemias, some of them can contribute, although not induce per se, to these disorders, such as the contribution of the age-related GFR reduction to the appearance of hypermagnesemia (reduced magnesium excretion) in a context of increased Mg supply and the contribution of the TALH functional reduction to the appearance of hypomagnesemia (reduced magnesium reabsorption) in a context of low magnesium intake or high magnesium excretion [1] (Table 4.1).

Hypomagnesemia (serum magnesium ˂1.7 mg/dl) can be mainly induced in the elderly by a reduced Mg intestinal absorption (malnutrition, malabsorption, etc.) and/or renal reabsorption (glucosuria, loop diuretics, thiazides, Fanconi syndrome, proton-pump inhibitors, etc.) [39, 53, 55, 56].

Moreover, hypomagnesemia can be caused by Mg intracellular shift (redistribution) as it occurs during refeeding syndrome in very malnourished old individuals. Hypomagnesemia can induce tachyarrhythmias which may be resistant to standard therapy and respond only to Mg supply. Even hypomagnesemia facilitates digoxin cardiotoxicity, neuromuscular irritability, tetany, delirium, and seizures. Furthermore, many of the cardiac and neurologic symptoms attributed to Mg deficiency may also be explained by the coexistence of hypokalemia or hypocalcemia. However, hypomagnesemia by itself can induce hypokalemia that corrects after Mg deficit is normalized [53, 54, 56].

Hypermagnesemia (serum magnesium >2.3 mg/dl) basically appears in two clinical settings: marked renal failure (GFR <20 ml/min/1.73 m^2), and excessive Mg supply, which is usually provided as antacids or cathartics [39]. However, hypermagnesemia symptoms (low blood pressure, vomiting, facial flushing, intestinal and/or urinary retention, and lethargy) appear when serum Mg level is above 4–6 mg/dl, and if untreated, it can progress to flaccid skeletal muscular paralysis (hyporeflexia), bradyarrhythmia, and even respiratory depression and cardiac arrest. Hypermanesemia can also be documented in some clinical conditions, usually found in the elderly, such as hypothyroidism, adrenal insufficiency, and lithium toxicity [39, 53, 54, 56].

Therefore, it is crucial to diagnose the dysmagnesemia-causing factor along with assessing the patient and his/her context in order to indicate the adequate prescription, rate of correction, and monitoring closely the patient's clinical status and laboratory values during his/her treatment. These treatments can be, for instance, Mg supply in hypomagnesia, or Mg discontinuation, intravenous calcium gluconate supply (Mg antagonist), and Mg loss measures (e.g., loop diuretics, dialysis) in hypermagnesemia [54].

Dysphosphatemia

Normal serum phosphorus range is 2.5–5.0 mg/dl in adults, with 1% of body phosphorus content placed in the extracellular compartment. The main phosphorus income is through the digestive tract, being absorbed in the small intestine (60%), in a process which can be increased by the vitamin D stimulus [56]. There is not a significant difference either in the serum phosphorus level or urine fractional excretion of phosphorus between young and old healthy people [52].

Regarding the nephrogeriatric giants' influence in dysphosphatemias, the one which can contribute, although not induced per se, to hyperphosphatemia is the age-related GFR reduction (reduced phosphorus excretion) in a context of increased phosphorus intake [1] (Table 4.1).

Hyperphosphatemia (serum phosphate level >5.0 mg/dl in adults) should be distinguished from spurious hyperphosphatemia which can be found in hemolyzed sample and from pseudohyperphosphatemia secondary to paraproteinemia, hyperlipidemia, or hyperbilirubinemia [56, 57].

The main pathophysiologic mechanism of hyperphosphatemia in this population is phosphorus retention due to a GFR reduction <25 ml/min/1.73 m^2, particularly in a setting of a high phosphorus diet. Besides, hyperphosphatemia can be caused in the elderly by phosphate shift from cells to the extracellular space secondary to massive cytolysis due to rhabdomyolysis (fall follows by hypothermia) or chemotherapy (bulky tumors) [56, 58]. Among the causes of hyperphosphatemia secondary to a reduced phosphorus renal excretion capability are the hypoparathyroidism and pseudohypoparathyroidism [58].

The symptoms of hyperphosphatemia are frequently in fact those from its accompanying hypocalcemia. Hyperphosphatemia can lead to secondary hypocalcemia by causing calcium precipitation (mainly when calcium-phosphorus product >70), vitamin D synthesis reduction, and reduced intestinal calcium absorption. Besides, hyperphosphatemia can induce secondary hyperparathyroidism [56, 58–60].

In dialysis patients, serum phosphorus >5.5 mg/dL is also associated with increased risk of all-cause and cardiovascular mortality, and this association can in part be due to vascular calcification. The pathophysiologic mechanisms by which high serum phosphorus contributes to vascular calcification consist, in part, of transforming vascular smooth muscular cells from a contractile to an osteochondrogenic phenotype and mineralization of their matrix through sodium-dependent phosphate cotransporters, reducing Klotho expression, and increasing fibroblast growth factor-23 levels and vascular calcification which is independently associated with adverse cardiovascular outcomes and mortality [59].

Hypophosphatemia (serum phosphate level <2.5 mg/dl in adult people) is usually asymptomatic until serum phosphate level is below 1 mg/dL. Malnutrition is one of the main causes of hypophosphatemia in the elderly [56]. Decreased intestinal phosphorus absorption can be observed in small intestine disorders, vitamin D deficiency and treatment based on corticosteroids or high doses of phosphate-binding drugs. Among other hypophosphatemia inducing mechanisms is an increased renal phosphorus excretion, as is the case of primary hyperparathyroidism, tubular dysfunction (e.g., post-obstructive polyuria), and hyperphosphaturia-inducing drugs (e.g., proximal diuretics, some antineoplastic agents) [58].

Hypophosphatemia can also be observed in refeeding syndrome (phosphorus intracellular shift), alcoholic patients, diabetic patients (poor phosphorus intake), acute leukemia and in the leukemic phases of lymphomas, sepsis, and heat stroke.

Regarding hypophosphatemia clinical consequences, erythrocytes experience a decrease in 2,3-diphosphoglycerate levels, thus hemolysis results from increased red cell rigidity [56]. Severe hypophosphatemia can also induce a dysfunction in the white cell phagocytosis, rhabdomyolysis, and altered renal tubular, heart, and respiratory functions. Moreover, prolonged phosphate depletion can lead to osteomalacia [61].

In dialysis patients, serum phosphorus level below 3.5 mg/dL is a mortality predictor, since it can reflect low protein intake and its associated death risk [58].

It is worth mentioning that it is very important to diagnose the dysphosphatemia-causing factor along with assessing the patient status and his/her context in order to indicate the adequate prescription, monitoring closely the patient clinical status and laboratory values during his/her treatment. This treatment can be, for instance, phosphorus supply in hypophosphatemia, or phosphorus supply discontinuation, phosphorus binders (reduced absorption), and/or phosphorus loss measures (e.g., dialysis) in hyperphosphatemia [58].

Dyscalcemias

Total serum calcium normal range is 9–10.5 mg/dl, and approximately 50% of serum calcium is bound to albumin, a small amount is complexed to anions, and the rest is as free ionized calcium [58]. Even though total serum calcium level and urine fractional excretion of calcium are similar between young and old individuals, in a volume expansion setting, there are a significant increase in urine calcium excretion and a significant serum calcium reduction in the elderly compared to the young. This phenomenon has been attributed to the reduced reabsorption capability in TALH (high calcium reabsorption segment) documented in the elderly [52] (Table 4.1).

Due to the fact that the calcium ionized form is the physiologically relevant one, if there is hypoalbuminemia, 0.8 mg/dl of calcium for every 1 mg reduction in serum albumin below 4 mg/dl should be added in order to correct the patient's calcemia to his/her albuminemia level. Serum ionized calcium increases in acidosis (lower albumin binding), while it reduces in alkalosis (higher albumin binding).

Healthy elderly people do not suffer from vitamin D deficiency; they do not have either hypercalciuria or its subsequent serum parathyroid hormone augment. However, since this population frequently have a low vitamin D diet, reduced sunlight exposure, decreased vitamin D renal hydroxylation (activation), and low serum sexual hormones levels, they have a predisposition to developing hypercalciuria. The latter phenomenon in addition to a poor calcium intestinal absorption leads this population to develop senile secondary hyperparathyroidism [62–64] (Table 4.1).

Regarding the nephrogeriatric giants' influence in dyscalcemia, some of them can contribute, although not induce per se, to these disorders. Since normally the kidney has a protective role against the development of hypercalcemia because of the extracellular calcium itself appears to have a calciuric effect on the renal tubule by its direct action on the TALH calcium-sensing receptor, two nephrogeriatric giants (the age-related GFR reduction and TALH dysfunction) could contribute to the appearance of hypercalcemia (reduced calcium excretion) in a context of increased calcium and/or vitamin D supply [1] (Table 4.1).

Among the main causes of hypocalcemia in the elderly are endocrine conditions (hypoparathyroidism, hypovitaminosis D), drugs (phenytoin, bisphosphonates, calcitonin), electrolyte disorders (chronic hypomagnesemia, acute hypermagnesemia, hyperphosphatemia), lifestyle (low sunlight exposure), digestive conditions (malabsorption, pancreatitis), chronic nephropathy, and massive cytolysis (rhabdomyolysis) [58].

Regarding hypocalcemia, clinical manifestations can be muscle cramps and finger numbness. Severe hypocalcemia may cause depression, cognitive capability reduction, laryngeal and carpopedal spasm, bronchospasm, seizures, prolonged QT interval in electrocardiogram, and cardiac arrhythmia [58]. The main cause of hypercalcemia in the elderly is an increase in the bone resorption, which can be induced by different causes such as immobility syndrome, high parathyroid hormone (primary hyperparathyroidism) or parathyroid hormone-related proteins levels (paraneoplastic syndrome), multiple myeloma, bone metastasis. Other hypercalcemia-inducing mechanisms are excessive active vitamin D levels, exogenous (medication) or endogenous (granulomatous diseases), which contribute to an increased calcium intestinal absorption, as well as a reduced urinary calcium excretion as is the case in thiazide treatment or, more rarely, in familial hypocalciuric hypercalcemia. Finally, hypercalcemia can also be documented in patients suffering from adrenal insufficiency and treatment based on lithium, vitamin A, estrogens, or antiestrogens [39, 58, 65].

Hypercalcemia can induce neuromuscular alterations (fatigue, weakness, depression), cardiac arrhythmia (QT interval shortening and heart block), digestive derangements (constipation, ulcus, pancreatitis), and renal disorders such as polyuria (nephrogenic insipidus diabetes), nephrolithiasis, and/or nephrocalcinosis [58, 65].

It is very important to diagnose the dyscalcemia-causing factor along with assessing the patient status and his/her context in order to indicate the adequate prescription, monitoring the patient's clinical status closely and laboratory values during his/her treatment. This treatment can consist of calcium and/or vitamin D supply for hypocalcemia, or calcium restriction, increased urine calcium excretion (hydration, furosemide, dialysis), and calcium redistribution (bisphosphonate, calcitonin) for hypercalcemia [58].

Acid-Base Disturbances

The kidney is the organ which maintains the acid-base equilibrium by means of the renal acid-base homeostasis roughly achieved by two processes, reabsorption of filtered bicarbonate (HCO_3^-) and excretion of fixed acids mediated by the same basic process: renal H^+ secretion (75). The reabsorption of HCO_3^- is mainly accomplished in the proximal tubule where the 70–90% of the filtered HCO_3^- is reabsorbed, whereas excretion of fixed acid, achieved through the acidification of urinary buffers and the excretion of ammonium ion, is mainly a distal tubular competence [35]. Renal threshold for bicarbonate is comparable in the aged and in the young [56].

Regarding distal acidification, it has been reported that titratable acid elimination behaves similarly in the young as in the aged, although one study reported that it is higher in subjects >60 years compared to the young. Conversely, there is an almost general agreement that ammonium elimination is lower in the aged than in the young subjects, except in one study in which differences between young and aged individuals were not found. However, in this study it was documented that the aged need more time to reach the peak acid excretion (between 6 and 8 h) (Table 4.1). In regard to the difference in renal tubular acidification between healthy young and old individuals, it could be attributed to the nephrogeriatric giant (tubular dysfunction) since, on one hand, the ammonium transport in the TALH could be reduced because of the reduced $Na^+ K^+2Cl^-$ tubular carriers' number documented in the aged kidney. On the other hand, there is a sort of aldosterone resistance in the distal tubules in the elderly, and this hormone stimulates the distal tubule acidification [56] (Table 4.1).

Acid-base imbalance generates different sort of internal milieu disorders as is the case of acidosis, alkalosis, or their combination (double or triple acid-base disorders). Acidosis is characterized by either a primary acid gain or alkali loss, while acidemia indicates an increased serum proton (H+) concentration (serum pH <7.36). On the contrary, alkalosis is characterized by either a primary acid loss or alkali gain, and alkalemia indicates a decreased serum H+ concentration (serum pH >7.44). In addition, acidosis is classified based on its inducing mechanism in respiratory acidosis (carbon dioxide retention), normochloremic or high anion-gap metabolic acidosis (bicarbonate conversion), and hyperchloremic or normal anion-gap metabolic acidosis (bicarbonate loss). Regarding alkalosis, it is usually classified based on its inducing mechanism in respiratory alkalosis (carbon dioxide high excretion) and metabolic alkalosis (bicarbonate gain) [66, 67].

Even though acid-base balance is remarkably well maintained in elderly people, who are generally able to maintain normal serum pH, bicarbonate, and carbon dioxide levels, aging-related renal tubular dysfunction (nephrogeriatric giant) and lung changes (senile lung) can contribute to easily induce acid-base disorders in the setting of different stressors [68] (Table 4.1).

In elderly patients the main cause of hyperchloremic (normal anion-gap) metabolic acidosis is bicarbonate loss through profuse diarrhea or renal tubule dysfunction induced by drugs (sparing potassium agents, ACEI, ARA, etc.), moderate renal damage (acute tubular necrosis, interstitial nephritis, etc.), and non-renal diseases which can induce tubular acidification disorders (adrenal insufficiency, etc.). Normal serum chlorine or high anion-gap metabolic acidosis has been documented in the elderly during severe renal failure (uremic acidosis), diabetic acidosis (ketoacidosis), and systemic inflammatory response syndrome mainly secondary to sepsis (hypoxic lactic acidosis: type A). Metabolic alkalosis can be induced by moderate volume contraction secondary to gastrointestinal (vomiting, diarrhea) or urinary losses (potent diuretics, polyuria, etc.). Moreover, respiratory compensation to metabolic acid-base disorders can be reduced. Finally, acute respiratory acidosis (<48 h) is usually documented secondary to central nervous system depression due to crane-encephalic trauma (falls) or benzodiazepines ingestion, while acute respiratory alkalosis (<48 h) is usually observed in hyperventilation secondary to sepsis. Finally, among the chronic respiratory disorders (>48 h), it deserves to be mentioned the chronic respiratory acidosis secondary to chronic obstructive pulmonary disease [66–70].

Internal Milieu Disorders and Frailty

Geriatrics has described four entities of its own, confusional syndrome, incontinence (fecal and/or urinary), gait disorders, and immobility syndrome, naming these geriatric syndromes as the "geriatric giants" because of their high prevalence and great impact on the geriatric health. These geriatric giants can appear as acute events or as an exacerbation of their already existing state, being often the only clinical expression of various diseases such as pneumonia, urinary infection, cardiac infarction, etc. It is worth pointing out that if the previously mentioned diseases appear in young people, they suffer from symptoms such as fever, cough, dysuria, chest pain, etc., while when these diseases appear in old people, there could be a lack of those symptoms but the appearance of the *geriatric giants*. This situation has led to the misconception that illnesses in the elderly are oligosyntomatic when in fact their symptomatology is very rich (the symptoms are the geriatric giants) but different compared to the one presented in young people [37].

In addition, as it was previously mentioned, aging process induces many changes in renal physiology which predispose old people to develop salt and water alterations (the nephrogeriatric giants). These changes consist of a reduction in GFR, diminution in water and sodium reabsorption, as well as in potassium secretion capability [1].

The geriatric syndromes (geriatric giants) and the aging-related renal function changes (nephrogeriatric giants) are clinical entities characteristic in the elderly that predispose and potentiate each other, leading to catastrophic events. For instance, an old person suffers from urinary sepsis, and because of that he develops a confusional syndrome. The accompanying fever causes him to lose water and also to reduce his water intake because of his confusion. Since old people have reduced water reabsorption ability, he develops severe dehydration and hypernatremia that worsen his confusional state leading to a catastrophic clinical event. This case represents an example of a geriatric giant (confusional syndrome) that is worsened by a nephrogeriatric giant (reduced water reabsorption capacity) [37] (Fig. 4.1).

Additionally, a nephrogeriatric giant can potentiate a geriatric giant leading to a catastrophic clinical event. For instance: an old person under the effect of very hot weather loses water (sweating), and since old people suffer primary hypodipsia and they have low salt and water reabsorption capacity, this patient develops hypotension that causes dizziness, altered gait and finally fall. This situation worsens his salt and water intake (water access restriction) leading him further to a severe

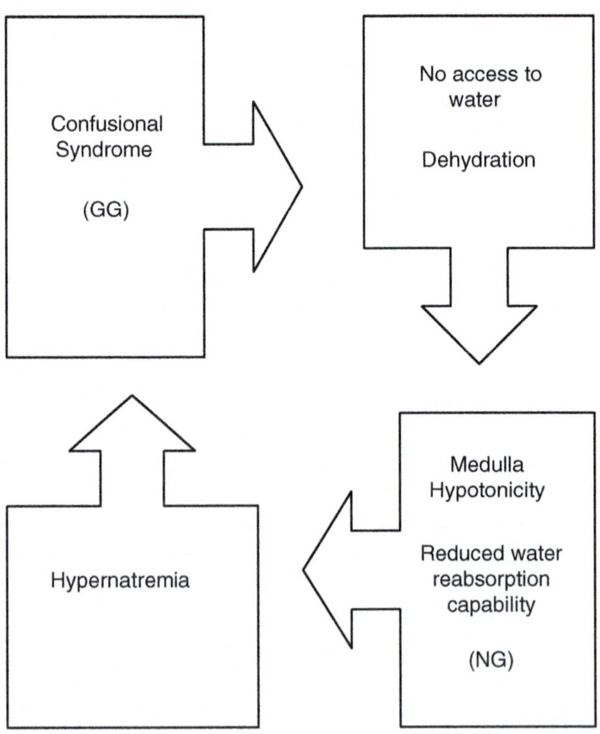

Fig. 4.1 Interdependence between geriatric giant (GG) and nephrogeriatric giant (NG)

volume contraction and acute renal failure. This is an example of a nephrogeriatric giant (reduced water intake and reabsorption) which is worsened by a geriatric giant (fall) [37].

Both cases described above are an example of what is named the feed-back between geriatric syndromes. The roots of this phenomenon are in the aging process, since it consists of loss of complexity. An organism is a system that is constituted by other small ones (cardiovascular, respiratory, etc.) which are named microsystem since they conform a bigger one: the organism or macrosystem. Then, complexity means all these microsystems working harmoniously. An organism functions due to coordination among their multiple microsystems. This coordination of systems or complexity makes the organism flexible and capable to overcome environmental changes. The senescence process weakens these microsystems and their coordination between them undermining complexity and making the person frail. They function normally under basal conditions, but they cannot handle extreme environmental changes, and therefore an otherwise insignificant event such as a hot weather or a urinary tract infection can lead old people to severe compromise or death [37, 70, 71] (Fig. 4.1).

Conclusion

Elderly individuals, and particularly those who are frail, are predisposed to suffer from different water, electrolyte, and acid-base disorders (sometimes with opposing effects), since these aged individuals are usually exposed to infectious, inflammatory, oncological, and pharmacological variables in a setting of an undermined homeostatic capability.

References

1. Musso CG. Geriatric nephrology and the 'nephrogeriatric giants'. Int Urol Nephrol. 2002;34(2):255–6.
2. Musso CG, Álvarez-Gregori J, Jauregui J, Macías-Núñez JF. Glomerular filtration rate equations: a comprehensive review. Int Urol Nephrol. 2016;48(7):1105–10. https://doi.org/10.1007/s11255-016-1276-1.
3. Musso CG, Belloso WH, Glassock RJ. Water, electrolytes, and acid-base alterations in human immunodeficiency virus infected patients. World J Nephrol. 2016;5(1):33–42. https://doi.org/10.5527/wjn.v5.i1.33.
4. Kugler JP, Hustead T. Hyponatremia and hypernatremia in the elderly. Am Fam Physician. 2000;61(12):3623–30.
5. Adrogué H, Wesson D. Salt & water. Houston: Libra & Gemini; 1993.
6. Hanotier P. Hyponatremia in the elderly: its role in frailty. Rev Med Brux. 2015;36(6):475–84.
7. Madsen CM, Jantzen C, Lauritzen JB, Abrahamsen B, Jorgensen HL. Hyponatremia and hypernatremia are associated with increased 30-day mortality in hip fracture patients. Osteoporos Int. 2016;27(1):397–404. https://doi.org/10.1007/s00198-015-3423-4.
8. Turgutalp K, Özhan O, Gök Oğuz E, Yılmaz A, Horoz M, Helvacı I, Kiykim A. Community-acquired hypernatremia in elderly and very elderly patients admitted to the hospital: clinical characteristics and outcomes. Med Sci Monit. 2012;18(12):CR729–34.

9. Ates I, Özkayar N, Toprak G, Yılmaz N, Dede F. Factors associated with mortality in patients presenting to the emergency department with severe hypernatremia. Intern Emerg Med. 2016;11(3):451–9. https://doi.org/10.1007/s11739-015-1368-4.
10. Liber M, Sonnenblick M, Munter G. Hypernatremia and copeptin levels in the elderly hospitalized patients. Endocr Pract. 2016;22(12):1429–35.
11. Toor MR, Singla A, DeVita MV, Rosenstock JL, Michelis MF. Characteristics, therapies, and factors influencing outcomes of hospitalized hypernatremic geriatric patients. Int Urol Nephrol. 2014;46(8):1589–94. https://doi.org/10.1007/s11255-014-0721-2.
12. Phillips PA, Rolls BJ, Ledingham DM, et al. Reduced thirst after water deprivation in healthy elderly men. N Engl J Med. 1984;311:753–9.
13. Andreucci V, Russo D, Cianciaruso B, Andreucci M. Some sodium, potassium and water changes in the elderly and their treatment. Nephrol Dial Transplant. 1996;11(Suppl 9):9–17.
14. Frangeskou M, Lopez-Valcarcel B, Serra-Majem L. Dehydration in the elderly: a review focused on economic burden. J Nutr Health Aging. 2015;19(6):619–27. https://doi.org/10.1007/s12603-015-0491-2.
15. Solomon LR, Lye M. Hypernatremia in the elderly patient. Gerontology. 1990;36:171–9.
16. Shannon RP, Minaker KL, Rowe JW. Aging and water balance in humans. Semin Nephrol. 1984;4:346–53.
17. Henriques M. Chronic hyponatremia: a new risk factor for fragility fractures in the elderly? Acta Reumatol Port. 2015;40(3):308–9.
18. Grundmann F. Elektrolytveränderungen im Alter mit Fokus auf Hyponatriämie. Z Gerontol Geriatr. 2016;49:477–82. https://doi.org/10.1007/s00391-016-1117-y.
19. Mannesse CK, Vondeling AM, van Marum RJ, van Solinge WW, Egberts TC, Jansen PA. Prevalence of hyponatremia on geriatric wards compared to other settings over four decades: a systematic review. Ageing Res Rev. 2013;12(1):165–73. https://doi.org/10.1016/j.arr.2012.04.006.
20. Lindner G, Pfortmüller CA, Leichtle AB, Fiedler GM, Exadaktylos AK. Age-related variety in electrolyte levels and prevalence of dysnatremias and dyskalemias in patients presenting to the emergency department. Gerontology. 2014;60(5):420–3. https://doi.org/10.1159/000360134.
21. Gefen S, Joffe E, Mayan H, Justo D. Recurrent hospitalizations with moderate to severe hyponatremia in older adults and its associated mortality. Eur J Intern Med. 2014;25(7):624–8. https://doi.org/10.1016/j.ejim.2014.06.020.
22. Schrier RW. Does 'asymptomatic hyponatremia' exist? Nat Rev Nephrol. 2010;6(4):185. https://doi.org/10.1038/nrneph.2010.21.
23. Gankam Kengne F, Andres C, Sattar L, Melot C, Decaux G. Mild hyponatremia and risk of fracture in the ambulatory elderly. QJM. 2008;101(7):583–8. https://doi.org/10.1093/qjmed/hcn061.
24. Renneboog B, Musch W, Vandemergel X, Manto MU, Decaux G. Mild chronic hyponatremia is associated with falls, unsteadiness, and attention deficits. Am J Med. 2006;119(1):71.e1–8.
25. Usala RL, Fernandez SJ, Mete M, Cowen L, Shara NM, Barsony J, Verbalis JG. Hyponatremia is associated with increased osteoporosis and bone fractures in a large US health system population. J Clin Endocrinol Metab. 2015;100(8):3021–31. https://doi.org/10.1210/jc.2015-1261.
26. Decaux G. Is asymptomatic hyponatremia really asymptomatic? Am J Med. 2006;119(7 Suppl 1):S79–82.
27. Barsony J, Manigrasso MB, Xu Q, Tam H, Verbalis JG. Chronic hyponatremia exacerbates multiple manifestations of senescence in male rats. Age (Dordr). 2013;35(2):271–88. https://doi.org/10.1007/s11357-011-9347-9.
28. Albabtain M, Brenner MJ, Nicklas JM, Hummel SL, McCormick MP, Pawlowski JL, Remington TL, Gure TR, Dorsch MP, Bleske BE. Hyponatremia, cognitive function, and mobility in an outpatient heart failure population. Med Sci Monit. 2016;22:4978–85.
29. Schafer JA. Renal water reabsorption: a physiologic retrospective in a molecular era. Kidney Int Suppl. 2004;66(91):S20–7.
30. Bevilacqua M. Hyponatraemia in AIDS. Bailliere Clin Endocrinol Metab. 1994;8(4):837–48.

31. Musso CG, Alvarez Gregori J, Jauregui JR, Macías Núñez JF. Creatinine, urea, uric acid, water and electrolytes renal handling in the healthy oldest old. World J Nephrol. 2012;1(5):123–6. https://doi.org/10.5527/wjn.v1.i5.123.
32. Roberts MM, Robinson AG. Hyponatremia in the elderly: diagnosis and management. Geriatr Nephrol Urol. 1993;3:43–50.
33. Musso CG, Macías Núñez JF, Imperiali N, Algranati L. Low fractional excretion of urea in hypothyroidism induced hyponatremia. Electron J Biomed. 2005;1:64–7.
34. Musso CG, Jauregui J. Hyponatremia secondary to reset osmostat in very old individual: a case report and pathophysiologic proposal. Electron J Biomed. 2016;3:49–51.
35. Rennke H, Denker B. Renal pathophysiology. The essentials. Philadelphia: Lippincott Williams & Wilkins; 2007.
36. Macías Núñez J, Musso CG, Rivera H, Imperiali N, Algranati L. Sodium loss induced hyponatremia in the elderly on low sodium diet. Electron J Biomed. 2006;2:60–4.
37. Musso CG, Jauregui J. Water and salt metabolism in the geriatric syndromes. Electron J Biomed. 2010;3:53–7.
38. Musso C, Liakopoulos V, Pangre N, DiTrolio J, Jauregui R, De Miguel R, Stefanidis I, Imperiali N, Algranati L. Renal physiology in elderly persons with severe immobility syndrome. Int Urol Nephrol. 2009;41(2):437–41. https://doi.org/10.1007/s11255-009-9551-z.
39. Lacy C, Armstrong L, Goldman M, Lance L. Drug information handbook. Hudson: Lexi-Comp; 2004.
40. Iwagaki H, Haruki N, Junichi N, Tamura M, Otsuji Y. Hyponatremia after initiation of angiotensin-converting enzyme inhibitor in a geriatric patient with chronic heart failure: a case of mineralocorticoid-responsive hyponatremia of the elderly. Geriatr Gerontol Int. 2017;17(5):847–8. https://doi.org/10.1111/ggi.12964.
41. Seyffart G. Drug dosage in kidney disease. Munich: Dustri-Verlag; 2011.
42. Lye M. Distribution of body potassium in healthy elderly subjects. Gerontologie. 1981;27:286–92.
43. Giordano M, Ciarambino T, Castellino P, Malatino L, Di Somma S, Biolo G, Paolisso G, Adinolfi LE. Diseases associated with electrolyte imbalance in the ED: age-related differences. Am J Emerg Med. 2016;34(10):1923–6. https://doi.org/10.1016/j.ajem.2016.05.056.
44. Tachi T, Yokoi T, Goto C, Umeda M, Noguchi Y, Yasuda M, Minamitani M, Mizui T, Tsuchiya T, Teramachi H. Hyponatremia and hypokalemia as risk factors for falls. Eur J Clin Nutr. 2015;69(2):205–10. https://doi.org/10.1038/ejcn.2014.195.
45. Kirkland JL, Lye M, Levy DW, Banerjee AK. Patterns of urine flow and electrolyte secretion in healthy elderly people. BMJ. 1983;285:1665–7.
46. Bardak S, Turgutalp K, Koyuncu MB, Harı H, Helvacı I, Ovla D, Horoz M, Demir S, Kıykım A. Community-acquired hypokalemia in elderly patients: related factors and clinical outcomes. Int Urol Nephrol. 2017;49(3):483–9. https://doi.org/10.1007/s11255-016-1489-3.
47. Koch CA, Fulop T. Clinical aspects of changes in water and sodium homeostasis in the elderly. Rev Endocr Metab Disord. 2017;18(1):49–66. https://doi.org/10.1007/s11154-017-9420-5.
48. Musso CG, Miguel R, Algranati L, Farias Edos R. Renal potassium excretion: comparison between chronic renal disease patients and old people. Int Urol Nephrol. 2005;37(1):167–70.
49. Eiam-Ong S, Sabatini S. Effect of ageing and potassium depletion on renal collecting tubule k-controlling ATPases. Nephrology. 2002;7:87–91.
50. Evans DB. Drugs and the kidney. Br J Hosp Med. 1980;24:244–51.
51. Turgutalp K, Bardak S, Helvacı I, İşgüzar G, Payas E, Demir S, Kıykım A. Community-acquired hyperkalemia in elderly patients: risk factors and clinical outcomes. Ren Fail. 2016;38(9):1405–12.
52. Musso CG, Juarez R, Vilas M, Navarro M, Rivera H, Jauregui R. Renal calcium, phosphorus, magnesium and uric acid handling: comparison between stage III chronic kidney disease patients and healthy oldest old. Int Urol Nephrol. 2012;44(5):1559–62. https://doi.org/10.1007/s11255-012-0230-0.
53. Musso CG. Magnesium metabolism in health and disease. Int Urol Nephrol. 2009;41(2):357–62. https://doi.org/10.1007/s11255-009-9548-7.

54. Spiegel D. Normal and abnormal magnesium metabolism. In: Schrier R, editor. Renal and electrolytes disorders. Philadelphia: Lippincott Williams & Wilkins; 2010. p. 229–50.
55. Musso CG, Belloso WH, Scibona P, Bellizzi V, Macías Núñez JF. Impact of renal aging on drug therapy. Postgrad Med. 2015;127(6):623–9. https://doi.org/10.1080/00325481.2015.1063957.
56. Musso CG, Macías Núñez JF. Renal acidification, calcium, phosphate and magnesium. In: Macías Núñez JF, Cameron S, Oreopoulos D, editors. Renal ageing: health and disease. New York: Springer; 2008. p. 155–71.
57. Aeberhard N, Schild C, Rodondi N, Roten-Joss C, Tänzler K. Phosphate disorders: hyperphosphatemia or pseudohyperphosphatemia? Praxis (Bern 1994). 2014;103(20):1203–6. https://doi.org/10.1024/1661-8157/a001792.
58. Popovtzer M. Calcium, phosphorus, vitamin D, and parathyroid hormone activity disorders. In: Schrier R, editor. Renal and electrolytes disorders. Philadelphia: Lippincott Williams & Wilkins; 2010. p. 166–228.
59. Lertdumrongluk P, Rhee CM, Park J, Lau WL, Moradi H, Jing J, Molnar MZ, Brunelli SM, Nissenson AR, Kovesdy CP, Kalantar-Zadeh K. Association of serum phosphorus concentration with mortality in elderly and nonelderly hemodialysis patients. J Ren Nutr. 2013;23(6):411–21. https://doi.org/10.1053/j.jrn.2013.01.018.
60. Carrivick SJ, Walsh JP, Brown SJ, Wardrop R, Hadlow NC. Brief report: does PTH increase with age, independent of 25-hydroxyvitamin D, phosphate, renal function, and ionized calcium? J Clin Endocrinol Metab. 2015;100(5):2131–4. https://doi.org/10.1210/jc.2014-4370.
61. Nachman B, Kleeman C. Hipofosfatemia, e hiperfosfatemia: aspectos clínicos y fisiopatológicos. In: Maxwell MH, Kleeman CR, Narins RG, editors. Transtornos clínicos hedroelectrolíticos. Buenos Aires: Panamericana; 1991. p. 688–723.
62. Plantalech L. Hiperparatiroidismo en ancianos. In: Sanchez A, Novelli JL, editors. Paratiroides. Rosario: Universidad de Rosario; 2000.
63. Fassi J, Russo Picasso MF, Furci A, Sorroche P, Jauregui R, Plantalech L. Variaciones estacionales de 25-hidroxivitamina D en jóvenes y ancianos de la ciudad de Buenos Aires. Medicina. 2003;63:215–20.
64. Plantalech L, Knoblovits P, Cambiazzo E, Balzaretti M, Oyamburu J, Bonetto A, Signorelli C, Faistein I, Gutman R. Hipovitaminosis D en ancianos institucionalizados de Buenos Aires. Medicina. 1997;57:29–35.
65. Matikainen N. Hypercalcemia. Duodecim. 2014;130(14):1404–12.
66. Ratnam S, Kaehny W, Shapiro J. Pathogeny and treatment of metabolic acidosis and alkalosis. In: Schrier R, editor. Renal and electrolytes disorders. Philadelphia: Lippincott Williams & Wilkins; 2010. p. 86–121.
67. Kaehny W. Pathophysiology and treatment of respiratory acid-base and mixed disorders. In: Schrier R, editor. Renal and electrolytes disorders. Philadelphia: Lippincott Williams & Wilkins; 2010. p. 122–36.
68. Anderson S. Fluid and electrolyte disorders in the elderly. In: Kokko J, Tannen R, editors. Fluids and electrolytes. Philadelphia: W.B. Saunders Company; 1996. p. 831–9.
69. Sica DA. Renal disease, electrolyte abnormalities, and acid-base imbalance in the elderly. Clin Geriatr Med. 1994;10(1):197–211.
70. Sobamowo H, Prabhakar SS. The kidney in aging: physiological changes and pathological implications. Prog Mol Biol Transl Sci. 2017;146:303–40. https://doi.org/10.1016/bs.pmbts.2016.12.018.
71. Musso CG. Clinical catastrophic events in geriatrics: is physiopathological bases. Electron J Biomed. 2005;2:912.

Hypertension in the Elderly

5

Ahmed H. Abdelhafiz, Rachel Marshall, Joseph Kavanagh, and Meguid El Nahas

Introduction

Globally, hypertension is the most prevalent cardiovascular risk factor increasing the risk of MACE [1]. In fact, it is likely that the majority of both CKD and cognitive dysfunction in older people are the reflection of underlying age-related vascular pathology [2]. Hypertension increases the risk of cardiovascular mortality and is responsible for about seven to eight million deaths worldwide every year [3]. The prevalence of hypertension increases with age and older people are likely to significantly benefit from BP reduction due to their high baseline cardiovascular risk [4]. However, older people are a functionally heterogeneous group ranging from a fit older person living independently in the community to a fully dependent frail individual residing in a care home. The concept of hypertension in older people does not differentiate between these groups. Moreover, with octogenarians becoming the fastest growing age group in our population [5], we can anticipate a significant rise in the prevalence of complex comorbid, frail, cognitively impaired patients rendering management of hypertension in this age group challenging. This chapter reviews the management challenges of hypertension in this rapidly growing and diverse sector of the population.

A. H. Abdelhafiz (✉)
Department of Geriatric Medicine, Rotherham General Hospital, Rotherham, UK

Department of Elderly Medicine, Rotherham General Hospital, Rotherham, UK

R. Marshall · J. Kavanagh
Department of Geriatric Medicine, Rotherham General Hospital, Rotherham, UK
e-mail: j.kavanagh@doctors.org.uk

M. El Nahas
Global Kidney Academy, Sheffield, UK
e-mail: m.el-nahas@sheffield.ac.uk

C. G. Musso et al. (eds.), *Clinical Nephrogeriatrics*,
https://doi.org/10.1007/978-3-030-18711-8_5

Pathogenesis

The pathogenesis of hypertension in old age is not very clear. In addition to the well-established primary and secondary causes of hypertension in the general population, stiffness and increased arterial wall thickness appear to play an increasing role with age. The aorta and large arteries have elastic properties that make them act as distensible tubes that transform the pulsatile cardiac strokes into a continuous stable blood flow to the peripheral circulation. With increasing age, there is a progressive loss of these elastic properties leading to increased vascular stiffness. This promotes the early return of reflected waves from the peripheral circulation amplifying the systolic, reducing the diastolic and widening the pulse pressures [6]. Systolic hypertension with a wide pulse pressure is characteristic of hypertension in the elderly. Factors associated with these vascular changes are likely to be genetic, inflammatory or neurohumoral early life events, exacerbated by exposure to smoking, high sodium intake or being sedentary and obese (Fig. 5.1). Utero-placental insufficiency or impaired lactation may have an adverse effect on the elastic properties of large arteries in later life [7]. It has also been postulated that birth weight and/or subsequent faster catch up growth for those born small for gestational age (SGA) may be a contributing factor for hypertension in older age. It has been argued that SGA may be associated with oligomeganephronia (reduced number of larger nephrons), that in turn may predispose to hypertension later in life. Aging itself is associated with alterations in a number of neuroendocrine pathways that predispose to hypertension including increased renin–angiotensin–aldosterone system (RAAS) and sympathetic nervous system (SNS) activities. Increased age-related inflammatory response leads to further vascular endothelial dysfunction and arterial stiffness [8], which is exacerbated by the reduced age-related nitric oxide bioavailability that alters the balance between vasodilation and vasoconstriction in favour of vasoconstriction, thus increasing vascular resistance and increasing BP [9]. Obesity is another factor that increases haemodynamic load on the aorta, induces chronic inflammation and increases the risk of metabolic syndrome and diabetes that promote arterial stiffness and vascular aging [10]. Of note, most of the older individuals have an age-related reduction in renal function that may contribute to water and salt retention and hypertension. Finally, sleep disturbances, due to a wide variety of pathology, are common with advanced age, and both sleep deprivation and obstructive sleep apnoea are associated with hypertension [11]. Undoubtedly, hypertension in older age is pathophysiologically complex and warrants targeted treatment.

Epidemiology

Hypertension occurs in about one billion people worldwide [11]. Framingham Heart Study data suggest at the age of 80 years, the lifetime risk of developing hypertension is 93% for men and 91% for women who were free of hypertension

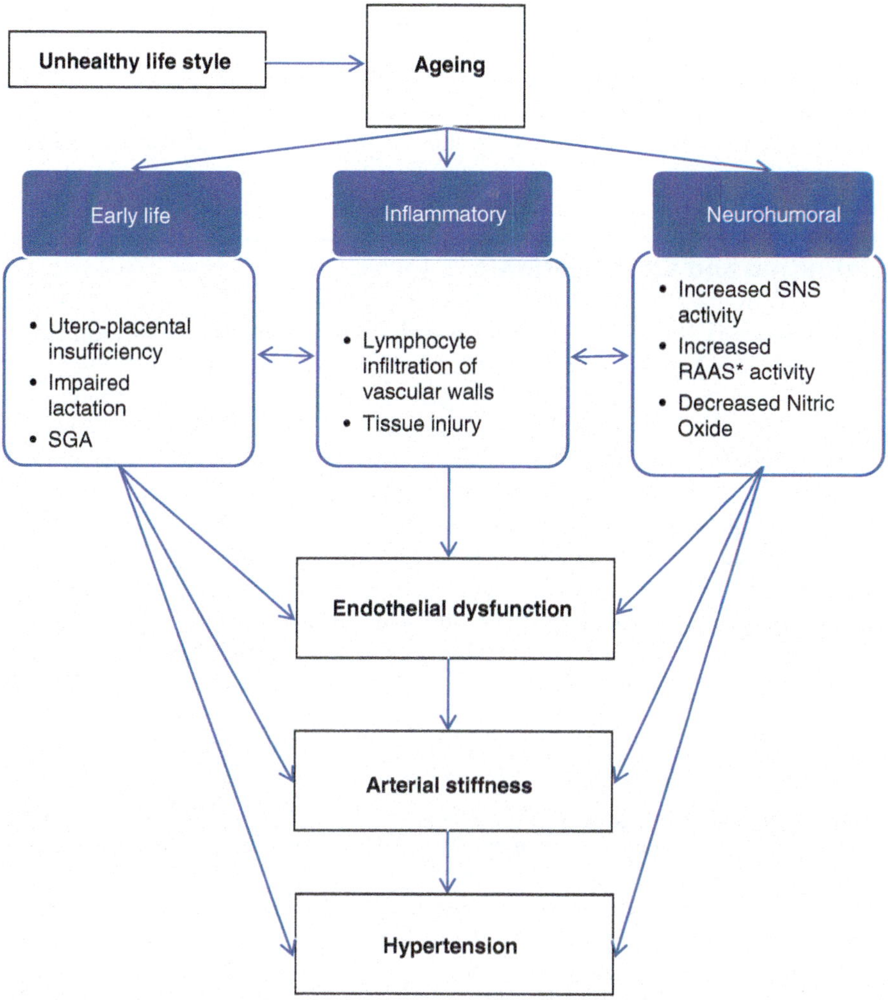

Fig. 5.1 Pathogenesis of hypertension in older people. RAAS (Renin Angiotensin Aldosterone System), SNS (Sympathetic Nervous System), SGA (born small for gestational age). Interaction between early life factors and aging-related inflammatory and neurohumoral changes is exacerbated by unhealthy lifestyle factors such as obesity and metabolic syndrome that lead to arterial wall stiffness and the development of hypertension

at the age of 55 years [12]. In Western countries, hypertension affects around 50% of community-dwelling older people (≥65 years of age), but in the low- and middle-income countries, the prevalence is higher reaching up to 78% [13, 14]. The prevalence of hypertension increases with increasing age affecting up to 75% of older people (>75 years) in the US [15, 16]. There are some gender differences in the prevalence of hypertension with more men affected than women under the age of 45 years, both genders equally affected between the ages of 45 and 64 years and more women affected than men above the age of 65 years [17]. Ageing, sedentary lifestyle, obesity and increased dietary salt appear to be the main driving forces for the increasing prevalence of hypertension in both developing and developed countries.

Definition and Classification

Hypertension is generally defined as a systolic blood pressure ≥140 mmHg or a diastolic blood pressure ≥90 mmHg based on ≥3 measurements at ≥2 visits to a medical practitioner [18]. Intriguingly, the definition of hypertension remains the same across all age groups, despite major and progressive changes in blood pressure with age. The severity of hypertension is classified into grades according to the task force statement of the European Society of Cardiology and the European Society of hypertension (ESC/ESH) or stages according to the Joint statement of the American Society of Hypertension and the International Society of Hypertension (ASH/ISH) [18, 19]. Recently, with the emergence of new evidence supporting the benefits of lower BP levels on cardiovascular and all-cause mortality, the American Heart Association (AHA) and the American College of Cardiology (ACC) have redefined hypertension at a lower level of BP>130/80 mmHg and the severity classification has been adjusted accordingly as detailed in Table 5.1 [20]. This has not been adopted by the American Academy of Family Physicians (AAFP), who felt that such a recommendation was not fully validated or justified. AAFP questioned the potential intellectual bias of investigators who were to a large extent involved in the clinical trials leading to such recommendations [21]. The lower target recommended by AHA/ACC was based on the emergence of new evidence from the cardioprotective effects of lower BP derived from the Systolic Blood Pressure Intervention Trial (SPRINT). However, on a careful appraisal of these results, intensive BP reduction actually failed to impact on MACE [22]. The observed benefit on overall cardiovascular and all-cause mortality seemed to be solely due to the impact of optimisation of antihypertensive therapy in heart failure.

Table 5.1 Classifications of hypertension

2014-ASH/ISH [15]		2017-ACC/AHA [17]	
Category	BP (mmHg)	Category	BP (mmHg)
Normal	<120/80	Normal	<120/80
Pre-hypertension	120–139/80–89	Elevated BP	<120–129/80
Hypertension	≥140/90	Hypertension	≥130/80
Stage 1	140–159/90–99	Stage 1	130–139/80–89
Stage 2	≥160/100	Stage 2	>140/90

Types of Hypertension in Old Age

Definitions of common types of hypertension in older people are summarised in Box 5.1. Isolated systolic hypertension (BP≥140/<90 mmHg) accounts for 60–80% of hypertension, the prevalence of which increases with age and is the most important determinant of cardiovascular risk in older people [23]. This has led some to advocate the use of systolic BP recording as the sole diagnostic and therapeutic marker of hypertension in older people [24]. White coat hypertension (high office but normal home BP) is common the prevalence of which can reach up to 72% of clinic BP readings [25]. Masked hypertension is the opposite of white coat hypertension (normal office but high home BP) and is associated with increased cardiovascular risk [26]. Both white coat and masked hypertension are best diagnosed with ambulatory BP monitoring. Resistant hypertension (BP uncontrollable on ≥3 antihypertensive medications including a diuretic) may be due to poor compliance with antihypertensive medications, concomitant use of medications that increase BP such as non-steroidal anti-inflammatory drugs or due to a secondary untreated cause of hypertension [27]. Pseudohypertension (high BP due to non-collapsing sclerotic arteries to cuff pressure) should be suspected in patients apparently having resistant hypertension but have no evidence of end-organ damage. It is best diagnosed by intra-arterial BP monitoring [28]. Orthostatic hypotension (BP drop by >20/10 mmHg within 3 minutes standing) is common affecting up to 20% of older people and is likely to be due to autonomic dysfunction, diminished baroreceptor sensitivity and reduced compensatory heart rate response to postural changes [29]. Nocturnal hypertension occurs when BP fails to physiologically drop (non-dipper patients) by 10–20% at night and is associated with end-organ damage. It often precedes the detection of daytime hypertension. Nocturnal hypotension occurs when BP drops by ≥20% at night increasing the risk of cerebral hypoperfusion (Box 5.1) [30].

Box 5.1 Common Types of Hypertension in Older People

Type	Definition
Isolated systolic hypertension	SBP≥140 mmHg with a DBP<90 mmHg
White coat hypertension	High office but normal home BP
Masked hypertension	Normal office but high home BP
Resistant hypertension	Failure of BP control on ≥3 antihypertensive medications including a diuretic
Pseudohypertension	Falsely high SBP due to sclerotic arteries that do not collapse with the cuff pressure
Orthostatic hypotension	A drop of >20 mmHg (SBP) or >10 mmHg (DBP) within 3 minutes of standing up
Nocturnal hypertension	BP does not physiologically drop by 10–20% at night (non-dippers)
Nocturnal hypotension	BP drops ≥20% at night (dippers)

BP blood pressure, *SBP* systolic blood pressure, *DBP* diastolic blood pressure

Diagnosis of Hypertension in Old Age

Measurement of BP in a resting and relaxed condition (empty bladder with no smoking, caffeine or exercise within 30 minutes of measurements) is required in order to diagnose hypertension. The cuff size should be adequate for mid-arm circumference. Measurements in both arms and the use of the higher reading with an average of two to three measurements taken on two to three separate occasions will minimise errors and provide a more accurate estimate [20]. Due to the variability of hypertension in older people, as described above, ambulatory BP readings may be required. Essential hypertension is the most common cause of hypertension but secondary causes should be screened for in patients with hypertension refractory to multiple drug therapy or in patients who lack a family history of hypertension (Box 5.2). It is important to note that due to the high prevalence of isolated systolic hypertension in the elderly, it is often appropriate to diagnose and treat hypertension based on systolic readings alone due to their correlation with cardiovascular risk [24].

Box 5.2 Secondary Causes of Hypertension in Older People

Cause	Clinical clues and initial screening[a]
Renal disease	
Renovascular	Abdominal bruit, worsening serum creatinine by >30% after use of ACEI or ARB, one kidney smaller than the other by >1.5 cm on renal ultrasound
Renoparenchymatous	Asymptomatic, impaired renal function, small kidneys on renal ultrasound, abnormal urine analysis
Adrenal disease	
Hyperaldosteronism	Persistent hypokalaemia, elevated aldosterone level
Hypercortisolism	Cushingoid facies, persistent hypokalaemia, elevated serum cortisol
Pheochromocytoma	Episodic sympathetic overactivity, elevated urinary metanephrines
Thyroid disease	
Hypothyroidism	Cold intolerance, constipation, bradycardia, high serum TSH and low serum thyroxine
Hyperthyroidism	Heat intolerance, diarrhoea, constipation, low serum TSH and high serum thyroxine
Hyperparathyroidism	Constipation, high serum calcium and PTH
Drugs	
Non-steroidal anti-inflammatory, steroids and alcohol	Medication history

[a]*ACEI* angiotensin-converting enzyme inhibitors, *ARB* angiotensin receptor blockers, *TSH* thyroid-stimulating hormone, *PTH* parathyroid hormone

Management of Hypertension in Old Age

Blood pressure control is essential to reduce the risk of cardiovascular events, mortality and slow decline in renal function. Management should begin with lifestyle modifications or non-pharmacological interventions. Such interventions may be the only treatments required in milder forms of hypertension. If BP targets are not achieved, the addition of pharmacological therapy should be considered. The threshold at which BP should be treated as recommended by the guidelines has been set at an SBP level ≥150–160 mmHg [18, 19]. It remains unclear whether older patients with mild hypertension (SBP >140 but <159 mmHg) will benefit from hypertension treatment. In 2002, the Prospective Studies Collaboration meta-analysis of 61 cohort studies between 1950 and 1990 has demonstrated a linear relationship between BP and mortality from ischaemic heart disease and stroke down to a BP of 115/75 mmHg in participants 40–89 years of age [31].

Recommended BP Targets

The European Society of Hypertension and the European Society of Cardiology recommend that older people with a systolic BP ≥160 mmHg should be treated to a level of 140–150 mmHg [19]. The American Society of Hypertension and the International Society of Hypertension recommend that older people aged ≥60 years with BP ≥150/90 mmHg should be treated to a blood pressure goal of <150/90 mmHg initially and if tolerated a systolic BP <140 mmHg [18]. However, recently the AHA and the ACC has set a new unified lower target at <130/80 mmHg for patients with various comorbidities such as diabetes, stroke, heart failure and CKD with or without albuminuria [20]. These guidelines, however, fail to differentiate between healthy older adults, frail older adults or those with significant comorbidities. Treatment decisions are generally left to the discretion of the treating physician based on the patient's response to treatment.

Lower BP Targets

As discussed above, recent evidence has shown that lower targets are more cardioprotective than those previously recommended by the guidelines. Results from the SPRINT study showed that treating to a SBP target of <120 mmHg compared with an SBP target <140 mmHg resulted in significantly lower rates of fatal and nonfatal major cardiovascular events (hazard ratio [HR] 0.66, 95% confidence interval [CI]0.51–0.85) and death from any cause in older people (≥75 years) (HR 0.67, 95%CI 0.49–0.91). These outcomes, however, were confined to an isolated beneficial effect on heart failure. The incidence of hypotension, acute kidney injury and CKD was higher in the intensive BP control arm of the study. Furthermore, the rate of progression of those with CKD was faster at lower BP levels. The exploratory analysis suggested that the benefit of intensive BP control was consistent among persons of the same age who were also frail or had reduced gait speed. However, this study did not enrol older people with diabetes, stroke, heart failure, dementia, limited life expectancy of <3 years, unintentional weight loss (>10% of body weight during the preceding 6 months) or those residing in nursing homes [22]. The exclusion of patients with such comorbidities is likely to represent a significant proportion of frail older adults. Individuals with these conditions may not benefit from such intensive BP reduction and may be at increased risk of adverse events. In a recent meta-analysis of 123 trials including 613,815 participants to investigate whether the benefits of BP reduction will differ by baseline BP levels, presence of comorbidities or by drug class, relative risk reductions were proportional to the magnitude of the blood pressure reductions down to <130 mmHg. BP reduction was significantly protective in individuals with a history of cardiovascular disease, coronary heart disease, stroke and heart failure with BP reductions demonstrating a modest benefit in individuals with diabetes or CKD. Every 10 mmHg reduction in SBP significantly reduced the risk of major cardiovascular disease events (relative risk [RR] 0·80, 95% CI 0·77–0·83), coronary heart disease (RR 0·83, 95% CI 0·78–0·88), stroke (RR0·73, 95% CI 0·68–0·77), and heart failure (RR0·72, 95% CI 0·67–0·78). This led to an overall 13% reduction in all-cause mortality (RR0·87,95% CI 0·84–0·91) [32]. In an updated meta-analysis of 19 trials including 44,989 participants, intensive BP lowering to a mean of 133/76 mmHg resulted in a reduction of major cardiovascular events (RR 14%, 95% CI 4–22%), myocardial infarction (RR13% 95% CI 0–24%), stroke (RR 22%, 95% CI10–32%), albuminuria (RR10%, 95% CI 3–16%) and retinopathy progression (RR19%, 95% CI 0–34%) compared with a mean BP of 140/81 mm Hg. However, there was no reduction of heart failure, cardiovascular death, total mortality or end-stage kidney disease. Whilst these analyses may have been strongly influenced by the inclusion of the SPRINT data, they suggest that there may be additional benefits from more intensive blood pressure lowering <140 mmHg in high-risk individuals. However, serious adverse events associated with intensive compared to less intensive BP lowering were high (1.2% v 0.9%, RR 1.35, 95% CI 0.93–1.97) [33] which included BP reduction-associated compromise of renal function. This in itself mitigates any potential benefit of aggressive BP management in older people with deteriorating renal function being associated with increased risk of cardiovascular morbidity and mortality.

Suggested BP Targets for Old Age

Due to the heterogeneity of older people, one BP target will not fit all. To achieve tight BP targets, the use of multiple antihypertensive medications will likely be required which will increase the treatment burden and the prevalence of side effects. It is best to base BP targets on the overall function, biological age and life expectancy taking into consideration patients' choice and putting the quality of life at the heart

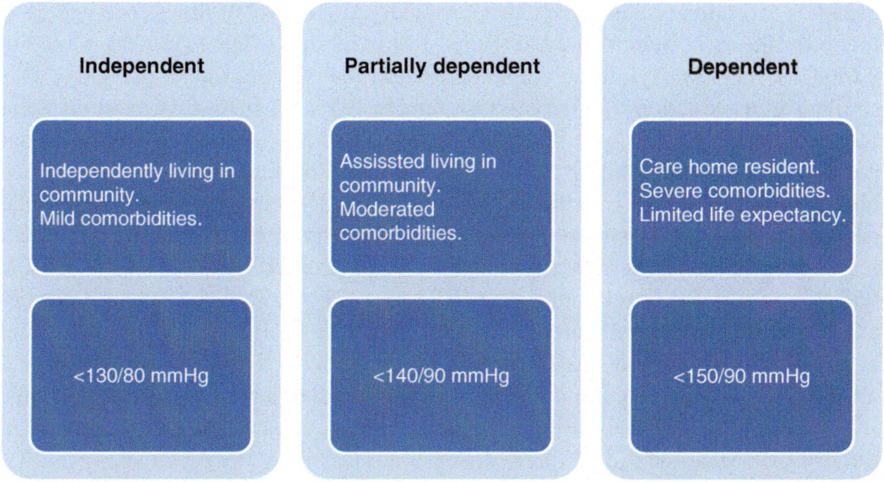

Fig. 5.2 Suggested BP targets based on patient's function. In the independent patients, there is evidence of extra cardiovascular benefits of lower BP <130/80 mmHg if well tolerated. In the partially dependent patients the competing comorbidities may increase the side effects of antihypertensive medications therefore, more tolerated higher targets are reasonable. In the dependent patients with limited life expectancy, the risks of side effects are higher especially injurious falls and fractures and the focus should be on the maintenance of quality of life rather than reducing cardiovascular risk

of care plans. In the dependent patients group, focus is on quality of life rather than on cardiovascular risk reduction. Therefore, individualised targets based on the net balance between cardiovascular risk reduction and the treatment burden as well as the quality of life should be considered for each patient. We suggest that older people could be viewed in three functional categories with different targets ranging from tighter BP control in the fit person to a more relaxed approach in the frail individual. Targets should not only be individualised but also be dynamic in order to follow the changing functional state of patients as they go through the aging process (Fig. 5.2).

Therapeutic Strategies

Non-pharmacologic BP Reduction Therapy

Non-pharmacological BP reduction interventions such as regular exercise, weight reduction in obese individuals, low sodium diet, low alcohol consumption and smoking cessation constitute a part of successful BP control in all patients [34]. Physical activity and fitness have been shown to be associated with lower mortality in older men with hypertension. In a Veterans Affairs prospective study of 2153 older men (mean age 75 years), who underwent routine and peak exercise tolerance testing, estimated in metabolic equivalents (METs), mortality risk was 11% lower (HR 0.89; 95% CI 0.86–0.93, [$P < 0.001$]) for every 1-MET increase in exercise capacity. Mortality risk improved proportionally to the level of fitness and was 48% lower for the most fit compared to the least fit individuals (HR 0.52, 95% CI 0.39–0.69, [$P < 0.001$]) [35]. In a systematic review, low sodium intake (<2 g/day) has resulted in a reduction of SBP by 3.47 mmHg (95% CI 0.76–6.18) and diastolic blood pressure (DBP) by 1.81 mmHg (95% CI 0.54–3.08) with no significant adverse effect on blood lipids, catecholamine levels or renal function compared to higher sodium intake (≥2 g/day). There were insufficient randomised controlled trials to assess the effects of reduced sodium intake on mortality and morbidity, but increased sodium intake was associated with an increased risk of stroke (RR 1.24, 95% CI 1.08–1.43), stroke mortality (RR1.63, 95% CI 1.27–2.10) and mortality associated with coronary heart disease (RR1.32, 95% CI 1.13–1.53) [36]. Smoking is another cardiovascular risk factor and whilst smoking cessation may not have a direct effect on BP reduction it will reduce the overall risk of cardiovascular events. In fact, smoking was one of the major determinants of cardiovascular mortality in the INTERSALT study [37].

Pharmacologic BP Reduction Therapy

The process of lowering BP, rather than the pharmacological agent used to lower BP, appears to be the main driver of cardiovascular risk reduction. In the collaborative meta-analysis of randomised trials, BP reduction reduced major cardiovascular events (stroke, myocardial infarction, heart failure, or cardiovascular death) and all-cause mortality irrespective of renal function or the antihypertensive drug class used [38]. Another meta-analysis has also shown equal effects of all drug classes in cardiovascular risk reduction [39]. However, some drug classes may have a preferential protective effect in different clinical situations. In a network meta-analysis of randomised controlled trials investigating BP-lowering agents in patients with diabetes and CKD, end-stage renal disease (ESRD) was significantly reduced by dual angiotensin-converting enzyme inhibitors (ACEI) and angiotensin receptor blockers (ARB) (OR 0.62, 95% CI 0.43–0·90) or ARB monotherapy (OR0.77, 95% CI 0.65–0.92). This benefit was independent of the BP-lowering effect and was recorded mainly in patients with type 2 diabetes mellitus and overt albuminuria. However, combined ACEI and ARB treatment increased the risk of acute kidney injury (AKI) and hyperkalaemia (OR 2.69, 95% CI 0.98–7.38 and OR2.69, 95% CI 0.97–7.47, respectively) [40]. Therefore, the efficacy of the dual blockade of the RAAS should be balanced with its safety, specifically in older patients who may depend on angiotensin II to maintain their glomerular filtration in the face of compromised renal blood flow, renovascular disease and ischemic nephropathy. It has been suggested that 1 year of dual ACEI and ARB treatment for 1000 patients with diabetes and CKD will prevent 3 cases of ESRD and regress 90 cases of albuminuria, but it will also lead to an extra 38 cases of AKI and 65 cases of hyperkalaemia [40]. This was initially shown in the ONTARGET (Ongoing Telmisartan Alone and in combination with Ramipril Global Endpoint Trial) trial which examined individuals at high cardiovascular or diabetes risk where dual blockade proved harmful; with increased risk of hypotensive symptoms (4.8%

vs.1.7%, [$P < 0.001$]), syncope (0.3% vs. 0.2%, [$P = 0.03$]), and renal dysfunction (13.5% vs. 10.2%, [$P < 0.001$]) [41]. In this study, the decline in CKD was faster in patients on dual RAAS blockade compared to those on either Ramipril or Telmisartan alone. These data have casted serious doubt and concern on dual RAAS blockade in individuals at high cardiovascular risk including the elderly. A retrospective analysis showed the prescription and use of RAAS inhibitors correlated best in the elderly with hospitalisation for AKI [42]. It has also been shown in a recent meta-analysis that calcium channel blockers and diuretics were superior to other drugs for the prevention of stroke and heart failure, respectively, whilst β-blockers were inferior to other drugs for the prevention of major cardiovascular disease events, stroke and renal failure [32].

Antihypertensive Agents in Old Age

The choice of antihypertensive class in old age should be influenced by individual comorbidity and the vulnerability of this group of the population to various side effects.

Diuretics Thiazide or loop diuretics are often necessary and well tolerated for those with volume overload or heart failure and have been shown to reduce cardiovascular morbidity and mortality in a number of studies. However, there is a significant risk of orthostatic hypotension, electrolyte imbalance and AKI, especially in states of volume depletion, so caution should be used in those at risk of dehydration or falls unless needed to control volume overload.

Calcium Channel Blockers (CCB) Dihydropyridines (such as amlodipine) are generally well tolerated, effective and safe in patients with renal dysfunction and variable oral intake making them probably the safest antihypertensives in the elderly and therefore the first choice if there is not an additional indication for an ACEI/ARB or diuretic [43]. Care should be taken in patients with chronic constipation or urinary problems (overactive bladder or outflow obstruction) due to constipating side effects. They can cause or worsen lower limb oedema and further impair those with poor mobility and chronic oedema or venous insufficiency. This side effect is however common to all vasodilators due to their effect on water and salt retention and can potentially be countered by increased diuretic therapy.

ACEI and ARB Drugs blocking RAAS offer significant prognostic benefit in those with ischemic heart disease, heart failure, diabetes with proteinuria and CKD [44]. Caution should be used in those with unreliable oral intake, previous or recurrent AKI and in older patients with advanced CKD. Dual treatment with ACEI and ARB significantly increases the risk of AKI and hyperkalaemia as well as accelerates the progression of established CKD [41]. Consider advising patients to omit ACEI/ARB if they become acutely unwell in order to reduce AKI risk (so-called sick day rules).

Beta-Blockers This class of antihypertensive are generally not very effective at lowering BP but may be used for a dual effect in ischemic heart disease, heart failure and atrial fibrillation or as an additive agent in resistant hypertension. Care should be taken in those with depression, fatigue and cognitive impairment due to exacerbating side effects. Beta-blockers can worsen lower degrees of heart block, which are common in the elderly, leading to bradycardia and cardiogenic syncope. Caution should be applied with beta-blockers which are renally excreted as a significant proportion of older individuals have reduced glomerular filtration rate.

Aldosterone Antagonists Such agents can augment diuretic therapy and offer prognostic benefit in heart failure but will increase the risk of hyperkalaemia, dehydration and AKI, so avoid in those with variable oral intake.

Alpha-Blockers Drugs such as doxazosin can be useful in those with significant renal impairment or as an additional agent in resistant hypertension. This class has variable tolerance in the elderly due to vasodilating effects resulting in orthostatic hypotension. However, doxazosin can reduce polypharmacy in certain circumstances such as benign prostatic hypertrophy by replacing other alpha-blockers (e.g. tamsulosin) for a dual effect.

Centrally Acting Agents Drugs such as Moxonidine can be used in patients with significant renal impairment or intolerance to other drugs but are best avoided in those with cognitive impairment due to central nervous system side effects. It can also exacerbate lower degrees of heart block and cause dry mouth and dizziness. Similar side effects can be attributed to other centrally acting antihypertensive agents such as methyldopa.

Vasodilators Drugs such as nitrates, hydralazine and nicorandil are generally reserved for use in co-existing heart failure or ischemic heart disease rather than as an isolated antihypertensive. They are likely to significantly worsen orthostatic hypotension due to vasodilating effects. As mentioned above, vasodilators are often associated with water and salt retention leading to peripheral oedema. This is not necessarily an indication to stop these agents if they are deemed beneficial but instead an indication to adjust and optimise the associated diuretic therapy. Advantages and disadvantages of individual antihypertensive medications in older people are summarised in Table 5.2.

Special Considerations for Antihypertensive Management in Older People

Older people are functionally heterogeneous and BP goals should be individualised and aimed at overall risk reduction based on patients' functional level, biological age and life expectancy rather than focused on a specific single target (Box 5.3). Common clinical conditions, which may require a more relaxed BP target, should be considered when treating hypertension in older people.

Table 5.2 Advantage and disadvantage of antihypertensive medications in older people

Category	Advantage	Disadvantage
Diuretics (thiazides and loop diuretics)	Cardioprotective Well tolerated Effective in systolic hypertension First choice in reducing exacerbation of heart failure	Hyponatremia Hypokalaemia Hyperuricaemia and gout Glucose intolerance Dehydration Aggravation of urinary incontinence
Calcium channel blockers	Cardioprotective Well tolerated Effective in systolic hypertension Useful in atrial fibrillation First choice in reducing stroke incidence	Peripheral oedema Negative inotropic effects Headache Dizziness Bradycardia Constipation
Angiotensin-Converting Enzyme Inhibitors (ACEI) and Angiotensin Receptor Blockers (ARB)	Effective in patients with: Heart failure Myocardial infarction Left ventricular hypertrophy Diabetes Chronic kidney disease Proteinuria Combination of ACEI and ARBs may delay the progression to ESRD	Chronic cough (ACEI) Hyperkalaemia Acute kidney injury (AKI) Accelerates CKD Contraindicated in patients with bilateral renal artery stenosis Angioedema Combined ACEI and ARB increases incidence of AKI and hyperkalaemia
β-blockers	Effective in patients with: Heart failure Myocardial infarction Left ventricular hypertrophy Angina pectoris Atrial fibrillation	Inferior to other drugs Bradycardia Hyperlipidaemia Glucose intolerance Bronchospasm Fatigue Depression Nightmares Confusion
Other agents:		
Renin inhibitors	Effective	Hyperkalaemia and AKI
Aldosterone antagonists	Suitable for patients with heart failure	Hyperkalaemia and gynaecomastia
Centrally acting agents, vasodilators and α-blockers	Suitable in patients with renal impairment	Dizziness, fatigue, orthostatic hypotension, confusion, dry mouth and syncope

CKD chronic kidney disease

Box 5.3 Considerations in Older People

Category	Consideration
Frailty	Frailty may have a U-shaped relation with cardiac outcomes
	Low BP could be related to malnutrition and comorbidities
	BP should not be lowered to <140/90 mmHg
Falls	Intensity of antihypertensive medications increases falls risk
	History of falls increases the risk of further falls
	All antihypertensive classes increase risk of falls
	Falls risk is highest shortly (30–45 days) after initiation of medications
Dementia	Significantly shortened life expectancy should be considered before deciding on preventative treatments
	Midlife hypertension is associated with increased risk of late-life dementia
	Relation between treated hypertension and incidence dementia is inconsistent
	Treating hypertension in patients with established dementia does not improve cognition
	SBP should not be lowered to <130 mmHg as it may contribute to more rapid cognitive decline
Systolic predominance	Systolic hypertension is related to increased arterial stiffness
	Systolic hypertension increases the risk of cardiovascular events and progression of kidney disease
	Current antihypertensive medications have limited effect on arterial stiffness
	When treating systolic hypertension, DBP should not be reduced to <70 mmHg to maintain coronary perfusion
Orthostatic hypotension	Found in up to a third of those over 75
	Associated with increased coronary heart disease and mortality
	More frequent in those with uncontrolled hypertension
	Decision on treating hypertension with orthostatic hypotension should be based on overall risk and patient symptoms
	Giving antihypertensives at night may exacerbate falls risk
Comorbidity and polypharmacy	A third of adults over 85 will have four or more comorbidities
	Overall burden of pathology, including subclinical, effects outcomes
	Those with comorbidity are often excluded from studies
	Prevalence of older people taking ≥3 antihypertensives is increasing
	Older people may be taking concomitant medications that increase BP such as non-steroidal anti-inflammatory drugs
	Polypharmacy may be associated with non-adherence but regular medications review, rationalisation and education may improve this

SBP systolic blood pressure, *DBP* diastolic blood pressure

Frailty The recent analysis of hypertension in the very elderly trial (HYVT) has shown that adjustment for frailty did not affect the benefit driven from antihypertensive treatment which may suggest that frailty is not a contraindication to treat older people (≥80 years) to a target BP of 150/80 mmHg. However, the population in the HYVT study was relatively healthier than the general population with a low prevalence of cognitive dysfunction [median (IQR) Mini-Mental State Examination 26.0 (22–28)]. The study also excluded those with major comorbidities such as stroke, heart failure and renal impairment who are likely to be frail [45]. Frailty may modify the relationship between BP and cardiovascular outcome. Whilst the meta-analysis of the prospective studies collaboration reported a linear relationship between BP reduction and cardiovascular outcome [34], prospective observational studies have shown an attenuated or even inverse association between BP and cardiovascular outcome in the very old (>75 years old) [46–50]. The explanation of this U-shaped phenomenon could be due to the presence of frailty as a confounding factor. Low BP in frail older people could be an expression of malnutrition, heart failure and other comorbidities that are associated with poor prognosis rather than being a direct consequence of antihypertensive therapy. The National Health and Nutrition Examination Survey (NHANES) has shown that in participants with faster walking speed, elevated SBP (>140 mm Hg) was associated with increased mortality, whilst among those with slower walking speed who are likely to be frail, the association was inverted. These results support the concept that frailty may modify the relationship between BP reduction and prognosis and suggest that overall individual function or biological age should be the determining factor in setting individualised BP targets [51]. It may also suggest that frailty is a useful surrogate marker of underlying comorbidities, the cardiovascular fitness of older individuals and consequently their tolerance for lower BP targets.

Falls Antihypertensive medications are associated with an increased risk of recurrent injurious falls. In a nationally representative sample of older people with multiple comorbidities moderate-intensity and high-intensity antihypertensive medication use (based on the standardised daily dose for each antihypertensive medication class) were associated with experiencing a serious fall injury (HR1.40 95% CI 1.03–1.90 and HR1.28 95% CI 0.91–1.80 respectively) compared with non-users. People who had experienced a fall with associated injury in the prior year have more than double the risk for subsequent serious fall injury (HR 2.31 95% CI 1.01–5.29 high-intensity antihypertensive group). No particular antihypertensive class was associated with the risk of fall injuries [52]. Therefore, the potential harms versus benefits of antihypertensive medications should be weighed in deciding whether to continue antihypertensive therapy in older people with multiple comorbidities, frailty and a history of previous falls. An Australian prospective study also demonstrated that higher doses of antihypertensive medications are independently associated with increased risk of falls in older people. In the 409 participants, mean

may be the main consideration rather than the intensive BP reduction of younger individuals with well-perfused organs and adequate vascular and organ perfusion autoregulation.

Systolic Predominance With increasing age, SBP begins to rise whilst DBP begins to plateau or decline [73]. These age-related changes, largely due to increased arterial stiffness, lead to increased pulse pressure and the predominance of systolic hypertension in older people. This is in contrast to younger people in whom hypertension is largely determined by increased peripheral arterial resistance. Systolic hypertension represents a major risk factor for cardiovascular and stroke events as well as CKD progression. The National Health and Nutrition Examination Survey (NHANES III, 1988–1991) has shown that <20% of hypertensive older individuals (>60 years of age) had an elevated DBP and this proportion declined steadily with the progression of age [74]. Systolic hypertension is largely due to increased arterial stiffness however, current antihypertensive medications work mainly by reducing peripheral vascular resistance with little effect on arterial stiffness making it difficult to control BP in older people. Increasing intensity of antihypertensive medications to reduce SBP may unduly reduce DBP compromising coronary artery filling and increasing the risk of cardiac events. In patients with systolic hypertension, DBP should not be reduced to levels <60 mmHg, or <65 mmHg in patients with known coronary artery disease or <70 mmHg in patients >80 years of age [75]. Therefore, a novel therapeutic approach is needed to specifically lower SBP, rather than DBP, by addressing arterial stiffness.

Orthostatic Hypotension Significant orthostatic hypotension, generally defined as a drop in systolic BP of ≥20 mmHg or diastolic BP of ≥10 mmHg at 1 or 3 minutes after standing, is common and was found in 34% of people 75 years or older in one population-based cohort study. The incidence increases for those on causative drugs (such as antihypertensives, sedatives and antidepressants) and multiple medications (regardless of their mechanisms), in residential care or with associated neurological conditions such as Parkinson's disease or autonomic neuropathies [76, 77]. Orthostatic hypotension is also a feature of the autonomic neuropathy that affects many older patients with CKD. Orthostatic hypotension itself has been linked to significantly increased risk of coronary heart disease (HR 1.35, 95% CI 1.08–1.57) and all-cause mortality (HR 1.22, 95% CI 1.09–1.36) although interestingly asymptomatic orthostatic hypotension has not been conclusively linked to falls risk [78]. Treatment of co-existing supine hypertension and orthostatic hypotension is a challenge for physicians and no consensus or significant data currently exists to guide treatment thresholds and targets. Pharmacological treatments for hypertension will reduce both supine and orthostatic BP and pharmacological treatments of orthostatic hypotension will increase both orthostatic and supine BP. In one prospective population-based study, the incidence of orthostatic hypotension was actually highest in those with uncontrolled hypertension (19%) compared to those with controlled hypertension (5%) and those without hypertension (2%) [78]. Such data can suggest that a general autonomic degenerative process underlies this condition and that the presence of asymptomatic orthostatic hypotension, in the absence of symptomatic orthostatic presyncope, postural instability or falls, should not necessarily prevent treatment of supine hypertension. Diurnal variations normally lead to the lowest BP at night and an associated increased natriuresis. Older people have a higher incidence of insomnia which can be exacerbated by conditions such as overactive bladder [11]. As such, the practice of giving antihypertensive agents just before going to sleep, which is currently recommended for younger patients in order to control night-time hypertension and to prevent orthostatic hypotension in the day time, may actually worsen the risk of nocturnal orthostatic hypotension and falls and should be used with caution in the elderly hypertensive. Adequate control of supine hypertension may actually improve orthostatic hypotension but patients should be closely observed for adverse effects such as presyncope and falls.

Comorbidity and Polypharmacy Patients naturally accumulate comorbidity with increased age, and population studies have previously suggested 31.4% of those over 85 years will have four or more chronic conditions [79]. Furthermore, there is likely to be the development of subclinical pathology in various organ systems, even in the absence of overt disease, which still contributes to a negative health outcome [80, 81]. Whilst frailty syndromes and specific conditions in the elderly are discussed separately, the accumulated burden of pathology, even subclinical, should be considered as part of a holistic assessment of the complex older patient. This burden of disease may shorten expected life span to the point where preventative cardiovascular treatment offers little benefit, or alternatively an accumulation of cardiovascular risk factors and MACE may suggest a more aggressive treatment strategy is appropriate. Whilst there is increasing research in patients in older age, those with multiple comorbidities are still often excluded from these data, such as in the SPRINT study [22]. As such there is a lack of consensus on the treatment of hypertension in those with extensive comorbidity, and individualised patient care plans are needed. In the US, the proportion of older people (≥80 years) taking ≥3 classes of antihypertensive medications has increased from 7% in 1988 to 30.9% in 2010 [16]. In 1127 care home residents ≥80 years old (mean age 87.6 years), participants with low SBP (<130 mmHg) and receiving ≥2 antihypertensive medications had a higher risk of mortality (HR, 1.78, 95% CI 1.34–2.37 [$P < 0.001$]) compared with other participants [82]. The findings of this study question the safety of using combination antihypertensive therapy in frail elderly patients with low SBP (<130 mmHg). Older people may also be taking regular medications that increase BP such as non-steroidal anti-inflammatory drugs, decongestants or glucocorticoids that may make BP control more challenging often resulting in a vicious circle of increased polypharmacy. Polypharmacy may also result in less medication adherence which is related to a greater perception of illness burden and loss of trust in medications [83]. Regular medication review and rationalisation, reducing medications that have hypertensive effects and educational programs may help reduce polypharmacy and improve adherence to BP treatment [84].

Conclusions

Older people are a heterogeneous group of individuals with varying degrees of comorbidity and functional level. Recent guidelines have suggested tighter BP control <130/80 mmHg which may offer more cardioprotective effects than relaxed targets. However, indiscriminate application of these guidelines may lead to overtreatment and polypharmacy, causing potential harm in older age groups especially in those with physical or cognitive functional disabilities and frailty. Therefore, management of hypertension in older people should be individualised considering tighter control in the biologically fit individuals and relaxed targets in the frail persons taking into consideration the overall patients' functional level, their preferences and putting their quality of life at the heart of care plans.

Key Points

- Prevalence of hypertension increases as the population ages.
- Tight targets suggested by recent guidelines may not be applicable to every individual.
- Targets and goals of therapy should be based on overall patients' functional level rather than age.
- Quality of BP control rather than quantity should be the primary objective in the older patient.
- Personalised treatment of hypertension is of utmost importance in older hypertensive individuals.

References

1. Kearney PM, Whelton M, Reynolds K, et al. Global burden of hypertension: analysis of worldwide data. Lancet. 2005;365:217–23.
2. Abdelhafiz AH, Ahmed S, El Nahas M. Microalbuminuria: marker or maker of cardiovascular disease. Nephron Exp Nephrol. 2011;119(suppl 1):e6–e10.
3. Danaei G, Finucane MM, Lin JK, et al. National, regional and global trends in systolic blood pressure since 1980: systematic analysis of health examination surveys and epidemiological studies with 786 country-years and 5.4 million participants. Lancet. 2011;377:568–77.
4. Mukhtar O, Jackson SHD. Risk: benefit of treating high blood pressure in older adults. Br J Clin Pharmacol. 2013;75(1):36–44.
5. Berrut G, Andrieu S, Araujo De Carvalho I, et al. Promoting access to innovation for frail old persons. IAGG (International Association of Gerontology and Geriatrics), WHO (World Health Organization) and SFGG (Societe Francaise de Geriatrie et de Gerontologie) workshop-Athens January 20–21, 2012. J Nutr Health Aging. 2013;17:688–93.
6. Laurent S, Cockcroft J, van Bortel L, et al. Expert consensus document on arterial stiffness: methodological issues and clinical applications. Eur Heart J. 2006;27:2588–605.
7. Mitchell GF. Arterial stiffness and hypertension. Hypertension. 2014;64:13–8.
8. Zubcevic J, Jun JY, Kim S, et al. Altered inflammatory response is associated with an impaired autonomic input to the bone marrow in the spontaneously hypertensive rat. Hypertension. 2014;63:542–50.

9. Walsh T, Donnelly T, Lyons D. Impaired endothelial nitric oxide bioavailability: a common link between aging, hypertension and atherogenesis? J Am Geriatr Soc. 2009;57:140–5.
10. Ferreira I, Beijers HJ, Schouten F, et al. Clustering of metabolic syndrome traits is associated with maladaptive carotid remodeling and stiffening: a 6-year longitudinal study. Hypertension. 2012;60:542–9.
11. Stepnowsky C, Ancoli-Israel S. Sleep and its disorders in seniors. Sleep Med Clin. 2008;3:281–93.
12. Vasan RS, Beiser A, Seshadri S, et al. Residual lifetime risk for developing hypertension in middle-aged women and men: the Framingham Heart Study. JAMA. 2002;287:1003–10.
13. Krause T, Lovibond K, Caulfield M, et al. Management of hypertension: summary of NICE guidance. BMJ. 2011;343:d4891.
14. Lloyd-Sherlock P, Beard J, Minicuci N, et al. Hypertension among older adults in low and middle-income countries: prevalence, awareness and control. Int J Epidemiol. 2014;43: 116–28.
15. Mozaffarian D, Benjamin EJ, Go AS, American Heart Association Statistics Committee and Stroke Statistics Subcommittee, et al. Heart disease and stroke statistics—2015 update: a report from the American Heart Association. Circulation. 2015;131:e29–e322.
16. Bromfield SG, Bowling CB, Tanner RM, et al. Trends in hypertension prevalence, awareness, treatment, and control among US adults 80 years and older, 1988–2010. J Clin Hypertens (Greenwich). 2014;16:270–6.
17. National Center for Health Statistics (US). Health, United States, 2007: with chart book on trends in the Health of Americans. Hyattsville: National Center for Health Statistics (US); 2007.
18. Weber MA, Schiffrin EL, White WB, et al. Clinical practice guidelines for the management of hypertension in the community: a statement by the American Society of Hypertension and the International Society of Hypertension. J Clin Hypertens (Greenwich). 2014;16:14–26.
19. Mancia G, Fagard R, Narkiewicz K, et al. 2013 ESH/ESC guidelines for the management of arterial hypertension: the task force for the management of arterial hypertension of the European Society of Hypertension (ESH) and of the European Society of Cardiology (ESC). J Hypertens. 2013;31:1281–357.
20. Whelton PK, Carey RM, Aronow WS, et al. ACC/AHA/AAPA/ABC/ACPM/AGS/APhA/ASH/ASPC/NMA/PCNA guideline for the prevention, detection, evaluation, and management of high blood pressure in adults: a report of the American College of Cardiology/American Heart Association Task Force on Clinical Practice Guidelines. J Am Coll Cardiol. 2017; https://doi.org/10.1016/j.jacc.2017.11.006.
21. Hauk L. Pharmacologic treatment of hypertension: ACP and AAFP release recommendations for adults 60 years and older. Am Fam Physician. 2017;95:588–9.
22. Williamson JD, Supiano MA, Applegate WB, et al. Intensive vs standard blood pressure control and cardiovascular disease outcomes in adults aged ≥75 years. A randomized clinical trial. JAMA. 2016;315:2673–82.
23. Safar H, Chahwakilian A, Boudali Y, et al. Arterial stiffness, isolated systolic hypertension, and cardiovascular risk in the elderly. Am J Geriatr Cardiol. 2006;15:178–82.
24. Williams B, Lacy PS, Thom SM, et al. Differential impact of blood pressure-lowering drugs on central aortic pressure and clinical outcomes: principal results of the Conduit Artery Function Evaluation (CAFE) study. Circulation. 2006;113:1213–25.
25. Yavuz BB, Yavuz B, Tayfur O, et al. White coat effect and its clinical implications in the elderly. Clin Exp Hypertens. 2009;31:306–15.
26. Cacciolati C, Hanon O, Alpérovitch A, et al. Masked hypertension in the elderly: cross-sectional analysis of a population-based sample. Am J Hypertens. 2011;24:674–80.
27. James PA, Oparil S, Carter BL, et al. 2014 evidence-based guideline for the management of high blood pressure in adults: report from the panel members appointed to the Eighth Joint National Committee (JNC 8). JAMA. 2014;311:507–20.
28. Spence JD. Pseudo-hypertension in the elderly: still hazy, after all these years. J Hum Hypertens. 1997;11:621–3.

29. Applegate WB, Davis BR, Black HR, et al. Prevalence of postural hypotension at baseline in the Systolic Hypertension in the Elderly Program (SHEP) cohort. J Am Geriatr Soc. 1991;39:1057–64.
30. Holt-Lunstad J, Jones BQ, Birmingham W. The influence of close relationships on nocturnal blood pressure dipping. Int J Psychophysiol. 2009;71:211–7.
31. Lewington S, Clarke R, Qizilbash N, Prospective Studies Collaboration, et al. Age-specific relevance of usual blood pressure to vascular mortality: a meta-analysis of individual data for one million adults in 61 prospective studies. Lancet. 2002;360:1903–13.
32. Ettehad D, Emdin CA, Kiran A, et al. Blood pressure lowering for prevention of cardiovascular disease and death: a systematic review and meta-analysis. Lancet. 2016;387:957–67.
33. Xie X, Atkins E, Lv J, et al. Effects of intensive blood pressure lowering on cardiovascular and renal outcomes: updated systematic review and meta-analysis. Lancet. 2016;387:435–43.
34. Ruixing Y, Weixiong L, Hanjun Y, et al. Diet, lifestyle, and blood pressure of the middle-aged and elderly in the Guangxi Bai Ku Yao and Han populations. Am J Hypertens. 2008;21:382–7.
35. Faselis C, Doumas M, Pittaras A, et al. Exercise capacity and all-cause mortality in male veterans with hypertension aged ≥70 years. Hypertension. 2014;64:30–5.
36. Aburto NJ, Ziolkovska A, Hooper L, et al. Effect of lower sodium intake on health: systematic review and meta-analyses. BMJ. 2013;346:f1326. https://doi.org/10.1136/bmj.f1326.
37. Intersalt: an international study of electrolyte excretion and blood pressure. Results for 24 hour urinary sodium and potassium excretion. Intersalt Cooperative Research Group. BMJ. 1988;297:319–28.
38. Blood Pressure Lowering Treatment Trialists' Collaboration. Blood pressure lowering and major cardiovascular events in people with and without chronic kidney disease: meta-analysis of randomised controlled trials. BMJ. 2013;347:f5680. https://doi.org/10.1136/bmj.f5680.
39. Thomopoulosa C, Paratib G, Zanchetti A. Effects of blood pressure lowering on outcome incidence in hypertension: 4. Effects of various classes of antihypertensive drugs-overview and meta-analyses. J Hypertens. 2015;33:195–211.
40. Palmer SC, Mavridis D, Navarese E, et al. Comparative efficacy and safety of blood pressure-lowering agents in adults with diabetes and kidney disease: a network meta-analysis. Lancet. 2015;385:2047–56.
41. The ONTARGET Investigators. Telmisartan, ramipril, or both in patients at high risk for vascular events. N Engl J Med. 2008;358:1547–59.
42. Tomlinson LA, Abel GA, Chaudhry AN, et al. ACE inhibitor and angiotensin receptor-II antagonist prescribing and hospital admissions with acute kidney injury: a longitudinal ecological study. PLoS One. 2013;8(11):e78465. https://doi.org/10.1371/journal.pone.0078465.
43. National Institute of Health and Clinical Excellence. Hypertension: clinical management of primary hypertension in adults. London: NICE; 2011.. NICE clinical guideline 127
44. HOPE Study Investigators. The HOPE study (heart outcomes prevention evaluation). J Renin-Angiotensin-Aldosterone Syst. 2000;1(1):18–20.
45. Warwick J, Falaschetti E, Rockwood K, et al. No evidence that frailty modifies the positive impact of antihypertensive treatment in very elderly people: an investigation of the impact of frailty upon treatment effect in the HYpertension in the Very Elderly Trial (HYVET) study, a double-blind, placebo-controlled study of antihypertensives in people with hypertension aged 80 and over. BMC Med. 2015;13:78.
46. van Bemmel T, Gussekloo J, Westendorp RG, et al. In a population based prospective study, no association between high blood pressure and mortality after age 85 years. J Hypertens. 2006;24:287–92.
47. Poortvliet RK, Blom JW, de Craen AJ, et al. Low blood pressure predicts increased mortality in very old age even without heart failure: the Leiden 85-plus study. Eur J Heart Fail. 2013;15:528–33.
48. Poortvliet RK, de Ruijter W, de Craen AJ, et al. Blood pressure trends and mortality: the Leiden 85-plus study. J Hypertens. 2013;31:63–70.
49. Mattila K, Haavisto M, Rajala S, et al. Blood pressure and five year survival in the very old. BMJ (Clin Res Ed). 1988;296:887–9.

50. Satish S, Freeman DH Jr, Ray L, et al. The relationship between blood pressure and mortality in the oldest old. J Am Geriatr Soc. 2001;49:367–74.
51. Odden MC, Peralta CA, Haan MN, et al. Rethinking the association of high blood pressure with mortality in elderly adults: the impact of frailty. Arch Intern Med. 2012;172:1162–8.
52. Tinetti ME, Han L, Lee DSH, et al. Antihypertensive medications and serious fall injuries in a nationally representative sample of older adults. JAMA Intern Med. 2014;174:588–95.
53. Callisaya L, Sharman JE, Close J, et al. Greater daily defined dose of antihypertensive medication increases the risk of falls in older people—a population-based study. J Am Geriatr Soc. 2014;62:1527–33.
54. Corrao G, Mazzola P, Monzio Compagnoni M, et al. Antihypertensive medications, loop diuretics, and risk of hip fracture in the elderly: a population-based cohort study of 81,617 Italian patients newly treated between 2005 and 2009. Drugs Aging. 2015;32:927–36.
55. Butt DA, Mamdani M, Austin PC, et al. The risk of hip fracture after initiating antihypertensive drugs in the elderly. Arch Intern Med. 2012;172:1739–44.
56. Fuller GF. Falls in the elderly. Am Fam Physician. 2000;61(7):2159–68.. 2173-4
57. Office for National Statistics. Deaths registered in England and Wales (series DR) 2016. London: ONS; 2017.
58. Alzheimer's Association. 2016 Alzheimer's disease facts and figures. Alzheimer's Dement. 2016;12(4):459–509.
59. Rait G, Walters K, Bottomley C, et al. Survival of people with clinical diagnosis of dementia in primary care: cohort study. BMJ. 2010;341:c3584.
60. Barnes DE, Cauley JA, Lui LY, et al. Women who maintain optimal cognitive function into old age. J Am Geriatr Soc. 2007;55:259–64.
61. Barnes DE, Yaffe K. The projected effect of risk factor reduction on Alzheimer's disease prevalence. Lancet Neurol. 2011;10:819–28.
62. Qiu C, Winblad B, Fratiglioni L. The age-dependent relation of blood pressure to cognitive function and dementia. Lancet Neurol. 2005;4:487–99.
63. Forette F, Seux ML, Staessen JA, et al. Prevention of dementia in randomised double-blind placebo-controlled Systolic Hypertension in Europe (Syst-Eur) trial. Lancet. 1998;352:1347–51.
64. Tzourio C, Anderson C, Chapman N, et al. Effects of blood pressure lowering with perindopril and indapamide therapy on dementia and cognitive decline in patients with cerebrovascular disease. Arch Intern Med. 2003;163:1069–75.
65. Lithell H, Hansson L, Skoog I, et al. The Study on COgnition and Prognosis in the Elderly (SCOPE); outcomes in patients not receiving add-on therapy after randomization. J Hypertens Engl. 2004;22:1605–12.
66. Peters R, Beckett N, Forette F, et al. Incident dementia and blood pressure lowering in the Hypertension in the Very Elderly Trial cognitive function assessment (HYVET-COG): a double-blind, placebo controlled trial. Lancet Neurol. 2008;7:683–9.
67. Di Bari M, Pahor M, Franse LV, et al. Dementia and disability outcomes in large hypertension trials: lessons learned from the systolic hypertension in the elderly program (SHEP) trial. Am J Epidemiol. 2001;153:72–8.
68. Beishon LC, Harrison JK, Harwood RH, et al. The evidence for treating hypertension in older people with dementia: a systematic review. J Hum Hypertens. 2014;28:283–7.
69. Sabayan B, Oleksik AM, Maier AB, et al. High blood pressure and resilience to physical and cognitive decline in the oldest old: the Leiden 85-plus study. J Am Geriatr Soc. 2012;60:2014–9.
70. Qiu C, Winblad B, Fratiglioni L. Low diastolic pressure and risk of dementia in very old people: a longitudinal study. Dement Geriatr Cogn Disord. 2009;28:213–9.
71. Ogliari G, Westendorp RG, Muller M, et al. Blood pressure and 10-year mortality risk in the Milan Geriatrics 75+ Cohort Study: role of functional and cognitive status. Age Ageing. 2015;44:932–7.
72. Mossello E, Pieraccioli M, Nesti N, et al. Effects of low blood pressure in cognitively impaired elderly patients treated with antihypertensive drugs. JAMA Intern Med. 2015;175:578–85.

73. Franklin SS, Jacobs MJ, Wong ND, et al. Predominance of isolated systolic hypertension among middle-aged and elderly US hypertensives. Hypertension. 2001;37:869–74.
74. Burt VL, Harris T. The third national health and nutrition examination survey: contributing data on aging and health. Gerontologist. 1994;34(4):486–90.
75. Denardo SJ, Gong Y, Nichols WW, et al. Blood pressure and outcomes in very old hypertensive coronary artery disease patients: an INVEST substudy. Am J Med. 2010;123:719–26.
76. Ooi WL, Hossain M, Lipsitz LA. The association between orthostatic hypotension and recurrent falls in nursing home residents. Am J Med. 2000;108:106–11.
77. Poon OI, Braun U. High prevalence of orthostatic hypotension and its correlation with potentially causative medications among elderly veterans. J Clin Pharm Ther. 2005;30:173–8.
78. Gangavati A, Hajjar I, Quach L, et al. Hypertension, orthostatic hypotension, and the risk of falls in a community-dwelling elderly population: the maintenance of balance, independent living, intellect, and zest in the elderly of Boston study. J Am Geriatr Soc. 2011;59(3):383–9.
79. Wolff JL, Starfield B, Anderson G. Prevalence, expenditures, and complications of multiple chronic conditions in the elderly. Arch Intern Med. 2002;162:2269–76.
80. Seeman TE, Singer BH, Rowe JW, et al. Price of adaptation–allostatic load and its health consequences. Arch Intern Med. 1997;157:2259–68.
81. Karlamangla AS, Singer BH, McEwen BS, Rowe JW, Seeman TE. Allostatic load as a predictor of functional decline: MacArthur studies of successful aging. J Clin Epidemiol. 2002;55:696–710.
82. Benetos A, Labat C, Rossignol P, et al. Treatment with multiple blood pressure medications, achieved blood pressure, and mortality in older nursing home residents the PARTAGE study. JAMA Intern Med. 2015;175:989–95.
83. Rajpura J, Nayak R. Medication adherence in a sample of elderly suffering from hypertension: evaluating the influence of illness perceptions, treatment beliefs, and illness burden. J Manag Care Pharm. 2014;20:58–65.
84. Ebrahim S, Fahey T, Schroeder K. How can we improve adherence to blood pressure-lowering medication in ambulatory care? Systemic review of randomized controlled trials. Arch Intern Med. 2004;164(7):722–32.

Urinary Tract Infections in the Elderly

6

Chrysoula Pipili and Eirini Grapsa

Epidemiology

Urinary tract infections (UTIs) are traditionally the most common type of infection in the elderly leading to impaired quality of life and increased morbidity and mortality (28-day mortality of 5%) [1–3]. Epidemiology of UTI varies between different settings, gender, season, and adults older than 85 years old. UTI is the first cause of infection among community dwellers and the second cause of infection among nursing home residents and hospitalized subjects [4–6]. In the oldest old and in women, the annual incidence is higher than men, ranging from 0.07 to 0.13 in women older than 85 in comparison to men in whom the incidence ranges from 0.05 per person-year to 0.08 in men aged 85 and older [7–9]. Interestingly, seasonal fluctuations of UTIs were noticed in individuals younger than 70 years in the UK. There was found an autumnal peak which faded progressively with the age until it disappears in adults older than 85, in whom UTIs were most common infection [10]. As the population ages, the prevalence of UTI in older adults is expected to grow, necessitating diagnostic, therapeutic, and preventive amelioration in order to improve the well-being of older adults.

Risk Factors

Healthy urinary tract is not a sterile environment but is colonized by a set of microorganisms which change throughout the time based on environmental and behavioral situations. Anatomical and physiologic changes caused by aging such as reduced innate immunity, general debility, malnutrition, and increase in residual

C. Pipili · E. Grapsa (✉)
Nephrology Department Aretaieio University Hospital,
National and Kapodistrian University of Athens, Athens, Greece
e-mail: egrapsa@aretaieio.uoa.gr

C. G. Musso et al. (eds.), *Clinical Nephrogeriatrics*,
https://doi.org/10.1007/978-3-030-18711-8_6

urine volume are the main specific features predisposing elderly to UTI. A number of coexisting chronic illnesses, foreign bodies (stone, catheter, prosthetic devices), polypharmacy, abnormalities of the renal tract (e.g., tumors, surgery, fistulae) and in renal function, and reduced self-hygiene result in more severe disease and challenges in therapeutic practice [11, 12]. All neurological conditions leading to incomplete bladder emptying such as Parkinson disease, Alzheimer's disease, and cerebrovascular disease are highly associated with UTIs [13, 14].

In community-dwelling elderly, the history of UTI is the strongest risk factor for UTI followed by diabetes mellitus, urinary incontinence, poor glycemic control, short-term and long-term urinary catheterization, and less frequent hematogenous spread from non-urinary source of bacteremia [15]. Decreased mobility also predisposes to UTI as increases the risk of hospitalization [16]. Elderly residing in nursing home facilities are more likely to have asymptomatic bacteriuria, due to higher incidence of cognitive and/or urinary and/or fecal impairment, use of catheters, and greater exposure to nosocomial pathogens leading to antibiotic-multiresistant pyelonephritis [13, 14, 17, 18]. Furthermore, hospital UTIs are more common among females and patients in rehabilitation, on immunosuppression, with acute urine retention or post-void residual urine and antecedents of UTI in the previous 6 months [19].

Older women are additionally susceptible to UTI because they do not have the protective estrogen effect in vaginal flora—since this hormone promotes the genitourinary acid pH by favoring the local colonization with protective lactobacilli. Besides, these patients are more likely to develop cystocele compared to their younger counterparts [15]. Moreover, sexual activity with no permanent partner along with the genetic background continues to be a contributing factor to symptomatic and recurrent UTI, even in the elderly [20–22]. Moore et al. found that the risk for UTI 2 days after intercourse increases almost 3.5 times in women aged 55–75 years old, while Nicolle et al. documented that the risk is extended within a 2-week period after sexual activity [20, 23]. In men, the prostatic hypertrophy and the urethral stricture can induce urinary obstruction. This phenomenon leads to urinary retention which promotes high post-void residual (bacteria reservoir), resulting in frequent UTIs relapses [12, 24]. Indeed, post-void residual greater than 180 ml are associated with bacteriuria in older men but not in postmenopausal women [23, 25]. Additionally, chronic bacterial prostatitis should be always a differential diagnosis in men as the presenting complains may be similar to recurrent UTI. Ultimately, renal transplant recipients are predisposed to UTIs especially the first-trimester post kidney transplantation. Female gender and surprisingly male kidney allografts are associated with higher occurrence of post-transplant UTIs [26].

Microbiology

Escherichia coli (*E. coli*) is the most commonly identified organism causing both cystitis and pyelonephritis in geriatric population dwelling either in community or in long-term care facilities. Nevertheless, *E. coli* cultures are found in lower percentage compared with the younger counterparts. Additionally, non-*E. coli* uropathogens (*Klebsiella pneumoniae*, *Proteus mirabilis*, and *Enterococcus faecalis*) are also found in urine cultures in this population [27–32]. Simultaneously, *Pseudomonas aeruginosa*, vancomycin-resistant enterococci, and *Candida* are highly documented in urine cultures of hospitalized patients [33]. *P. mirabilis* and *E. faecalis* are isolated in urine more often in men than women [34]. Furthermore, the majority of urinary cultures show a steady rise of resistant uropathogens that prompt toward the use of broader empiric antibiotic therapy [6]. The prevalence of extended-spectrum beta-lactamase (ESBL)-producing *E. coli* is 27% in community and is associated with hospital admission [35]. Interestingly, UTI secondary to non-typhoidal Salmonella without concomitant gastroenteritis has been identified in the geriatric population, being related to urologic malignancies [36].

Finally, Fagan et al. pointed out that separate recommendations should be considered for men and women in regards to empiric antimicrobial treatment as they noticed gender differences in resistance rates. In men, *E. coli* showed frequently high resistance to ciprofloxacin, tetracyclines, and sulphonamides and *Klebsiella pneumoniae* and *P. mirabilis* to mecillinam, whereas in women, *E. coli* was highly resistant to trimethoprim [37, 38].

Patients with chronically placed catheters present some remarkable unique microbial features [41–44]:

1. Biofilm-associated organisms which most of them are urease-producing bacterial species (e.g., *P. mirabilis*, *Morganella morganii*, *Providencia stuartii*, and *K. pneumoniae*). By hydrolyzing urea, they increase the urine pH and therefore predispose to urinary stone formation and catheter obstruction [39, 40].
2. Polymicrobial urine cultures, where the pathogens usually found, vary among the subsequent urine cultures. Conversely, a single microorganism is typically cultured in patients with short-term catheterization.
3. Yeasts in urine cultures, usually *Candida* species (13–32% of cultures).

Definitions

The clinical spectrum of UTIs in the elderly ranges from asymptomatic bacteriuria, symptomatic uncomplicated or complicated UTI (benign cystitis to pyelonephritis), recurrent UTIs, to sepsis associated with UTI requiring hospitalization. The definition of common terms includes:

Asymptomatic Bacteriuria (ASB)

Positive urine cultures (bacteria or yeasts) are growing at least 10^5 colony-forming units/ml in the absence of symptoms or signs of UTI. For men, one urine sample is adequate, while for women two consecutive samples are required which would grow no more than two pathogen species, and no urinary catheter would have been inserted within the last 7 days (after first urine culture) [45]. ASB is observed in almost all patients with urine catheters, in 50% of hospitalized patients, in nursing home residents, and in 16–50% in geriatric women [45, 46]. Increasing age and female gender are the strongest predictors for asymptomatic bacteriuria. Patients with diabetes mellitus have also increased incidence of asymptomatic bacteriuria, often containing fungi, associated with poor glycemic control and neurogenic bladder [47]. Data indicate that 16 percentage (16%) evolve to symptomatic UTI [11, 45].

It is worth mentioning that when ASB combined with chronic urinary incontinence is difficult to be differentiated from symptomatic UTI. Generally, it does not require any treatment, and the repeated use of antibiotics should be avoided as it might promote antibiotic resistance and recurrent infections, *Clostridium difficile*, or noninfectious diarrhea, nausea, cachexia, and worsening of renal function [11, 15, 45, 48]. In particular, patients with diabetes mellitus, institutionalized patients, renal transplant recipients, patients prior to joint replacement, or patients with recurrent urinary tract infections have no additional benefit of ASB treatment [48]. However, preemptive antibiotics should be applied for patients with ASB who are undergoing invasive urologic procedures with a high risk of bleeding into urinary tract, such as transurethral prostate resection. Antibiotic treatment before procedure prevents symptomatic disease and sepsis post procedure, compared to no prophylactic treatment [46, 48].

Symptomatic UTI

No universally accepted definitions for symptomatic UTI in elderly exist [49–51]. Typically, it is determined by the presence of at least two of the following criteria [6]: fever (>37.9 °C), new or worsening incontinence, voiding urgency, suprapubic tenderness, costovertebral tenderness or any pain not explained by other diagnoses, pyuria (defined as more than ten white blood cells (WBC)/μL per high-power field of unspun urine or more than four per high-power field × 400 to a sediment centrifuged urine), and bacteriuria (defined as more than 10^5 colony-forming units/ml with no more than two species of microorganisms).

- *Uncomplicated UTI*: symptomatic UTI in a normal genitourinary tract with no prior instrumentation.
- *Complicated UTI*: Symptomatic UTI in patients with [52]:
  1. Urine retention due to (a) functional abnormalities such as ureteric reflux; (b) structural abnormalities such as obstruction of the urethra, cystocele, urethral stricture, prostatic hypertrophy, stones, tumors, and cancers; (c) neurological conditions such as brain or spinal cord infections or injuries, diabetes, stroke, multiple sclerosis, pelvic injury, or trauma; and (d) weakened bladder muscle, progressing with the aging.
  2. Antecedents of urinary instrumentation (urethral or suprapubic catheter, stent, nephrostomy tube) or systemic disease, renal insufficiency, renal

transplantation, polycystic kidneys, and immunocompromised (systemic steroid, HIV infection).

UTIs in elderly men need special consideration and should be managed as complicated due to potential prostate source [52].

Catheter-Associated (CA) Bacteriuria/UTI

The definition for CA bacteriuria is the same with ASB, and similarly treatment is not recommended. Bacteriuria occurs almost universally after 3–4 days of catheter insertion [53]. CA UTI is observed when the urine of a symptomatic UTI patient, with no other source of infection, grows more than 10^3 CFU/ml with of more than a single uropathogen. The same criteria should be applied to symptomatic patients who had their catheter removed 48 h before the urine sample was collected [54]. In case of recently placed catheter, a count of more than 10^2 CFU/ML is adequate for the diagnosis of UTI. Furthermore, women who continue to present CA bacteriuria despite catheter removal before more than 48 h should be considered for treatment [23]. Bacteremia could be a potential complication of CA bacteriuria in 40% of gram-negative bacteremia in nursing home residents [55]. It has been observed that in-and-out catheter procedure for bladder emptying and/or sample obtaining carries a small risk of infection (around 1%) and is well tolerated by patients [11].

Recurrent UTI

It is defined as more than three symptomatic UTIs within a year or more than two UTIs within 6 months. It may correspond to a reinfection, which is a new uropathogen or a previously isolated strain, or a relapse, which means a persistent infection with the same uropathogen even after adequate therapy. Generally, reinfection is responsible for the majority (75%) of recurrent UTIs which are usually observed in the outpatient setting and are associated with increased ambulatory visits, increased therapeutic and prophylactic antibiotic use, anxiety, and demoralization [23, 56, 57]. Epidemiologically, women with genetic predisposition and diabetes mellitus are even more affected by recurrent UTIs [21, 22].

Diagnostic Considerations in Geriatric Population

The common diagnostic urinary dilemmas in elder population refer to atypical presentation of infection, nursing home residents, chronic urine catheter, fever, and delirium. The notions and proportion cited in this passage are based on expert opinions and guidelines recommendations [45, 49, 55, 58].

Evaluation of urine is a crucial step in establishing a diagnosis of UTI. In general, the detection of nitrite and leucocyte esterase in urine dipstick has a high predictive value of UTI, but it is not enough to diagnose it, compared to the sensitivities for nitrite (25%) and leucocyte esterase (75–96%) [59, 60]. Conversely, a negative urine dipstick is enough to rule out a urinary cause of infection as both leucocyte esterase test and nitrite test have a very high specificity, which is about 94–98% and 92–100%, respectively [59, 60]. Interestingly, recent literature demonstrated dipstick sensitivity of 97% in the geriatric population; however, since there are multiple difficulties (e.g., miscommunication, dementia, and difficult to obtain clean catch urine), urine culture should be obtained when UTI suspicion is high in this group [61].

In addition, combined point-of-care test (POCT) for urine culture and susceptibility testing was not found to improve the UTI diagnosis or the appropriate antibiotic prescription for patients with suspected uncomplicated UTI [62]. Nitrite in urine means gram-negative bacteriuria but could be absent if the causing pathogen is *Pseudomonas*, *Staphylococcus*, or *Streptococcus* [6, 59], and it could show false positive in dilute urine [11]. Furthermore, false-negative leucocyte esterase in urine may be observed when glucose, ketones, albumin, and certain antibiotics (e.g., doxycycline, gentamycin, and cephalexin) are present, while false-positive results ("sterile pyuria") could be observed on vaginal contamination, chronic interstitial nephritis, nephrolithiasis, uroepithelial tumors, tuberculosis, and sexually transmitted disease and when meropenem, imipenem, and clavulanic acid are present in urine [6, 11, 63].

When there are UTI-specific symptoms, such as fever, acute painful urination (dysuria), new or worsening urinary incontinence, frequent suprapubic or costovertebral angle pain or tenderness, and positive urine sample for pyuria and/or bacteriuria ($>10^5$ CFU/ml), empiric treatment should be started undeniably. Later, the antibiotic treatment should be adjusted based on the culture result. However, the cutoff point of bacteriuria should be lowered to $>10^3$ in patients harboring *E. coli* and in male patients with *Klebsiella* species and *E. faecalis* and symptoms of UTI, such as positive nitrite or leucocyte esterase dipstick, voiding urgency or dysuria [64].

Patients with atypical urinary symptoms and signs, such as vague changes in habitual mental status (confusion, lethargy, disorganized speech, disparate perception) and in urine characteristics (malodorous, dark-colored urine), with no localizing symptoms and sign, should be observed for at least 24–48 h providing supportive and symptomatic management. These actions consist of providing an adequate oral or intravenous hydration, topical vaginal estrogen in women with history of recurrent UTI, stopping medication which cause urinary retention (antihistamines, anticholinergics/antispasmodics, tricyclic antidepressants, decongestants, opioid analgesics, nonsteroidal anti-inflammatory drugs), or dehydration (diuretics, etc.) [45, 51]. If the patient is clinically well and his/her symptoms are mild, the evaluation and treatment can be delayed until culture results are available. Sufficient data have demonstrated recovery in 25–50% of women presenting UTI symptoms without antibiotics within a week showing no adverse outcomes [65, 66]. Nonetheless, frail elderly patients with persistent altered mental status and urine changes (as the frequency and the color) should be assessed for UTI in case of newly confirmed pyuria without bacteriuria and treated with short-term antibiotics. Acute delirium is frequent in the elderly, and many experts interpreted it as UTI except there are evidence against it [45, 65, 66]. However, delirium includes many predisposing (dehydration, polypharmacy, constipation, alcohol excess, surgery) and precipitating factors (general anesthesia, malnutrition, benzodiazepine withdrawal) which should be considered prior checking urinalysis and culture [67].

Great challenges and controversies complicate the diagnosis of UTI among nursing home residents with or without chronic catheterization. Debilitating conditions such as urinary incontinence, cognitive impairment, advanced age with limited mobility, extensive comorbidities, and multiple indwelling catheters are far more prevalent among institutionalized elder population [37, 68].

In view of that, manifestations of infection are non-specific; hence, difficult to interpret and cooperation for clinical examination and urine sample collection is problematic. Pyrexia in patients with indwelling catheters is not indicative of UTI, and other sources of infection should be ruled out first [69]. Signs of sepsis imply absolutely UTI among this elderly category, and ideally catheter should be removed with culture obtained from a newly inserted catheter before administering antibiotics [54, 69, 70].

Literature review revealed that symptomatic patients with urinary catheters should be treated with antimicrobials when low-level bacteriuria, CA-associated bacteriuria/UTI, pyrexia (axillary temperature >37.9 °C or 1.5 °C above baseline temperature), costovertebral tenderness without obvious cause, or new onset delirium are detected [49]. In nursing home residents without indwelling catheter, the assessment for detecting UTI is required when:

1. They start having fever or leukocytosis plus a new or a worsening urinary symptom or signs (urgency, frequency, incontinence, gross hematuria, costovertebral/suprapubic pain/tenderness) or
2. They start suffering from dysuria plus gross hematuria or change in mental status [51].

Special treatment is recommended for geriatric men. Urine testing (urinalysis plus culture) is necessary when they have urinary symptoms or acute pain/tenderness of the testes, epididymis, or prostate [51, 69]. If some of the previous manifestations are present, differential diagnosis with prostatitis, epididymitis, and chlamydial infection is required. In this case, the presence of fever implies a complicated UTI.

It is worth to be mentioned that fever response to serious infection may be blunted or absent in 20–30% of the elderly population. In this sense, antipyretic or anti-inflammatory medications should be continuously reviewed since they can mask an early infectious process [6, 71].

Treatment

The proper antibiotic selection and the UTI treatment duration should be based on guidelines, gender, local pathogens resistance patterns, and severity of the infection (cystitis, pyelonephritis, complicated, uncomplicated, worsening sepsis). In men, the duration of antimicrobial treatment is often extended for a 7–14-day course. Additional considerations focused on the aged population are evaluation of baseline well-being, comorbidities, living location (community, institutionalized), and chronic catheter insertion. The threshold for hospitalization in the elderly is low as general clinical decompensation comes easier in the context of hemodynamic instability, antibacterial intolerance or no response, and inability to cope in the community.

Overall, urologic evaluation is mandatory once there is suspicion of obstruction or intrarenal abscess and failure of antibacterial response after 72 h treatment. Furthermore, patients on warfarin who commenced on antibiotic need warfarin dose modification. This could be performed either by testing INR a week after antibiotic initiation or preemptively decreasing warfarin dose by 15–20% when antibiotics are introduced [72, 73].

Interestingly, Mody and Juthani-Mehta do not recommend to obtain urinalysis or culture after antimicrobial therapy due to the high incidence of transient and recurrent bacteriuria in the elderly. Instead of that, they suggest to evaluate clinical response only based on general status and symptoms improvement [45].

Prophylaxis

The majority of prevention schemes applied in younger adults have been extrapolated to the elderly population. Long-term antibiotic prophylaxis and postcoital antibiotic prophylaxis for women who have UTI associated with sexual intercourse carry on to be the most commonly used prevention strategies. However, as the risk of antibacterial resistance expands, alternative measures including cranberry, D-mannose extracts, methenamine salts, and topical estrogen have been applied. Unfortunately, the natural products have not been found to limit recurrent infections associated with urinary catheters, and as most natural supplements pharmacokinetic studies are still required to demonstrate its potency, dosing, and active ingredient patterns. Future novel preventive approaches that have scientific basis and are underway are Lactobacillus probiotics and vaccines, made from combinations of dead uropathogenic strains delivered by injection or by vaginal suppository [74].

Cranberry Supplements

Even though the cranberry effect in reducing the recurrent UTIs is not verified in young patients with or without urinary catheter, the studies are very favorable in the elderly population [6, 68, 75, 76]. Cranberry effect depends on its ingredient proanthocyanidin which interrupts *E. coli* adhesion to bladder epithelium [77, 78]. The optimal cranberry dose is not clear yet, and most of the studies have used doses ranging from 100 to 500 mg of cranberry juice or concentrated capsules provided once daily. Due to potential extent of warfarin action, cranberry extract is not recommended for patients on warfarin [79].

D-mannose

This is a pineapple extract which hampers bacterial adherence to the uroepithelium by blocking FimH adhesion, which is positioned at the tip of the type 1 fimbria of enteric bacteria [80]. Preclinical data support its favorable effect in the UTI prevention, but similar to the cranberries, there is no consensus at which dose and schedule should be commenced [81].

The D-mannose powder used in the randomized controlled study of Kranjčec et al. demonstrated equal prophylactic effect to nitrofurantoin [82]. However, the participants were only 100; hence, more studies are necessary to confirm this result.

The effect of methylamine salt (hippurate or mandelate) in UTI prevention has already been known for a long time [6, 81, 84]. In the elderly, this beneficial effect is certified by few studies applying mainly methenamine hippurate [6, 84, 85]. This dose may be adjusted depending on the urine pH, targeting a urine ph < 6. Methylamine can be associated with minor gastrointestinal tract adverse effects and is contraindicated in patients suffering from severe renal and/or hepatic failure and severe dehydration or who are receiving urine-alkalinizing drugs [6, 83–85].

Vaginally Applied Estrogens

Topical vaginal estrogens prevent infection by reparation of the normal vaginal flora and promoting a local acid pH [68, 86]. Conversely, oral estrogens have not demonstrated any similar effect and should not be used for preventing bacteriuria in women [87].

Catheter: Related UTIs

Urinary catheters should be placed when they are absolutely indicated and removed as soon as possible. An aseptic technique and the smallest possible catheter caliber helps to minimize the risk of infection.

In parallel, the use of all condom/silver-coated/hydrophilic-coated/chlorhexidine-coated urethral catheter and intermittent catheterization are associated with infection and bacteriuria reduction [23, 39, 54, 88]. Prophylactic antibiotics do not minimize CA infection, nor the time of catheter removal or replacement, even it can lead to select resistant microorganisms [54, 88–90].

Conclusion

Urinary tract infections (UTIs) are the most common type of infection in the elderly. The most important risk factors are a number of coexisting chronic illnesses, foreign bodies (stone, catheter, prosthetic devices), polypharmacy, abnormalities of the renal tract (e.g., tumors, surgery, fistulae) and in renal function, and reduced self-hygiene. *Escherichia coli* (*E. coli*) is the most commonly identified organism. The prevalence of UTI in older adults is expected to grow, necessitating diagnostic, therapeutic, and preventive amelioration in order to improve the well-being of older adults.

References

1. Wagenlehner F, Wullt B, Ballarini S, Zingg D, Naber KG. Social and economic burden of recurrent urinary tract infections and quality of life: a patient web-based study (GESPRIT). Expert Rev Pharmacoecon Outcomes Res. 2018;18(1):107–17. https://doi.org/10.1080/14737167.2017.1359543.
2. Tal S, Guller V, Levi S, Bardenstein R, Berger D, Gurevich I, Gurevich A. Profile and prognosis of febrile elderly patients with bacteremic urinary tract infection. J Inf Secur. 2005;50(4):296–305. PMID:15998090
3. Koch AM, Eriksen HM, Elstrøm P, Aavitsland P, Harthug S. Severe consequences of healthcare-associated infections among residents of nursing homes: a cohort study. J Hosp Infect. 2009;71(3):269–74. https://doi.org/10.1016/j.jhin.2008.10.032. PMID:19147254
4. Garibaldi RA, Brodine S, Matsumiya S. Infections among patients in nursing homes: policies, prevalence, problems. N Engl J Med. 1981;305(13):731–5. PMID:7266615
5. Nicolle LE, SHEA Long-Term-Care-Committee. Urinary tract infections in long-term-care facilities. Infect Control Hosp Epidemiol. 2001;22(3):167–75. PMID:11310697
6. Matthews SJ, Lancaster JW. Urinary tract infections in the elderly population. Am J Geriatr Pharmacother. 2011;9(5):286309. https://doi.org/10.1016/j.amjopharm.2011.07.002. PMID:21840265
7. Jackson SL, Boyko EJ, Scholes D, Abraham L, Gupta K, Fihn SD. Predictors of urinary tract infection after menopause: a prospective study. Am J Med. 2004;117(12):903–11. PMID:15629728
8. Caljouw MA, den Elzen WP, Cools HJ, Gussekloo J. Predictive factors of urinary tract infections among the oldest old in the general population. A population-based prospective follow-up study. BMC Med. 2011;9:57. https://doi.org/10.1186/1741-7015-9-57. PMID:21575195
9. Griebling TL. Urologic diseases in america project: trends in resource use for urinary tract infections in men. J Urol. 2005;173(4):1288–94. PMID:15758784
10. Rosello A, Pouwels KB, Domenech DE Cellès M, van Kleef E, Hayward AC, Hopkins S, Robotham JV, Smieszek T, Opatowski L, Deeny SR. Seasonality of urinary tract infections in the United Kingdom in different age groups: longitudinal analysis of The Health Improvement Network (THIN). Epidemiol Infect. 2018;146(1):37–45. https://doi.org/10.1017/S095026881700259X.
11. Durso SC. Oxford American handbook of geriatric medicine. Oxford University Press. 2010; p. 654–62.
12. High KP. Infection in the elderly. In: Halter JB, Ouslander JG, Tinetti ME, Studenski S, High KP, Ashana S, editors. Hazzard's geriatric medicine and gerontology. 6th ed. New York: McGraw-Hill; 2009. p. 333–67.
13. Nicolle LE. Urinary tract infection in geriatric and institutionalized patients. Curr Opin Urol. 2002;12(1):51–5. PMID:11753134
14. Nicolle LE. Urinary tract infection in long-term-care facility residents. Clin Infect Dis. 2000;31(3):757–61. PMID:11017826
15. Escobar C, Bhatia S, Wajnberg A. Urinary tract infection. In: Hayashi J, Leff B, editors. Geriatric home-based medical care. Switzerland: Springer International Publishing; 2016. p. 174–81.

16. Rogers MA, Fries BE, Kaufman SR, Mody L, McMahon LF Jr, Saint S. Mobility and other predictors of hospitalization for urinary tract infection: a retrospective cohort study. BMC Geriatr. 2008;8:31. https://doi.org/10.1186/1471-2318-8-31. PMID:19032784
17. Juthani-Mehta M, Quagliarello VJ. Infectious diseases in the nursing home setting: challenges and opportunities for clinical investigation. Clin Infect Dis. 2010;51(8):931–6. https://doi.org/10.1086/656411. PMID:20822459
18. Nicolle LE. Urinary tract pathogens in complicated infection and in elderly individuals. J Infect Dis. 2001;183(Suppl 1):S5–8. PMID:11171003
19. Girard R, Gaujard S, Pergay V, Pornon P, Martin-Gaujard G, Bourguignon L, UTIC Group. Risk factors for urinary tract infections in geriatric hospitals. J Hosp Infect. 2017;97(1):74–8. https://doi.org/10.1016/j.jhin.2017.05.007.
20. Moore EE, Hawes SE, Scholes D, Boyko EJ, Hughes JP, Fihn SD. Sexual intercourse and risk of symptomatic urinary tract infection in post-menopausal women. J Gen Intern Med. 2008;23(5):595–9. https://doi.org/10.1007/s11606-008-0535-y. PMID:18266044
21. Zaffanello M, Malerba G, Cataldi L, Antoniazzi F, Franchini M, Monti E, Fanos V. Genetic risk for recurrent urinary tract infections in humans: a systematic review. J Biomed Biotechnol. 2010;2010:321082. https://doi.org/10.1155/2010/321082. PMID:20379347
22. Renko M, Tapanainen P, Tossavainen P, Pokka T, Uhari M. Meta-analysis of the significance of asymptomatic bacteriuria in diabetes. Diabetes Care. 2011;34(1):230–5. https://doi.org/10.2337/dc10-0421. PMID:20937688
23. Nicolle LE, Bradley S, Colgan R, Rice JC, Schaeffer A, Hooton TM, Infectious Diseases Society of America, American Society of Nephrology, American Geriatric Society. Infectious Diseases Society of America guidelines for the diagnosis and treatment of asymptomatic bacteriuria in adults. Clin Infect Dis. 2005;40(5):643–54. PMID:15714408
24. Nicolle LE. Urinary tract infections in the elderly. Clin Geriatr Med. 2009;25(3):423–36. https://doi.org/10.1016/j.cger.2009.04.005. PMID:19765490
25. Allan WR, Kumar A. Prophylactic mezlocillin for transurethral prostatectomy. Br J Urol. 1985;57(1):46–9.
26. Thölking G, Schuette-Nuetgen K, Vogl T, Dobrindt U, Kahl BC, Brand M, et al. Male kidney allograft recipients at risk for urinary tract infection? PLoS One. 2017;12(11):e0188262. https://doi.org/10.1371/journal.pone.0188262.
27. Katsarolis I, Poulakou G, Athanasia S, Kourea-Kremastinou J, Lambri N, Karaiskos E, Collaborative Study Group on Antibiotic Resistance in Community-acquired Urinary Tract Infections, et al. Acute uncomplicated cystitis: from surveillance data to a rationale for empirical treatment. Int J Antimicrob Agents. 2010;35(1):62–7. https://doi.org/10.1016/j.ijantimicag. PMID:19906513
28. Czaja CA, Scholes D, Hooton TM, Stamm WE. Population-based epidemiologic analysis of acute pyelonephritis. Clin Infect Dis. 2007;45(3):273–80. PMID:17599303
29. Chen Y, Nitzan O, Saliba W, Chazan B, Colodner R, Raz R. Are blood cultures necessary in the management of women with complicated pyelonephritis? J Infect. 2006;53(4):235–40. PMID:16434102
30. van Nieuwkoop C, van't Wout JW, Spelt IC, Becker M, Kuijper EJ, Blom JW, Assendelft WJ, van Dissel JT. Prospective cohort study of acute pyelonephritis in adults: safety of triage towards home based oral antimicrobial treatment. J Inf Secur. 2010;60(2):114–21. https://doi.org/10.1016/j.jinf.2009.11.008.
31. Kofteridis DP, Papadimitraki E, Mantadakis E, Maraki S, Papadakis JA, Tzifa G, Samonis G. Effect of diabetes mellitus on the clinical and microbiological features of hospitalized elderly patients with acute pyelonephritis. J Am Geriatr Soc. 2009;57(11):2125–8. https://doi.org/10.1111/j.1532-5415.2009.02550.x. PMID: 20121956
32. Marques LP, Flores JT, Barros Junior Ode O, Rodrigues GB, Mourão Cde M, Moreira RM. Epidemiological and clinical aspects of urinary tract infection in community-dwelling elderly women. Braz J Infect Dis. 2012;16(5):436–41. https://doi.org/10.1016/j.bjid.2012.06.025.

33. Nicolle LE. Resistant pathogens in urinary tract infections. J Am Geriatr Soc. 2002;50(7 Suppl):S230–5. PMID:12121518
34. Nicolle LE. Asymptomatic bacteriuria in the elderly. Infect Dis Clin N Am. 1997;11(3):647–62.
35. Artero A, Esparcia A, Alberola J, Madrazo M, Nogueira JM, Eiros JM. Prospective cohort study of risk factors for extended-spectrum ß-lactamase-producing *Escherichia coli* urinary tract infections in elderly patients admitted to hospital. Int J Clin Pract. 2017;71(9). doi: https://doi.org/10.1111/ijcp.13001.
36. Gorelik Y, Paul M, Geffen Y, Khamaisi M. Urinary tract infections due to Nontyphoidal salmonella. Am J Med Sci. 2017;353(6):529–32. https://doi.org/10.1016/j.amjms.2017.03.010.
37. Fagan M, Lindbæk M, Grude N, Reiso H, Romøren M, Skaare D, et al. Antibiotic resistance patterns of bacteria causing urinary tract infections in the elderly living in nursing homes versus the elderly living at home: an observational study. BMC Geriatr. 2015;15:98. https://doi.org/10.1186/s12877-015-0097-x. PMID:26238248
38. Delcaru C, Podgoreanu P, Alexandru I,Popescu N, Măruţescu L, Bleotu C, et al. Antibiotic resistance and virulence phenotypes of recent bacterial strains isolated from urinary tract infections in elderly patients with prostatic disease. Pathogens. 2017;6(2):22. pii: E22. https://doi.org/10.3390/pathogens6020022.
39. Tenke P, Kovacs B, Jäckel M, Nagy E. The role of biofilm infection in urology. World J Urol. 2006;24(1):13–20. PMID:16402262
40. Kunin CM. Blockage of urinary catheters: role of microorganisms and constituents of the urine on formation of encrustations. J Clin Epidemiol. 1989;42(9):835–42. PMID:2778465
41. Tambyah PA, Maki DG. Catheter-associated urinary tract infection is rarely symptomatic: a prospective study of 1,497 catheterized patients. Arch Intern Med. 2000;160(5):678–82. PMID: 10724054
42. Tambyah PA, Halvorson KT, Maki DG. A prospective study of pathogenesis of catheter-associated urinary tract infections. Mayo Clin Proc. 1999;74(2):131–6. PMID: 10069349
43. Matsukawa M, Kunishima Y, Takahashi S, Takeyama K, Tsukamoto T. Bacterial colonization on intraluminal surface of urethral catheter. Urology. 2005;65(3):440–4. PMID:15780351
44. Tenke P, Köves B, Johansen TE. An update on prevention and treatment of catheter-associated urinary tract infections. Curr Opin Infect Dis. 2014;27(1):102–7. https://doi.org/10.1097/QCO.0000000000000031. PMID: 24345923
45. Mody L, Juthani-Mehta M. Urinary tract infections in older women: a clinical review. JAMA. 2014;311(8):844–54. https://doi.org/10.1001/jama.2014.303.
46. Monane M, Gurwitz JH, Lipsitz LA, Glynn RJ, Choodnovskiy I, Avorn J. Epidemiologic and diagnostic aspects of bacteriuria: a longitudinal study in older women. J Am Geriatr Soc. 1995;43(6):618–22. PMID:7775718
47. Zhanel GG, Nicolle LE, Harding GK. Prevalence of asymptomatic bacteriuria and associated host factors in women with diabetes mellitus. The Manitoba Diabetic Urinary Infection Study Group. Clin Infect Dis. 1995;21(2):316–22. PMID:8562738
48. Köves B, Cai T, Veeratterapillay R, Pickard R, Seisen T, Lam TB, et al. Benefits and harms of treatment of asymptomatic bacteriuria: a systematic review and meta-analysis by the European Association of Urology urological infection guidelines panel. Eur Urol. 2017;72(6):865–8. https://doi.org/10.1016/j.eururo.2017.07.014.
49. Loeb M, Bentley DW, Bradley S, Crossley K, Garibaldi R, Gantz N, et al. Development of minimum criteria for the initiation of antibiotics in residents of long-term-care facilities: results of a consensus conference. Infect Control Hosp Epidemiol. 2001;22(2):120–4.
50. Stone ND, Ashraf MS, Calder J, Crnich CJ, Crossley K, Drinka PJ, Society for Healthcare Epidemiology Long-Term Care Special Interest Group, et al. Surveillance definitions of infections in long-term care facilities: revisiting the McGeer criteria. Infect Control Hosp Epidemiol. 2012;33(10):965–77. https://doi.org/10.1086/667743. PMID:22961014
51. Rowe TA, Juthani-Mehta M. Diagnosis and management of urinary tract infection in older adults. Infect Dis Clin N Am. 2014;28(1):75–89. https://doi.org/10.1016/j.idc.2013.10.004. PMID: 24484576

52. Lipsky BA. Urinary tract infections in men. Epidemiology, pathophysiology, diagnosis, and treatment. Ann Intern Med. 1989;110(2):138–50. PMID: 2462391
53. Beveridge LA, Davey PG, Phillips G, McMurdo ME. Optimal management of urinary tract infections in older people. Clin Interv Aging. 2011;6:173–80. https://doi.org/10.2147/CIA.S13423.
54. Hooton TM, Bradley SF, Cardenas DD, Colgan R, Geerlings SE, Rice JC, Infectious Diseases Society of America, et al. Diagnosis, prevention, and treatment of catheter-associated urinary tract infection in adults: 2009 International Clinical Practice Guidelines from the Infectious Diseases Society of America. Clin Infect Dis. 2010;50(5):625–63. PMID:20175247
55. Ryan S, Gillespie E, Stuart RL. Urinary tract infection surveillance in residential aged care. Am J Infect Control. 2018;46(1):67–72. https://doi.org/10.1016/j.ajic.2017.07.002.
56. Eriksson I, Gustafson Y, Fagerström L, Olofsson B. Do urinary tract infections affect morale among very old women? Health Qual Life Outcomes. 2010;8:73. https://doi.org/10.1186/1477-7525-8-73. PMID: 20650004
57. Litman HJ, Steers WD, Wei JT, Kupelian V, Link CL, McKinlay JB, Boston Area Community Health Survey Investigators. Relationship of lifestyle and clinical factors to lower urinary tract symptoms: results from Boston Area Community Health survey. Urology. 2007;70(5):916–21. PMID:17919693. https://doi.org/10.1016/j.urology.2007.06.1117.
58. McGeer A, Campbell B, Emori TG, Hierholzer WJ, Jackson MM, Nicolle LE, et al. Definitions of infection for surveillance in long-term care facilities. Am J Infect Control. 1991;19(1):1–7. PMID:1902352
59. Wilson ML, Gaido L. Laboratory diagnosis of urinary tract infections in adult patients. Clin Infect Dis. 2004;38(8):1150–8. PMID: 15095222
60. Rahn DD, Boreham MK, Allen KE, Nihira MA, Schaffer JI. Predicting bacteriuria in urogynecology patients. Am J Obstet Gynecol. 2005;192(5):1376–8.
61. Shimoni Z, Glick J, Hermush V, Froom P. Sensitivity of the dipstick in detecting bacteremic urinary tract infections in elderly hospitalized patients. PLoS One. 2017;12(10):e0187381. https://doi.org/10.1371/journal.pone.0187381.
62. Holm A, Cordoba G, Møller Sørensen T, Rem Jessen L, Frimodt-Møller N, Siersma V. Effect of point-of-care susceptibility testing in general practice on appropriate prescription of antibiotics for patients with uncomplicated urinary tract infection: a diagnostic randomised controlled trial. BMJ Open. 2017;7(10):e018028. https://doi.org/10.1136/bmjopen-2017-018028.
63. Juthani-Mehta M, Tinetti M, Perrelli E, Towle V, Quagliarello V. Role of dipstick testing in the evaluation of urinary tract infection in nursing home residents. Infect Control Hosp Epidemiol. 2007;28(7):889–91. PMID:17564998
64. Sundvall PD, Gunnarsson RK. Evaluation of dipstick analysis among elderly residents to detect bacteriuria: a cross-sectional study in 32 nursing homes. BMC Geriatr. 2009;9:32. https://doi.org/10.1186/1471-2318-9-32. PMID:19635163
65. Christiaens TC, De Meyere M, Verschraegen G, Peersman W, Heytens S, De Maeseneer JM. Randomised controlled trial of nitrofurantoin versus placebo in the treatment of uncomplicated urinary tract infection in adult women. Br J Gen Pract. 2002;52(482):729–34. PMID:12236276
66. Ferry SA, Holm SE, Stenlund H, Lundholm R, Monsen TJ. Clinical and bacteriological outcome of different doses and duration of pivmecillinam compared with placebo therapy of uncomplicated lower urinary tract infection in women: the LUTIW project. Scand J Prim Health Care. 2007;25(1):49–57. PMID:17354160. https://doi.org/10.1080/02813430601183074.
67. Delirium HJ. In: Cooper N, Forrest K, Mulley G, editors. ABC of geriatric medicine. Oxford: Blackwell Publishing Ltd; 2009. p. 11–5.
68. Detweiler K, Mayers D, Fletcher SG. Bacteruria and urinary tract infections in the elderly. Urol Clin N Am. 2015;42(4):561–8. https://doi.org/10.1016/j.ucl.2015.07.002.
69. Scottish Intercollegiate Guidelines Network [SIGN]. Management of suspected bacterial urinary tract infection in adults: a national clinical guideline. SIGN; 2006. Available at: www.sign.ac.uk.

70. HPA. Diagnosis of UTI. Quick reference guide for primary care; 2009. Available at: http://www.hpa.or.uk/web/HPAwebfile/HPAweb(C/1194947330877
71. High KP, Bradley SF, Gravenstein S, Mehr DR, Quagliarello VJ, Richards C, Infectious Diseases Society of America, et al. Clinical practice guideline for the evaluation of fever and infection in older adult residents of long-term care facilities: 2008 update by the Infectious Diseases Society of America. J Am Geriatr Soc. 2009;57(3):375–94. https://doi.org/10.1111/j.1532-5415.2009.02175.x. PMID:19278394
72. Baillargeon J, Holmes HM, Lin YL, Raji MA, Sharma G, Kuo YF. Concurrent use of warfarin and antibiotics and the risk of bleeding in older adults. Am J Med. 2012;125(2):183–9. https://doi.org/10.1016/j.amjmed.2011.08.014. PMID:22269622
73. Ahmed A, Stephens JC, Kaus CA, Fay WP. Impact of preemptive warfarin dose reduction on anticoagulation after initiation of trimethoprim-sulfamethoxazole or levofloxacin. J Thromb Thrombolysis. 2008;26(1):44–8. PMID:17985084
74. Vicariotto F. Effectiveness of an association of a cranberry dry extract, D-mannose, and the two microorganisms *Lactobacillus plantarum* LP01 and *Lactobacillus paracasei* LPC09 in women affected by cystitis: a pilot study. J Clin Gastroenterol. 2014;48(Suppl 1):S96–101. https://doi.org/10.1097/MCG.0000000000000224.
75. McMurdo ME, Argo I, Phillips G, Daly F, Davey P. Cranberry or trimethoprim for the prevention of recurrent urinary tract infections? A randomized controlled trial in older women. J Antimicrob Chemother. 2009;63(2):389–95. https://doi.org/10.1093/jac/dkn489. PMID:19042940
76. Jepson RG, Williams G, Craig JC. Cranberries for preventing urinary tract infections. Cochrane Database Syst Rev. 2012;10:CD001321. https://doi.org/10.1002/14651858.CD001321.pub5. PMID:23076891
77. Gupta K, Chou MY, Howell A, Wobbe C, Grady R, Stapleton AE. Cranberry products inhibit adherence of p-fimbriated *Escherichia coli* to primary cultured bladder and vaginal epithelial cells. J Urol. 2007;177(6):2357–60. PMID:17509358
78. Howell AB, Vorsa N, Der Marderosian A, Foo LY. Inhibition of the adherence of P-fimbriated *Escherichia coli* to uroepithelial-cell surfaces by proanthocyanidin extracts from cranberries. N Engl J Med. 1998;339(15):1085–6.
79. Committee on Safety of Medicines and the Medicines and Healthcare products Regulatory Agency. Interactions between warfarin and cranberry juice: new advice. MHRA/CSM current problems in pharmacovigilance. 2004;30:10. Available at: http://www.mhra.gov.uk/Howweregulate/Medicines/Herbalmedicines/HerbalSafetyNews/Currentsafetyissues/con1004343
80. Mydock-McGrane LK, Cusumano ZT, Janetka JW. Mannose-derived FimH antagonists: a promising anti-virulence therapeutic strategy for urinary tract infections and Crohn's disease. Expert Opin Ther Pat. 2016;26(2):175–97. https://doi.org/10.1517/13543776.2016.1131266.
81. Altarac S, Papeš D. Use of D-mannose in prophylaxis of recurrent urinary tract infections (UTIs) in women. BJU Int. 2014;113(1):9–10. https://doi.org/10.1111/bju.12492.
82. Kranjčec B, Papeš D, Altarac S. D-mannose powder for prophylaxis of recurrent urinary tract infections in women: a randomized clinical trial. World J Urol. 2014;32(1):79–84. https://doi.org/10.1007/s00345-013-1091-6.
83. Lee BB, Simpson JM, Craig JC, Bhuta T. Methenamine hippurate for preventing urinary tract infections. Cochrane Database Syst Rev. 2007;(4):CD003265. Review. Update in: *Cochrane Database Syst Rev*. 2012;10:CD003265.PMID:17943785.
84. Kasanen A, Junnila SY, Kaarsalo E, Hajba A, Sundquist H. Secondary prevention of recurrent urinary tract infections. Comparison of the effect of placebo, methenamine hippurate, nitrofurantoin and trimethoprim alone. Scand J Infect Dis. 1982;14(4):293–6.
85. Cronberg S, Welin CO, Henriksson L, Hellsten S, Persson KM, Stenberg P. Prevention of recurrent acute cystitis by methenamine hippurate: double blind controlled crossover long term study. Br Med J (Clin Res Ed). 1987;294(6586):1507–8. PMID:3111615

86. Eriksen B. A randomized, open, parallel-group study on the preventive effect of an estradiol-releasing vaginal ring (Estring) on recurrent urinary tract infections in postmenopausal women. Am J Obstet Gynecol. 1999;180(5):1072–9. PMID:10329858
87. Perrotta C, Aznar M, Mejia R, Albert X, Ng CW. Oestrogens for preventing recurrent urinary tract infection in postmenopausal women. Cochrane Database Syst Rev. 2008;2:CD005131. https://doi.org/10.1002/14651858.CD005131.pub2. PMID:18425910
88. Morton SC, Shekelle PG, Adams JL, Bennett C, Dobkin BH, Montgomerie J, Vickrey BG. Antimicrobial prophylaxis for urinary tract infection in persons with spinal cord dysfunction. Arch Phys Med Rehabil. 2002;83(1):129–38. PMID:11782843
89. Rutschmann OT, Zwahlen A. Use of norfloxacin for prevention of symptomatic urinary tract infection in chronically catheterized patients. Eur J Clin Microbiol Infect Dis. 1995;14(5):441–4.
90. Mohler JL, Cowen DL, Flanigan RC. Suppression and treatment of urinary tract infection in patients with an intermittently catheterized neurogenic bladder. J Urol. 1987;138(2):336–40. PMID:3496470

Glomerulopathies in the Elderly

7

Arunraj Navaratnarajah and Michelle Willicombe

Introduction

Precise data on the prevalence of glomerular disease in the elderly is lacking as elderly patients have often been poorly represented in biopsy registries. In addition, interpretation of the available data is complicated by the differing age definitions utilised by research groups worldwide, together with disparities in the ethnic predisposition associated with glomerular disease. The growing elderly population, together with the appreciation that directed therapy for glomerular disease in this age group may improve renal outcomes, is altering this paradigm.

In this chapter we describe how glomerular disease is diagnosed in the elderly, the common renal histopathological findings reported in elderly patients and the recognised management strategies reported in the literature.

Diagnosing Glomerular Disease in the Elderly

The Ageing Glomerulus

Even in healthy individuals, the glomerulus undergoes physiological changes associated with ageing. A study performing renal histological evaluation of elderly living transplant donors with normal renal function demonstrated that there is a development of focal and global glomerulosclerosis associated with age [1]. As the percentage of sclerosed glomeruli increases with age, this in turn leads to a reduction in the number of functional glomeruli. These glomerular changes are often accompanied by other age-related changes including tubular atrophy, interstitial

A. Navaratnarajah (✉) · M. Willicombe (✉)
West London Renal and Transplant Centre, Hammersmith Hospital,
Imperial NHS Healthcare Trust, London, UK
e-mail: a.navaratnarajah@nhs.net; michelle.willicombe@nhs.net

C. G. Musso et al. (eds.), *Clinical Nephrogeriatrics*,
https://doi.org/10.1007/978-3-030-18711-8_7

fibrosis and arteriosclerosis [1, 2]. This physiological ageing is associated with a decline in glomerular filtration rate (GFR) which occurs at approximately 0.75 ml/min/year [3]. The proportion of glomeruli with global sclerosis will increase in the presence of non-age related glomerular pathology, and this has been shown to be associated with a poorer renal prognosis.

Renal Biopsies in the Elderly

In the correct clinical setting, as in young patients, the nature of glomerular pathology needs to be diagnosed by renal biopsy, and age alone should not pose a contraindication. Complication rates following a renal biopsy are low, with no recognised increased risk in elderly patients [4]. A biopsy will not only allow diagnostic confirmation, it can also provide prognostic information guiding appropriate therapeutic interventions and there have now been many studies which have shown the benefit of biopsies in the elderly [5–14]. However, despite the low risk, consideration is also required as to the suitability of therapy guided by the differential diagnosis in the elderly, as relative contraindications to immunotherapy are higher in the old. Therefore, a renal biopsy should be offered to elderly patients with suspected glomerular pathology providing there are no contraindications to either the biopsy (e.g. coagulation abnormalities) or the treatment of the underlying disease process (e.g. immunotherapy).

Before a biopsy can be considered, there must be recognition that an underlying glomerular pathology may be present. This may be considered more challenging in the elderly population due to the physiological decline in glomerular filtration rate (GFR) with age, the increased prevalence of co-morbidities associated with CKD and proteinuria (e.g. hypertension and diabetes), the increased prevalence of albuminuria on urinalysis and increased susceptibility to AKI from intercurrent illnesses.

Acute kidney injury is common in hospitalised patients, and the incidence increases in elderly patients [15]. Epidemiological studies have shown that prerenal and acute tubular necrosis are the commonest cause of AKI [16]. Therefore, consideration of glomerular disease in the context of AKI may be overlooked. Furthermore, in order to appropriately detect glomerular disease in patients, urinalysis is a prerequisite and this may not be universally performed in AKI cases believed to be related to prerenal causes [17]. Adjusting for the age-related physiological decline in GFR which occurs after the age of 40, glomerular disease in the elderly may present with preserved GFR and urinary abnormalities ranging from low grade proteinuria with or without haematuria to nephrotic syndrome. However, it is important to highlight that elderly patients with nephrotic syndrome have a higher predisposition to developing co-existing AKI compared with younger patients. Therefore, for all elderly patients, a thorough clinical history and examination, together with urinalysis, renal imaging and serological markers are vital to determine the correct differential diagnosis and identify a subgroup of patients who require a renal biopsy for suspected glomerular disease.

Consideration of Urinalysis Interpretation in the Elderly

Proteinuria

Proteinuria is an important biomarker for glomerular disease. Albuminuria predicts ESRD, cardiovascular disease and death across all age groups. Whilst the prevalence of albuminuria increases with age, it has not been shown to occur as part of the natural ageing process, and interpretation of albuminuria needs careful consideration [1]. Firstly, scrutiny of the method used to detect and define the level of albuminuria is required. The spot urinary albumin:creatinine (UACR) and protein:creatinine (UPCR) ratios are proportional to the daily excretion of creatinine, which may be reduced in females and older patients with less muscle mass therefore leading to an overestimation of albuminuria [18]. Twenty-four hour urinary collections would be more accurate to evaluate the degree of albuminuria in older patients, although they are often impractical for most patients. Newer equations have been developed to calculate the estimated UACR and UPCR, which may provide a more practical and accurate estimation of albuminuria and proteinuria than previous methods in the elderly population [19]. The second consideration required in assessing glomerular proteinuria in older patients is the relevant contribution posed by co-morbidities. This is an important consideration when deciding on obtaining a renal biopsy. In these patients a biopsy may not change management, and the risks of the procedure although low, may outweigh any benefits. Diabetes represents one such challenging co-morbidity. The incidence of diabetes increases with age, and albuminuria is one of the earliest manifestations of diabetic nephropathy. It has been shown that a significant proportion of non-diabetic glomerular lesions may be found on biopsy of diabetic patients, who would otherwise have been denied tailored treatment [20]. However, extrapolation of these findings specifically to the elderly population has not been performed. Determination of which diabetic patients may benefit from biopsy remains a challenge across all age groups [21].

Haematuria

Microscopic haematuria in conjunction with proteinuria is suggestive of glomerular disease. Both dysmorphic red blood cells (RBCs) and red cell casts are suggestive of glomerular pathology. Elderly patients presenting with isolated haematuria must have a urinary tract malignancy excluded. Isolated haematuria of glomerular origin, in the absence of dysfunction or proteinuria is likely to have a benign course in the elderly.

Serological Testing

Serological testing may aid with diagnosing the aetiology of an underlying glomerular disease in the elderly, which is particularly helpful in situations where a renal biopsy is contraindicated. Serological tests required will be determined by the clinical presentation and most likely differential. Pauci-immune glomerulonephritis (granulomatosis with polyangiitis and microscopic polyangiitis) is one of the commonest histological diagnoses of glomerular disease found on renal biopsy in the elderly. Therefore, performing a serological ANCA screen (including MPO and PR3) in elderly patients with evidence of glomerular disease is important, especially in the setting of rapidly deteriorating function. Elderly patients with nephrotic syndrome are frequently found to have membranous glomerulonephritis and amyloidosis, with primary light chain amyloidosis the most common form of amyloid described. Therefore, testing for anti-phospholipase 2 receptor antibody (anti-PLA2R), screening serum and urine with protein electrophoresis and immunofixation together with serum for free light chains should be considered for all elderly patients with nephrotic syndrome. Other serological tests may also be justified when assessing elderly patients with evidence of glomerular disease and include serum complement, anti-GBM, ANA, dsDNA, cryoglobulins, rheumatoid factor and virology screens. Appropriate additional screening will depend upon the clinical presentation. Although a positive serological test will be supportive of a diagnosis in most cases, a renal biopsy remains necessary for confirmation and to guide appropriate treatment. Figure 7.1 summarises an approach to diagnosing glomerular disease in elderly patients.

Frequency of Presentation and Histological Findings in Renal Biopsies in the Elderly

A list of publications over the last 15 years which have analysed the indications and histological findings in renal biopsies performed in patients over the age of 65 is summarised in Table 7.1. Acute kidney injury and nephrotic syndrome are the most commonly reported indications for biopsies in this age group. Nephrotic syndrome is the reported clinical presentation in approximately 1/3 of cases described in each biopsy series. The definition of AKI varies between series but often includes the clinical picture of a rapidly progressive glomerulonephritis. The most common histological diagnoses found in biopsies performed for nephrotic syndrome include membranous glomerulonephritis, amyloidosis (predominantly primary amyloid), FSGS and minimal change disease. When considering biopsies undertaken for all causes, similar diagnoses are seen, however there is a predominance of pauci-immune glomerulonephritis. In the studies comparing biopsy findings in the elderly compared with a control group, there appears to be a lower proportion of biopsies with a diagnosis of secondary glomerulonephritides such as lupus, diabetes and secondary FSGS or minor glomerular abnormalities in the elderly population [6, 9, 10, 13]. This may reflect the overall frequency in elderly patients (e.g. lupus) but may also reflect the higher threshold for performing biopsies in elderly patients.

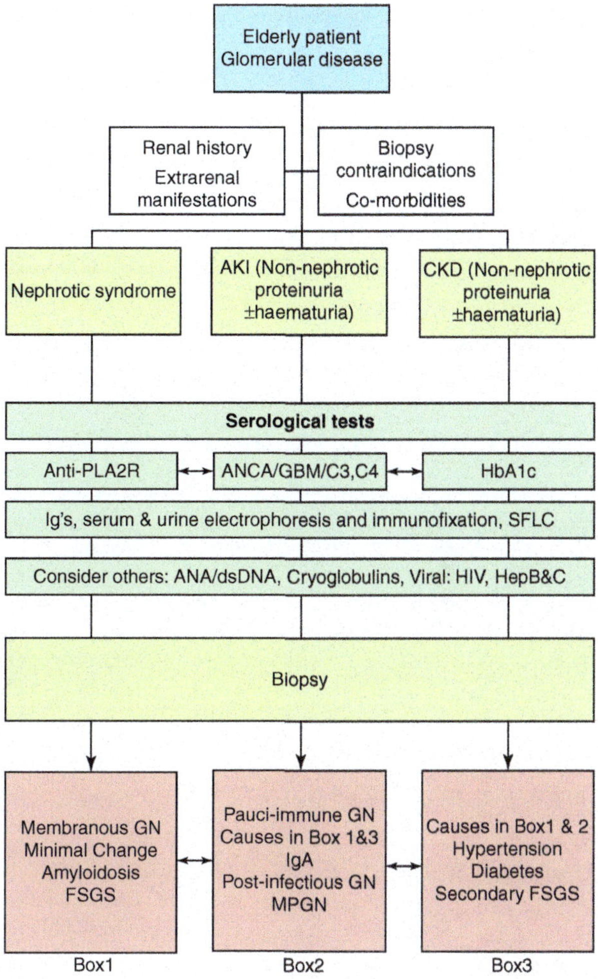

Fig. 7.1 Management of an elderly patient with suspected glomerular disease by presentation and likely diagnosis

Common Glomerular Diseases in the Elderly

Membranous Glomerulonephritis

Membranous nephropathy is one of the commonest histological findings for biopsies performed for nephrotic syndrome in the elderly, and occurs more frequently in males. Membranous nephropathy may be primary (idiopathic) or secondary, and it is important to distinguish between the two as there are implications for treatment. Differentiating between the primary and secondary forms can be aided by history and examination, serology and to a lesser degree histological features.

Histopathological features of membranous nephropathy include normal glomerular cellularity, glomerular basement membrane thickening with subepithelial

Table 7.1 Summary of the spectrum of glomerular disease from biopsy series in patients over the age of 65

Author	Country	Year	Number of biopsies (% overall series)	Age criteria	Indications for biopsy (%)	Glomerular diseases (in order of frequency)	Biopsy findings by nephrotic syndrome indication
Nair et al[a]	US	2004	100 (3.2)	>80	NS (33) AKI (23) ANS (20)	Crescentic GN FSGS MCD	Benign nephrosclerosis MCD FSGS
Nair et al[a]	US	2004	413 (4.6)	66–79	AKI (41) NS (33) ANS (12)	Crescentic GN MGN FSGS	Benign nephrosclerosis MGN DM
Verde et al	Spain	2012	71 (0.4)	>85	AKI (47) NS (32) CKD (13)	Amyloidosis Crescentic GN MGN	Amyloidosis MGN MCD
Pincon et al	France	2010	150 (–)	>70	AKI (31) NS (30) CKD (19)	Pauci-immune GN MPGN MGN	MCD MPGN MGN
Moutzouris et al	US	2009	235 (3.1)	>80	AKI (46) CKI (24) NS (13.2)	Pauci-immune GN FSGS (secondary) Hypertensive nephrosclerosis	MGN Amyloidosis MCD
Rollino et al	Italy	2014	131 (11.1)	>75	–	MGN Crescentic GN IgA	–
Yokoyama et al[a]	Japan	2012	276 (2.7)	>80	NS (50.7) CNS (17.4) AKI (22.5)	'Primary GN' except IgA Pauci-immune GN Amyloidosis	MGN MCD Amyloid
Yokoyama et al[a]	Japan	2012	2802 (27)	>65–79	NS (36.2) CNS (31.0) AKI (18.6)	MGN Pauci-immune GN IgA	MGN MCD DM
Brown et al	Ireland	2012	236 (17)	>65	AKI (31.8) NS (25) Proteinuria (7.6)	Pauci-immune GN MGN IgA	–
Perkowska-Ptasinska et al	Poland	2016	352 (13.7)	>65	Nephrotic proteinuria (55.6) Non-nephrotic proteinuria (39.6)	MGN FSGS Amyloid	MGN FSGS Amyloid

[a]Reported from same study. *NS* nephrotic syndrome, *AKI* acute kidney injury, *ANS* acute nephritic syndrome, *CNS* chronic nephritic syndrome, *CKI* chronic progressive kidney injury, *MCD* minimal change disease, *MGN* membranous glomerulonephritis, *GN* glomerulonephritis, *FSGS* focal and segmental glomerulosclerosis, *MPGN* membranoproliferative glomerulonephritis

immune complexes of IgG and complement deposition. On silver stain, the deposits may be detected by 'holes' early in the disease which may develop into 'spikes' at later stages. Granular capillary wall IgG ± C3 is visible on immunofluorescence, and extensive foot process effacement and subepithelial deposits are present on electron microscopy [22]. It has been reported that in primary membranous, IgG4 deposition dominates, whilst in secondary membranous, the other Ig subclasses are more prominent [23].

A useful marker that points to idiopathic membranous nephropathy is the presence of circulating IgG4 antibodies to the M-type phospholipase A2 receptor [24]. The anti-PLA2R antibody may be seen in up to 70% of idiopathic membranous cases, and as well as aiding diagnosis, may provide a useful tool to monitor disease activity [25]. In the elderly, secondary causes of membranous nephropathy are more common, especially malignancies [26]. One study demonstrated advancing age as an independent risk factor for cancer associated membranous nephropathy. In this cohort, 10% of 240 patients with membranous nephropathy had an underlying malignancy. There was an age-related difference, and cancer was diagnosed in one in every four patients with membranous nephropathy over the age 65 compared with 1 of every 50 patients under age 55 [27]. It is therefore important that appropriate investigations to exclude secondary malignancies are conducted. The commonest malignancies encountered with include lung and prostate. Other secondary causes of membranous though less likely include lupus, chronic hepatitis B, and drugs including non-steroidal anti-inflammatory agents.

Patients with membranous nephropathy usually present with nephrotic syndrome, and elderly patients usually have significantly worse function and co-existing hypertension compared with their younger counterparts [26]. It is unknown whether the renal outcomes in membranous nephropathy are worse in the elderly, and if the natural history differs from younger patients. It is likely that increased malignancy-associated membranous and increased chronic histological changes in this age group may impact on patient and renal survival, respectively.

In general, patients with membranous and non-nephrotic range proteinuria have a good prognosis, whilst approximately one third of patients with heavy proteinuria will progress to end stage renal disease [28]. Although some patients will also undergo an unpredictable spontaneous remission, which complicates therapeutic decisions. Nevertheless, all patients should have their symptoms of nephrotic syndrome managed supportively, particularly in view of reducing the risk of associated complications [28, 29]. Oedema should be treated with diuretics and salt-restriction. Hypertension and proteinuria should be addressed with drugs modulating the renin-angiotensin-aldosterone axis, i.e. angiotensin-converting enzyme inhibitors or angiotensin receptor blockers. Management of hyperlipidaemia with statin therapy aids cardiovascular risk reduction. Patients with membranous who have a low serum albumin (<25 g/l) are at increased risk of thrombosis, it is therefore recommended that these patients receive anti-coagulation therapy [29]. Besides supportive therapy, patients with secondary associations should have management focusing on treating the underlying cause. For elderly patients with primary membranous, it is important to risk-stratify when tailoring therapy, especially considering potential adverse effects of treatments in this co-morbid group. In the elderly, immunosuppressive therapy should be reserved for those at high risk of progression to ESRD, and balanced against overall life expectancy.

Corticosteroids have shown no benefit above supportive therapy in the treatment of membranous nephropathy. It is therefore recommended that in selected cases, initial therapy with a 6-month course of an alkylating agent (cyclophosphamide) in combination with corticosteroids is used in cases where heavy proteinuria persist despite supportive therapy. Although this regimen has been shown to have superior outcomes compared with supportive treatment alone in the treatment of membranous glomerulonephritis, it is also associated with a significantly higher adverse event rate [28, 30]. Malignancy, infection and bone marrow suppression are all recognised adverse effects of this immunosuppression protocol, which may exacerbate the independent higher risk of these complications seen in elderly people. In patients who meet the criteria for treatment but in whom an alkylating agent is contraindicated or has failed to induce remission, a calcineurin inhibitor (CNI) can be used. There have been several small randomized clinical trials (RCTs) which have suggested potential efficacy of CNI therapy in treating membranous glomerulonephritis [28, 31–33]. Evidence suggests CNI therapy should be used for a minimum of 6–12 months. Relapse occurs following treatment withdrawal and maintaining patients on long term low CNI treatment may prevent relapse, but presently there is no high quality safety data on long term use for this indication [29]. Although CNI inhibitors have a favourable safety profile compared with alkylating agents in the elderly, consideration of the nephrotoxicity of CNIs are required, which may compound the nephrosclerosis seen in elderly patients. The identification of PLA2R antibodies have resulted in the use of B-cell directed agents, for example, rituximab, an anti-CD20 chimeric monoclonal antibody, emerging as alternative treatment option for idiopathic membranous nephropathy [28]. The efficacy of such agents has not been proven in a RCT setting yet and whether the safety profile of such agents may be preferential over alkylating agents or CNIs in the treatment of membranous in the elderly needs to be determined [28].

Minimal Change Disease

Minimal change disease (MCD) has been reported to account for between 10% and 25% of nephrotic syndrome in adults, and is a relatively common cause of nephrotic syndrome from biopsy series in the elderly. The majority of cases are idiopathic but MCD has also been associated with drugs, infections, cancer (particularly haematological malignancies) and an underlying history of allergy [34]. Minimal change nephropathy in the elderly is associated with a higher prevalence of renal dysfunction and hypertension [35, 36]. Concurrent AKI has been reported in about a third of MCD in the elderly usually with acute tubular injury.

Minimal change disease is characterised by the absence of glomerular lesions by light microscopy, no staining on immunofluorescence, and foot-process effacement but no electron-dense deposits on electron microscopy. When examining by light microscopy alone, it can be difficult to make the diagnosis of minimal change nephropathy in the elderly given the frequently co-existing superimposed lesions of nephrosclerosis. MCD and FSGS are both podocytopathies which have traditionally been considered as part of the same disease process. As such, FSGS should also be considered in MCD cases resistant to therapy and repeat biopsy is often indicated, particularly as the focal lesions of FSGS may have been missed with the first biopsy.

In addition to supportive care, treatment with corticosteroids is recommended for an initial episode of minimal change disease [29, 34]. Traditionally, response to steroids in adults is slower and less predictable, with estimated response rate of 75% by 3 months [35]. However, in another case series comparing older with younger Chinese patients with biopsy proven minimal change disease, steroid response was comparable, and furthermore elderly patients had fewer relapses [36]. Although, it is possible that ethnic differences may underlie steroid responsiveness in adult minimal change disease. Generally however, the older individual should not be considered resistant until after 4 months of therapy. In patients who remit, corticosteroids should be tapered slowly over a total period of 6 months after achieving remission. For patients who frequently relapse or are steroid resistant, KDIGO currently recommends treatment with either cyclophosphamide or a calcineurin inhibitor [29]. The overall renal prognosis in adult patients with minimal change disease is good. Elderly patients may be considered to have a worse prognosis, as they are more likely to present with dialysis-requiring AKI, have underlying chronic kidney disease and experience complications associated with immunotherapy. However, it is recommended that these patients still receive therapy even if on dialysis as recovery is possible.

Focal and Segmental Glomerulosclerosis

Focal and segmental glomerulosclerosis (FSGS) defines a histopathological lesion rather than a disease, and approximately 80% of cases are considered primary (idiopathic). Secondary causes include familial or genetic (e.g. podocin, nephrin mutations), viral (e.g. HIVAN, parvovirus B19), drug-induced (e.g. heroin, interferon-α) or adaptive, mediated by glomerular hypertrophy or hyperfiltration in response to states with either reduced kidney mass (renal agenesis, dysplasia, reflux nephropathy, nephrectomy) or normal kidney mass (hypertension, obesity or sickle cell anaemia).

FSGS is defined by scarring (sclerosis) in parts (segmental) of some (focal) glomeruli by light microscopy, which represent segmental obliteration of glomerular capillaries by extracellular matrix [37]. The Columbia Classification describes five variants based on light microscopy findings and include; FSGS not-otherwise-specified, perihilar, cellular, tip and collapsing disease [37, 38]. These variants represent the differing location of the glomerular lesions, degree of glomerular hypercellularity and presence of tuft collapse. Despite differences in the light microscopy findings, the electron microscopy reveals diffuse foot process effacement in all. The pathology alone in elderly patients may be difficult to separate from minimal change given co-existing global glomerulosclerosis and vascular lesions in the elderly kidney.

Elderly patients with FSGS can present with acute nephrotic syndrome, they typically have an insidious onset of nephrosis, often presenting with a degree of renal impairment and hypertension. Though secondary FSGS is common in the elderly patient with proteinuria, particularly in the Afro-Caribbean population (likely with mutations of the Apolipoprotein L1 [*APOL1*] gene), the primary lesion is uncommon in the very elderly [6, 39]. It is also thought that primary FSGS in elderly, in contrast to the young, is not driven by pre-existing gene mutations.

Untreated primary FSGS usually follows a progressive course to ESRD. Poor prognostic factors in the elderly include severe proteinuria, marked renal dysfunction at presentation, significant interstitial fibrosis on initial biopsy, collapsing variant, and initial poor response of proteinuria to therapy. Renal survival is worse in patients who do not reach remission, and FSGS has the worst renal prognosis of all the primary glomerulonephritides [38].

In the elderly it is important to distinguish between primary and secondary FSGS, as the primary lesion is often responsive to immunosuppressive therapy, whereas in secondary FSGS, treatment should be directed at the predisposing aetiology. Specific immunosuppressive treatment should be restricted to those with persistent nephrotic range proteinuria, as patients with non-nephrotic proteinuria are at low risk for progressive kidney failure and ESRD. All patients merit optimisation of blood pressure and proteinuria with renin-angiotensin system (RAS) blockade [29]. There is a paucity of data on long-term outcomes in managing elderly patients with primary FSGS. Such patients if able to tolerate are usually treated with a prolonged course of corticosteroids for at least 4 months. Corticosteroid trials can be given to those who relapse late after remission (>2 months). In cases of steroid-resistance defined by persisting nephrotic syndrome 4 months after treatment, or steroid-dependence (relapse within 2 months of steroid wean), a calcineurin inhibitor, cyclosporine or tacrolimus, can be given for approximately 12 months with or without low dose steroid [29]. In those whom CNI therapy is contraindicated, the combination of MMF and high-dose dexamethasone can be trialled. Rituximab may be considered in steroid-dependent cases, but evidence in the form of controlled trials is lacking.

Crescentic Glomerulonephritis

Three distinct mechanisms of crescentic glomerulonephritis are described, and all occur in elderly patients. The mechanisms are pauci-immune (absence of immunoglobulins), which is frequently associated with ANCA-associated vasculitis (AAV), anti-glomerular basement membrane (which has a linear deposit of IgG along the capillary walls) and immune complex (which has a granular pattern of immunoglobulins along the capillary wall).

ANCA-Associated Vasculitis

ANCA associated vasculitis (AAV) encompasses the small vessel vasculitides characterised by the presence of anti-neutrophil cytoplasmic antibodies, and include microscopic polyangiitis (MPA), granulomatosis with polyangiitis (GPA), eosinophilic granulomatosis (eGPA) and renal limited vasculitis (RLV). Both MPA and GPA are considered diseases of the elderly, with a peak age at presentation of between 65 and 75 years [40]. There is an equal gender distribution, but there does appear to be an ethnic predisposition with AAV being diagnosed more frequently in Caucasians [40].

Microscopic polyangiitis and GPA are considered systemic diseases and may present with extra-renal manifestations. Patients may present with non-specific symptoms including fever, weight loss, lethargy, arthralgia with or without renal, pulmonary, skin and neurological involvement. Granulomatosis with polyangiitis has a specific association with upper airway, ear and ophthalmic disease, with granulomas seen in effected tissue if biopsied. The renal presentation may range from mild dysfunction with blood and protein on urinalysis, to a rapidly progressive glomerulonephritis with dialysis dependence.

Serological testing in suspected cases of AAV should be performed. Proteinase 3 (PR3) and myeloperoxidase (MPO) are the target antigens in AAV, and PR3-ANCA and MPO-ANCA antibodies detected by ELISA usually correspond to the c-ANCA and p-ANCA staining patterns seen on immunofluorescence. Approximately 90% of patients with GPA and MPA are ANCA positive. In ANCA+ GPA patients, up to 90% will have PR3 antibodies, whilst in ANCA+ MPA patients nearly all patients will have MPO antibodies. For patients with RLV, up to 80% have MPO antibodies. The sensitivity and specificity of ANCA serologies in patients is dependent upon the clinical presentation [41]. For patients presenting with a rapidly progressive glomerulonephritis, the positive predictive value of ANCA was 99%, whilst for those with mild renal dysfunction with proteinuria and haematuria the positive predictive value was much lower at 66%. This information will help decide on therapeutic management for those patients who present with systemic disease who are otherwise unfit for a biopsy.

For patients in whom a renal biopsy is not contraindicated, a biopsy will confirm the diagnosis of a suspected AAV with renal involvement and will also provide prognostic information [42]. The histological features of an AAV by light microscopy show a necrotizing and crescentic glomerulonephritis. ANCA-associated vasculitides are characterised by the absence of staining for immunoglobulins or complement on immunofluorescence, or the 'pauci-immune' staining pattern. The first histopathological classification of AAV was described in 2010 by an international working group. The classification separates four categories of glomerular lesions: focal (≥50% of the glomeruli are normal), crescentic (≥50% of the glomeruli have crescents), sclerotic (≥50% of the glomeruli are globally sclerotic) and mixed (combination of features with <50% glomeruli being normal or globally sclerotic or having crescents) [42]. Patients classified in the focal group have the best renal outcome, whilst sclerotic patients have the worst renal outcomes. This is an important tool to consider when deciding on therapeutic management in elderly patients.

ANCA-associated vasculitis is associated with high morbidity and mortality, and the prognosis is even worse in elderly patients [43]. Treatment protocols usually depend on the clinical presentation and immediate risk of organ or life-threatening involvement. An exception to this is in some patients with severe RLV already requiring dialysis at the time of presentation, in whom immunotherapy is not always appropriate, a clinical scenario where access to histological findings may be helpful in guiding management. In elderly patients, further modifications to treatment approaches have been made, likely due to perceived frailty and intolerance to standard treatment regimens. However, as well as the age and degree of renal impairment at presentation, the treatment received in elderly patients with AAV, has been shown to influence overall survival [43]. Deviations from standard immunotherapy protocols in the elderly, which often involved a reduction in immunosuppression burden, have had a detrimental impact on patient survival. Therefore, it may be argued that elderly patients with organ-threatening or life-threatening involvement should be treated by standard protocols.

The mainstay of induction immunotherapy consists of oral or intravenous cyclophosphamide and glucocorticoids [40]. Rituximab has shown equivalence compared with cyclophosphamide in achieving remission in patients [40], though its efficacy compared with cyclophosphamide has not been reported in patients with severe renal impairment or pulmonary haemorrhage. Plasmapheresis is used in AAV cases which present with acutely advanced renal impairment and in cases of pulmonary haemorrhage. Approximately 60% of patients of patients with AAV will achieve remission by 3 months [44]. Once remission is achieved, maintenance immunotherapy will be required, for which azathioprine is recommended as first line [29].

Anti-Glomerular Basement Membrane Disease

Anti-glomerular basement membrane disease is a rare pulmonary-renal syndrome which may present with a rapidly progressive glomerulonephritis and pulmonary haemorrhage which without treatment, survival is unlikely [45]. It is characterised by the presence of antibodies against the $\alpha3$ chain of type IV collagen. Anti-GBM antibodies may be detected in most patients with the disease. It has a bimodal age distribution, with peak incidences in the 20–30 age group and then in patients >60 years. Up to 40% of patients with anti-GBM disease are ANCA positive and the ANCA is usually directed against MPO [45]. Double positivity has been correlated with risk of relapse, and these patients require maintenance immunotherapy, and therefore it is important to test for a co-existing ANCA. Renal biopsy shows a crescentic glomerulonephritis, with linear IgG staining of the capillary walls on immunofluorescence. Treatment involves plasmapheresis together with cyclophosphamide and glucocorticoids [29, 45]. A prolonged course of plasmapheresis is recommended, for up to 14 days or until the anti-GBM antibody is no longer detected. Treatment using this protocol has been shown to be effective at treating lung haemorrhage in most cases, whilst successful treatment of the renal inflammation depends on level of function at presentation. Given the poor outcome if left untreated, age alone should not pose a contraindication to treating anti-GBM disease.

Mesangioproliferative Glomerulonephritis Including IgA Nephropathy

Membranoproliferative glomerulonephritis (MPGN) is characterised by mesangial hypercellularity, endocapillary proliferation and thickened glomerular basement membrane on light microscopy, with immune-complex or complement deposition by immunofluorescence. As such, MPGN may be considered either an immune-complex mediated glomerulonephritis (e.g. associated with infections, autoimmune disease or monoclonal immunoglobulins) or a complement-mediated glomerulonephritis (e.g. C3 glomerulonephritis).

In elderly patients, staphylococcus-associated glomerulonephritis is more common than post-streptococcal glomerulonephritis [46]. In cases of post-streptococcal glomerulonephritis, the renal biopsy demonstrates an acute endocapillary glomerulonephritis with mesangial and capillary granular immune deposition. Although much less common in the elderly, when it does occur, post-streptococcal glomerulonephritis is not benign, with mortality as high as 20%. Unlike in the young where progression to ESRD is rare, the long-term renal prognosis in the elderly is poor, especially in patients with persistent proteinuria [47]. The elderly are particularly vulnerable in view of co-morbidity, likely pre-existing glomerulosclerosis, and age-related immune paresis. Unlike post-streptococcal glomerulonephritis, in cases of staphylococcal associated glomerulonephritis renal dysfunction occurs when the infection is active rather than following recovery [46]. Staphylococcal associated glomerulonephritis has been shown to occur more commonly in males and in those who are immunocompromised. The prognosis of staphylococcus associated glomerulonephritis is poor, with 44% of elderly patients failing to recover renal function in one series [46]. In patients with staphylococcal associated glomerulonephritis there is often IgA deposition on immunofluorescence, which if present portends to a worse prognosis [48]. The management in all cases involves treatment of the underlying infection.

IgA is the commonest primary glomerulonephritis worldwide and is frequently reported in biopsy series from elderly patients with a prevalence ranging from 5% to 10% of all diagnoses. It is more common in Caucasian and Asian ethnicities. IgA nephropathy is characterised by IgA dominant mesangial staining by immunofluorescence, with light microscopy examination commonly showing mesangial hypercellularity and increased mesangial matrix, which may be focal and segmental. Although most cases are primary IgA, mesangial IgA deposition may also be seen secondary to cirrhosis, coeliac disease, inflammatory bowel disease, dermatitis herpetiformis, seronegative arthropathies including ankylosing spondylitis and HIV infection.

The mode of presentation of IgA nephropathy in the elderly is wide ranging from isolated asymptomatic microscopic haematuria to rapidly progressive glomerulonephritis. Elderly patients with IgA nephropathy often have hypertension, AKI and nephrotic range proteinuria at the time of presentation [49]. They also tend to have a higher degree of tubulointerstitial fibrosis and vasculopathy on biopsy.

There is a graded association between rate of decline in renal function and degree of proteinuria beyond 1 g a day, with those patients with little or no proteinuria having a low risk of progression. Other factors important in determining prognosis include hypertension, GFR at presentation and histological parameters. The Oxford classification of IgA nephropathy now incorporates five features which can be utilised to predict outcomes: mesangial hypercellularity, endocapillary hypercellularity, segmental glomerulosclerosis, tubulointerstitial fibrosis and crescent formation or the MEST-C score [50]. Elderly patients with IgA nephropathy have faster progression to ESRD, with 40% reaching ESRD in one study by 10 years [49]. Higher mortality rates are also observed when compared with their younger counterparts.

No specific treatment protocols have been highlighted for the elderly population and management where appropriate should follow the published guidelines for managing IgA in the adult population. Treatment for proteinuric IgA nephropathy should begin with RAS blockade to optimise blood pressure and limit proteinuria [29]. Patients with persistent proteinuria of >1 g a day despite maximal RAS blockade for 3–6 months and relatively good function could receive a 6-month course of corticosteroids [29]. More potent combined immunosuppressive regimens incorporating cyclophosphamide or azathioprine should be reserved for those with rapidly progressive disease or histological evidence of severe active inflammation, particularly the presence of crescents.

Glomerular Disease Associated with Monoclonal Immunoglobulins Including Myeloma

Monoclonal gammopathies are characterised by the proliferation of a clone of B cells or plasma cells which synthesise monoclonal immunoglobulin or monoclonal immunoglobulin fragments. The term monoclonal gammopathy of renal significance (MGRS) differentiates monoclonal gammopathies that result in renal disease compared with the more benign monoclonal gammopathy of undetermined significance (MGUS). Patients with MGRS do not reach the criteria for myeloma, although they are at risk of progression to overt myeloma [51]. Patients with myeloma and glomerular disease, should have their myeloma managed accordingly. However, for those patients with MGRS, who do not reach the criteria for myeloma, the spectrum of renal pathology is wide, and given that the incidence of monoclonal gammopathies increase with age, any elderly patient with unexplained AKI or clinical evidence of glomerular disease should have their serum and urine screened for a MGRS with protein electrophoresis and immunofixation, and their serum tested for free light chains. Recognition of MGRS is important as it will influence therapeutic management and subsequent renal prognosis [52].

Light chain cast nephropathy (LCCN) is the most frequent complication of multiple myeloma, and LCCN may be diagnosed by the clinical presentation of AKI, high serum free light chains (SFLC) and light chains in the urine. That said, the heterogeneity of renal lesions and glomerular pathology seen with MGRS means a renal biopsy is often necessary to determine the nature of renal injury, which may in turn help to guide treatment [52]. The exception to this is in the case of light chain amyloidosis where a biopsy of alternative tissue (e.g. abdominal wall fatty tissue) is sufficient to diagnose the renal lesion in the relevant clinical setting. Similar to myeloma, in patients with monoclonal gammopathy and proteinuria or nephrotic syndrome, the most frequently associated glomerular pathology is primary (AL) amyloidosis or monoclonal immunoglobulin deposition disease (MIDD) [52]. However other glomerular lesions may be seen and present with varying degrees of proteinuria, haematuria and renal dysfunction. These lesions include proliferative glomerulonephritis with monoclonal immunoglobulin deposition (PGNMID), membranoproliferative glomerulonephritis, type I cryoglobulinaemia, fibrillary glomerulonephritis, immunotactoid glomerulopathy and C3 glomerulonephritis associated with monoclonal gammopathy. The renal classification of MGRS may be categorised by their ultrastructural appearance of whether the deposits are organised or not [52]. Table 7.2 shows a summary of the spectrum of MGRS renal glomerular pathology together with clinical features. Given that the term MGRS was only coined in 2012, this is a developing field and it is likely that the clinical relevance and definitions of the renal lesions seen with MGRS will evolve considerably.

Therapeutic strategies for MGRS have been extrapolated from treatments used in overt myeloma and include proteasome inhibitors (bortezomib, carfilzomib and ixazomib), immunomodulatory agents (e.g. thalidomide and lenalidomide), alkylating agents (e.g. cyclophosphamide and melphalan) and monoclonal antibodies (e.g. daratumumab [anti-CD38]) [53]. Like in myeloma itself treatment depends in part on the age and co-morbidities of patients. Collaborative trials will be required to determine the optimal therapeutic combinations for specific renal pathologies associated with MGRS, especially in elderly patients over the years to come.

Treatment Considerations in the Elderly

Treatment of elderly patients with glomerulopathies needs co-ordination and collaboration between geriatricians, family practitioners and nephrologists. There are nuances to the older patient that should affect prescribing practices. A lot of morbidity in this cohort can be as much attributable to drug effects than the primary pathology. Consideration must be given to frailty, poly-pharmacy, and the alterations in drug pharmacodynamics and pharmacokinetics with ageing that can affect the distribution, metabolism, and excretion of drugs. The relative proportion of fat increases with age, and overall, there is reduction in lean body mass as well as diminished renal and hepatic clearance. Reduced renal clearance is particularly important in clearance of water-soluble drugs. There is also diminished tolerance and increased sensitivity to some of the adverse effects associated with medicines.

Table 7.2 Distribution of MGRS associated glomerular disease

Deposits		Glomerular disease	Renal presentation	Extra-renal involvement	Laboratory testing (where reported)
Organised	Fibrils	Amyloidosis	Proteinuria, NS CKD	Yes (heart, liver, nerves)	λ LC most common Serum EP ≤80% (AL) Urine EP ≤67% (AL) SFLC ≤88% (AL)
		Fibrillary GN	Proteinuria, NS Haematuria CKD	No	Serum EP ~17% Urine EP ~17% SFLC (K> λ)
	Microtubules	Immunotactoid GN	Proteinuria, NS Haematuria CKD	Uncommon	Low complement ~30% Serum EP ≤67% Urine EP ≤53% SFLC ~20%
		Type I Cryoglobulinaemia	Proteinuria, NS Haematuria CKD/AKI	Yes (skin, joints, nerves)	Low complement Serum EP: 76%
Non-organised		Monoclonal Ig deposition disease	Proteinuria, NS Haematuria CKD	Yes (heart, liver, lung)	K LC most common Serum EP (HC>LC) Urine EP (HC>LC) SFLC: 100%
		Proliferative GN with monoclonal Ig deposits	Proteinuria, NS Haematuria CKD	No	Low complement ~30% Serum EP 30% Urine EP 30%
		Monoclonal Ig C3 GN	Proteinuria, NS Haematuria CKD	No	Low C3 common Serum/urine EP 100%

Adapted from Bridoux et al.

Once the primary glomerular disorder has been defined, this should guide therapy. As in younger adults, symptoms and complications of CKD should be managed, and there is convincing evidence in support of use of common drugs like ACE-inhibitors and statins in older people [54, 55]. There is no clear consensus in this age group however, on appropriate treatment targets. Due to lack of outcomes data in patients aged greater than 70 with GFR <60 ml/min, there is no recommendation on target BP range [29]. There is also a paucity of controlled trials including older patients with CKD taking several key drugs together. It is known that older patients have an increased sensitivity to diuretics and may develop pre-renal uraemia, particularly with concurrent RAS blockade.

As well as pharmacotherapy for risk factor modification, immunosuppressive therapies in the elderly confers additional hazard. For instance, ANCA-associated vasculitis is one such example of a common glomerulopathy in the elderly with high death rate in the 1st year, particularly in the first 3 months, with majority of patients dying from complications of therapy, especially infection, as opposed to underlying pathology. However, this needs to be balanced against the inferior outcomes associated with modifying standard treatment protocols [43]. High-dose corticosteroids are poorly tolerated with complications of infection, diabetes, hypertension, sleep disturbance, easy bruising and myalgia common in the elderly. Recent growing evidence for equivalent outcomes with low-dose or no steroid-regimens in glomerular disease exists, and steroid-minimisation may be particularly of value in this age group. Rituximab may prove to be an optimal immune therapy for elderly patients [56].

Careful attention should be paid to tailoring the prescription to the older individual, particularly given the marked heterogeneity among elderly individuals. Even when the risk of progression to ESRD is less a concern given short life expectancy, aiming to preserve residual renal function can alleviate and facilitate management of complications of other health-related issues in the elderly. Some misconceptions about age may result in optimal therapies being unnecessarily withheld from older patients. Overall, the evidence base supports the notion that carefully selected elderly patients can benefit from immunosuppressive therapy in glomerular disease, accepting a higher risk of adverse effects. Meticulous attention to monitoring, prophylaxis, and dose adjustment for age and GFR can negate some of this extra risk.

Conclusion

The wide spectrum of glomerular disease occurring in the elderly is becoming more evident with the increased inclusivity of older patients in published renal biopsy series. Importantly, age itself should not pose a contraindication to pursuing renal tissue in elderly patients with suspected glomerular disease. Specific diagnoses are more common in the elderly and include pauci-immune glomerulonephritis and AL amyloidosis. In some cases, serological investigations may help in determining the diagnosis, but histology may provide additional prognostic information which may inform appropriateness of treatment, especially when immunotherapy is required. Careful consideration must be given in treating glomerular disease in older patients as they are a co-morbid group where evidence to guide optimal management is lacking.

References

1. Rule AD, Amer H, Cornell LD, Taler SJ, Cosio FG, Kremers WK, et al. The association between age and nephrosclerosis on renal biopsy among healthy adults. Ann Intern Med. 2010;152(9):561–7.
2. Glassock RJ, Rule AD. The implications of anatomical and functional changes of the aging kidney: with an emphasis on the glomeruli. Kidney Int. 2012;82(3):270–7.
3. Lindeman RD, Tobin J, Shock NW. Longitudinal studies on the rate of decline in renal function with age. J Am Geriatr Soc. 1985;33(4):278–85.
4. Hogan JJ, Mocanu M, Berns JS. The native kidney biopsy: update and evidence for best practice. Clin J Am Soc Nephrol. 2016;11(2):354–62.
5. Zhu P, Zhou FD, Zhao MH. The renal histopathology spectrum of elderly patients with kidney diseases: a study of 430 patients in a single Chinese center. Medicine (Baltimore). 2014;93(28):e226.
6. Yokoyama H, Sugiyama H, Sato H, Taguchi T, Nagata M, Matsuo S, et al. Renal disease in the elderly and the very elderly Japanese: analysis of the Japan Renal Biopsy Registry (J-RBR). Clin Exp Nephrol. 2012;16(6):903–20.
7. Verde E, Quiroga B, Rivera F, Lopez-Gomez JM. Renal biopsy in very elderly patients: data from the Spanish registry of glomerulonephritis. Am J Nephrol. 2012;35(3):230–7.
8. Rollino C, Ferro M, Beltrame G, Quattrocchio G, Massara C, Quarello F, et al. Renal biopsy in patients over 75: 131 cases. Clin Nephrol. 2014;82(4):225–30.
9. Nair R, Bell JM, Walker PD. Renal biopsy in patients aged 80 years and older. Am J Kidney Dis. 2004;44(4):618–26.
10. Moutzouris DA, Herlitz L, Appel GB, Markowitz GS, Freudenthal B, Radhakrishnan J, et al. Renal biopsy in the very elderly. Clin J Am Soc Nephrol. 2009;4(6):1073–82.
11. Harmankaya O, Okuturlar Y, Kocoglu H, Kaptanogullari H, Yucel SK, Ozkan H, et al. Renal biopsy in the elderly: a single-center experience. Int Urol Nephrol. 2015;47(8):1397–401.
12. Haas M, Spargo BH, Wit E-JC, Meehan SM. Etiologies and outcome of acute renal insufficiency in older adults: a renal biopsy study of 259 cases. Am J Kidney Dis. 2000;35(3):433–47.
13. Brown CM, Scheven L, O'Kelly P, Dorman AM, Walshe JJ. Renal histology in the elderly: indications and outcomes. J Nephrol. 2012;25(2):240–4.
14. Perkowska-Ptasinska A, Deborska-Materkowska D, Bartczak A, Stompor T, Liberek T, Bullo-Piontecka B, et al. Kidney disease in the elderly: biopsy based data from 14 renal centers in Poland. BMC Nephrol. 2016;17(1):194.
15. Liangos O, Wald R, O'Bell JW, Price L, Pereira BJ, Jaber BL. Epidemiology and outcomes of acute renal failure in hospitalized patients: a national survey. Clin J Am Soc Nephrol. 2006;1(1):43–51.
16. Liano F, Pascual J. Epidemiology of acute renal failure: a prospective, multicenter, community-based study. Madrid Acute Renal Failure Study Group. Kidney Int. 1996;50(3):811–8.
17. Death NCEiPOa. NCEPOD acute kidney injury: adding insult to injury report. 2009. Available from: http://www.ncepod.org.uk/2009.
18. Carter CE, Gansevoort RT, Scheven L, Heerspink HJ, Shlipak MG, de Jong PE, et al. Influence of urine creatinine on the relationship between the albumin-to-creatinine ratio and cardiovascular events. Clin J Am Soc Nephrol. 2012;7(4):595–603.
19. Fotheringham J, Campbell MJ, Fogarty DG, El Nahas M, Ellam T. Estimated albumin excretion rate versus urine albumin-creatinine ratio for the estimation of measured albumin excretion rate: derivation and validation of an estimated albumin excretion rate equation. Am J Kidney Dis. 2014;63(3):405–14.
20. Sharma SG, Bomback AS, Radhakrishnan J, Herlitz LC, Stokes MB, Markowitz GS, et al. The modern spectrum of renal biopsy findings in patients with diabetes. Clin J Am Soc Nephrol. 2013;8(10):1718–24.
21. Dhaun N, Bellamy CO, Cattran DC, Kluth DC. Utility of renal biopsy in the clinical management of renal disease. Kidney Int. 2014;85(5):1039–48.

22. Fogo AB, Lusco MA, Najafian B, Alpers CE. AJKD atlas of renal pathology: membranous nephropathy. Am J Kidney Dis. 2015;66(3):e15–7.
23. Ohtani H, Wakui H, Komatsuda A, Okuyama S, Masai R, Maki N, et al. Distribution of glomerular IgG subclass deposits in malignancy-associated membranous nephropathy. Nephrol Dial Transplant Off Publ Eur Dial Transpl Assoc – Eur Ren Assoc. 2004;19(3):574–9.
24. Beck LH Jr, Bonegio RG, Lambeau G, Beck DM, Powell DW, Cummins TD, et al. M-type phospholipase A2 receptor as target antigen in idiopathic membranous nephropathy. N Engl J Med. 2009;361(1):11–21.
25. Hofstra JM, Beck LH Jr, Beck DM, Wetzels JF, Salant DJ. Anti-phospholipase A(2) receptor antibodies correlate with clinical status in idiopathic membranous nephropathy. Clin J Am Soc Nephrol. 2011;6(6):1286–91.
26. Deegens JK, Wetzels JF. Membranous nephropathy in the older adult: epidemiology, diagnosis and management. Drugs Aging. 2007;24(9):717–32.
27. Lefaucheur C, Stengel B, Nochy D, Martel P, Hill GS, Jacquot C, et al. Membranous nephropathy and cancer: epidemiologic evidence and determinants of high-risk cancer association. Kidney Int. 2006;70(8):1510–7.
28. Ruggenenti P, Fervenza FC, Remuzzi G. Treatment of membranous nephropathy: time for a paradigm shift. Nat Rev Nephrol. 2017;13(9):563–79.
29. KDIGO. KDIGO clinical practice guidelines for glomerulonephritis. Kidney Int. 2012; Suppl 2.
30. Perna A, Schieppati A, Zamora J, Giuliano GA, Braun N, Remuzzi G. Immunosuppressive treatment for idiopathic membranous nephropathy: a systematic review. Am J Kidney Dis. 2004;44(3):385–401.
31. Praga M, Barrio V, Juarez GF, Luno J, Grupo Espanol de Estudio de la Nefropatia M. Tacrolimus monotherapy in membranous nephropathy: a randomized controlled trial. Kidney Int. 2007;71(9):924–30.
32. Chen M, Li H, Li XY, Lu FM, Ni ZH, Xu FF, et al. Tacrolimus combined with corticosteroids in treatment of nephrotic idiopathic membranous nephropathy: a multicenter randomized controlled trial. Am J Med Sci. 2010;339(3):233–8.
33. Cattran DC, Greenwood C, Ritchie S, Bernstein K, Churchill DN, Clark WF, et al. A controlled trial of cyclosporine in patients with progressive membranous nephropathy. Canadian Glomerulonephritis Study Group. Kidney Int. 1995;47(4):1130–5.
34. Vivarelli M, Massella L, Ruggiero B, Emma F. Minimal change disease. Clin J Am Soc Nephrol. 2017;12(2):332–45.
35. Waldman M, Crew RJ, Valeri A, Busch J, Stokes B, Markowitz G, et al. Adult minimal-change disease: clinical characteristics, treatment, and outcomes. Clin J Am Soc Nephrol. 2007;2(3):445–53.
36. Tse KC, Lam MF, Yip PS, Li FK, Choy BY, Lai KN, et al. Idiopathic minimal change nephrotic syndrome in older adults: steroid responsiveness and pattern of relapses. Nephrol Dial Transpl Off Publ Eur Dial Transpl Assoc – Eur Ren Assoc. 2003;18(7):1316–20.
37. D'Agati VD, Kaskel FJ, Falk RJ. Focal segmental glomerulosclerosis. N Engl J Med. 2011;365(25):2398–411.
38. Rosenberg AZ, Kopp JB. Focal segmental glomerulosclerosis. Clin J Am Soc Nephrol. 2017;12(3):502–17.
39. Genovese G, Friedman DJ, Ross MD, Lecordier L, Uzureau P, Freedman BI, et al. Association of trypanolytic ApoL1 variants with kidney disease in African Americans. Science. 2010;329(5993):841–5.
40. Shi L. Anti-neutrophil cytoplasmic antibody-associated vasculitis: prevalence, treatment, and outcomes. Rheumatol Int. 2017;37(11):1779–88.
41. Jennette JC, Wilkman AS, Falk RJ. Diagnostic predictive value of ANCA serology. Kidney Int. 1998;53(3):796–8.
42. Berden AE, Ferrario F, Hagen EC, Jayne DR, Jennette JC, Joh K, et al. Histopathologic classification of ANCA-associated glomerulonephritis. J Am Soc Nephrol. 2010;21(10):1628–36.

43. Tanna A, Guarino L, Tam FW, Rodriquez-Cubillo B, Levy JB, Cairns TD, et al. Long-term outcome of anti-neutrophil cytoplasm antibody-associated glomerulonephritis: evaluation of the international histological classification and other prognostic factors. Nephrol Dial Transpl Off Publ Eur Dial Transpl Assoc – Eur Ren Assoc. 2015;30(7):1185–92.
44. Nachman PH, Hogan SL, Jennette JC, Falk RJ. Treatment response and relapse in antineutrophil cytoplasmic autoantibody-associated microscopic polyangiitis and glomerulonephritis. J Am Soc Nephrol. 1996;7(1):33–9.
45. McAdoo SP, Pusey CD. Anti-glomerular basement membrane disease. Clin J Am Soc Nephrol. 2017;12(7):1162–72.
46. Nasr SH, Fidler ME, Valeri AM, Cornell LD, Sethi S, Zoller A, et al. Postinfectious glomerulonephritis in the elderly. J Am Soc Nephrol. 2011;22(1):187–95.
47. Rodriguez-Iturbe B, Musser JM. The current state of poststreptococcal glomerulonephritis. J Am Soc Nephrol. 2008;19(10):1855–64.
48. Nasr SH, D'Agati VD. IgA-dominant postinfectious glomerulonephritis: a new twist on an old disease. Nephron Clin Pract. 2011;119(1):c18–25. discussion c6
49. Oshima Y, Moriyama T, Itabashi M, Takei T, Nitta K. Characteristics of IgA nephropathy in advanced-age patients. Int Urol Nephrol. 2015;47(1):137–45.
50. Trimarchi H, Barratt J, Cattran DC, Cook HT, Coppo R, Haas M, et al. Oxford classification of IgA nephropathy 2016: an update from the IgA Nephropathy Classification Working Group. Kidney Int. 2017;91(5):1014–21.
51. Steiner N, Gobel G, Suchecki P, Prokop W, Neuwirt H, Gunsilius E. Monoclonal gammopathy of renal significance (MGRS) increases the risk for progression to multiple myeloma: an observational study of 2935 MGUS patients. Oncotarget. 2018;9(2):2344–56.
52. Bridoux F, Leung N, Hutchison CA, Touchard G, Sethi S, Fermand JP, et al. Diagnosis of monoclonal gammopathy of renal significance. Kidney Int. 2015;87(4):698–711.
53. Kumar SK, Rajkumar V, Kyle RA, van Duin M, Sonneveld P, Mateos MV, et al. Multiple myeloma. Nat Rev Dis Primers. 2017;3:17046.
54. Mangoni AA, Jackson SH. The implications of a growing evidence base for drug use in elderly patients. Part 1. Statins for primary and secondary cardiovascular prevention. Br J Clin Pharmacol. 2006;61(5):494–501.
55. Mangoni AA, Jackson SH. The implications of a growing evidence base for drug use in elderly patients part 2. ACE inhibitors and angiotensin receptor blockers in heart failure and high cardiovascular risk patients. Br J Clin Pharmacol. 2006;61(5):502–12.
56. Timlin H, Lee SM, Manno RL, Seo P, Geetha D. Rituximab for remission induction in elderly patients with ANCA-associated vasculitis. Semin Arthritis Rheum. 2015;45(1):67–9.

Acute Kidney Injury in the Elderly

8

Myrto Giannopoulou, Stefanos Roumeliotis, Theodoros Eleftheriadis, and Vassilios Liakopoulos

Introduction

The elderly represent the fastest growing subgroup of the general population in the developed countries. It is projected that in the United States and Western Europe alone there will be an increase in individuals older than 60 years from 231 million in 2000 to approximately 400 million by 2050 [1]. Therefore, it is important to understand the impact of the aging process on normal physiology, the risk factors and etiology of AKI in this frail group of patients as well as the accompanying clinical consequences that these physiologic alterations can have.

Histologic and Physiology Alterations in Elderly Individuals (Table 8.1)

The histological alterations that occur in the aging kidney, start after the third decade of life and lead to intimal thickening of both the afferent and efferent renal arterioles [2]. This leads to renovascular dysautonomy resulting to impaired ability to maintain renal function in both hypotensive (due to hypovolemia, changes in cardiac output or medication effects, i.e., nonsteroidal anti-inflammatory drugs) and hypertensive states. The aging kidney has a decreased production of vasodilatory prostaglandins, leading to an altered balance in arteriolar tone regulation [3, 4]. Inflammatory cell accumulation and fibroblast deposition in the interstitial matrix result to interstitial fibrosis [5, 6]. Glomerular tissue is slowly replaced by fibrous tissue over time [7], ending up in glomerulosclerosis which is manifested by an average loss of approximately 4500 nephrons per kidney per year during the aging

M. Giannopoulou · S. Roumeliotis · T. Eleftheriadis · V. Liakopoulos (✉)
Division of Nephrology and Hypertension, 1st Department of Internal Medicine, AHEPA Hospital, Medical School, Aristotle University of Thessaloniki, Thessaloniki, Greece
e-mail: liakopul@otenet.gr

C. G. Musso et al. (eds.), *Clinical Nephrogeriatrics*,
https://doi.org/10.1007/978-3-030-18711-8_8

Table 8.1 Histologic and physiologic alterations in elderly individuals

Intimal thickening of both the afferent and efferent renal arterioles
Renovascular dysautonomy
Decreased production of vasodilatory prostaglandins
Increased glomerulosclerosis
Decreased tubular number and length
Renal medullary hypotonicity
Sodium and water wasting secondary to a reduced tubular reabsorption

process and a yearly average decrease in glomerular filtration rate (GFR) of 0.8–1.0 mL/min/1.73m^2 [8]. Nephrosclerosis has been found to progressively increase with age, reaching 58% for 60 to 69-year-olds and 73% for 70 to 77-year-olds [9], whereas renal mass reaches approximately 75–80% of young adulthood weight by the age of 80–90 years [10].

The renal tubules are also affected by aging, with decreased tubular number and length leading to increased tubular frailty especially in nephrotoxic or hypoxic conditions [11, 12]. Renal medullary hypotonicity resulting in subsequent decreased response to antidiuretic hormone and reduction in water reabsorption, causes a reduced capacity to maximally concentrate urine and predisposes elderly patients to dehydration [13, 14]. Furthermore, in elderly patients, a decrease in thirst regulation in combination to the aforementioned blunted response of arginine vasopressin release in hypovolemic states, result in more pronounced alterations in water equilibrium. Sodium reabsorption by the thick ascending loop of Henle is also affected in the aging kidney and is believed to be secondary to a decreased availability of functional sodium-potassium-chloride transporters [15]. As a result, hyponatremia secondary to senile sodium leakage and water disequilibrium is common in geriatric patients. In summary, the most important of renal changes that make old people prone to AKI are (1) disturbance in the autoregulatory vascular defense, (2) reduction in the number of glomeruli and glomerular capillaries, and (3) renal tubular frailty and salt and water wasting secondary to a reduced tubular reabsorption capability.

Epidemiology of AKI in the Elderly

Significant proportions of the population both in USA and Western Europe are older than 65 years of age (approximately 17.5% in Italy, 16% in the UK, 16% in Spain, and 12.5% in USA) [16]. In China, patients aged 80 years or older are the age group of population in which the incidence of AKI has been reported to increase most rapidly [17]. The relative risk of AKI in the elderly has been reported to be increased from a 3.5- to 10-fold compared to younger individuals. The incidence of AKI in elderly hospitalized patients in the United States was 3.1% in 2000 [18], whereas in another study AKI has been estimated to occur in 2–7% of all hospital admissions and at even higher rates in elderly patients [13]. Groenveld et al. showed that the age-related yearly incidence of AKI rose from 17 per million in adults under the age of 50 years to 949 per million in the 80–89 years age group [19]. A systematic review and meta-analysis of recovery of kidney function after AKI in the elderly has shown that recovery after AKI is approximately 28% less likely to occur in patients older than 65 years [20]. Long-term recovery is also less likely and it is believed that AKI in the elderly results more often in CKD [20]. Acute kidney injury has consistently been associated with increased morbidity and mortality [18], and multiple studies have demonstrated worse outcomes in the elderly [20].

Risk Factors for Acute Kidney Injury in the Elderly

Several risk factors have been associated with AKI in the elderly population and can be broadly divided into three categories: presence of comorbidities, for instance, diabetes mellitus (DM), chronic kidney disease (CKD), congestive heart failure, and atherosclerosis; use of nephrotoxic medications, aminoglycosides, angiotensin-converting enzyme inhibitors (ACEI), nonsteroidal anti-inflammatory drugs (NSAIDs), vancomycin, amphotericin B, cyclosporine, tacrolimus, etc; and genetic profile. Preexisting DM, hypertension, and proteinuria have been determined to be independent risk factors for developing AKI during hospitalization in elderly patients [21]. There is a correlation between increasing severity of preoperative proteinuria and development of AKI as well as with the need for renal replacement therapy (RRT) in patients undergoing coronary artery bypass grafting surgery [22]. Elderly patients with an eGFR between 45 and 59 mL/min/1.73 m^2 have approximately two times the risk of AKI compared with matched cohorts with an eGFR of 60 mL/min/1.73 m^2 or greater. In patients with baseline eGFR less than 60 mL/min/1.73 m^2, the presence of DM further augments the risk for AKI [23]. Elderly patients taking ACEI, angiotensin receptor blockers (ARB), or NSAIDs before their hospitalization also seem to be at an increased risk of developing AKI, secondary to the effects that those medications have on the autoregulatory ability of the aging kidney in times of stress and hemodynamic changes. Furthermore, decreased body mass, altered medication clearance, and the long half-lives of certain medications (such as NSAIDs) have a detrimental effect and augment the risk for AKI. Within the intensive care unit (ICU), the most frequent specific adverse drug reaction in the elderly is drug-induced AKI; common offending agents include aminoglycosides, ACE inhibitors, NSAIDs, vancomycin, amphotericin B, cyclosporine, and tacrolimus [24]. Recent research has suggested that a variety of genetic factors are involved in mechanisms affecting the development and recovery from AKI, including the expression of specific microRNA, degree of telomere shortening, heme-oxygenase modulated autophagy, and chordin 1–regulated expression of bone morphogenic protein 7 in restoring tubular epithelium after injury [9]. Other age-related factors, such as the telomere shortening [25], the relationship between autophagy and heme-oxygenase-1 [26] and Klotho deficiency [27], are thought to be involved in mechanisms predisposing to AKI or its recovery [28]. Prediction models for postoperative AKI and RRT, based on the clinical risk factors, have been suggested and externally validated [29].

Causes of AKI in the Elderly

Approximately 35% of AKI cases have prerenal causes, 40% have intrarenal (intrinsic) causes, and 25% are secondary to postrenal (obstructive) causes [29]. Alterations in renal structure and physiology with aging lead to some potential differences in the distribution of frequency of etiologies of AKI in this population, when compared to general population.

Prerenal

As in the general population, prerenal AKI is most commonly a result of volume depletion, which can be secondary to gastrointestinal losses, renal losses, or intravascular losses. Elderly patients are particularly prone to the development of dehydration during times of physiologic stress and have a decreased adaptive ability to maintain renal blood flow and GFR. Diuretic use exacerbates the underlying predisposition to volume depletion and may contribute in up to 25–40% of cases of prerenal AKI in elderly patients [30]. The use of NSAIDs by approximately 10–25% of the elderly [31], has been associated with an absolute risk of prerenal AKI of 13% in a nursing home cohort [32]. Factors like prolonged NSAID half-life, decreased body mass and the age-related physiologic changes make this age group more susceptible to AKI, as they are more dependent on prostaglandin production to maintain afferent arteriolar vasodilation [33]. Diminished effective arterial blood volume states (i.e., congestive heart failure, nephrotic syndrome, or cirrhosis) can also lead to the development of AKI [34]. Profound hypercalcemia, often secondary to an underlying malignancy, can likewise lead to a state of volume depletion in the elderly patient. Diuretics are frequently prescribed medications in the elderly population and have been estimated to contribute to volume depletion in approximately 25–40% of the cases of prerenal AKI in elderly patients [30]. As mentioned earlier, ACE inhibitors, ARBs, and NSAIDs all can alter renal hemodynamics and lead to a prerenal state especially when combined with volume depletion, underlying chronic kidney disease, bilateral renal artery stenosis (or unilateral renal artery stenosis with a solitary kidney), CHF, and concomitant diuretic use [31].

Renal

The most prevalent form of intrinsic AKI in the elderly patient is acute tubular necrosis (ATN), which can be caused by nephrotoxic agents (drugs, i.e., aminoglycosides, amphotericin, *cis*-platinum, and heme-pigment deposition), ischemia, sepsis, and prolonged volume depletion with delayed resuscitation. Risk factors for ischemic ATN like pre-existing chronic kidney disease, diabetes, atherosclerosis, active malignancy, and low serum albumin are more prevalent among the elderly [35]. In the elderly, due to loss of lean body mass, serum creatinine can overestimate renal function, leading to inappropriate dosing of medications and other nephrotoxic agents (e.g., radiocontrast agents) [33]. Contrast-induced nephropathy (CIN) is a major cause of AKI in hospitalized elderly patients, due to a higher prevalence of chronic kidney disease [36], which is a major risk factor for CIN. Surgical interventions, with cardiac surgery and aortic aneurism repair being the most common procedures, are associated with almost one third of cases of ischemic ATN in the elderly [37]. The available data suggest that elderly patients are at an increased risk of developing CIN compared with younger patients [38]. Septic ATN results from endotoxemia-induced renal vasoconstriction and is the underlying cause of approximately one-third of cases of ATN in elderly patients. Sepsis has been linked to 30% of ATN cases in the elderly and endotoxemia-triggered renal vasoconstriction may heighten the elderly patient's susceptibility to ATN [39]. Another cause of intrinsic AKI in the elderly patient is acute interstitial nephritis (AIN), implicated in approximately 5% of cases [8]. Some common medications leading to AIN are sulfonamides, penicillin-based antibiotics, cephalosporins, proton-pump inhibitors, and NSAIDs. Due to the fact that over-the-counter medications (e.g., NSAIDS) are more frequently taken by the elderly, AIN seems to be more common in this population than young patients [40]. Furthermore, age is a well-known risk factor for the development of aminoglycoside nephrotoxicity [41]. Atheroembolic disease that leads to showering of cholesterol plaques into the microcirculation and renal occlusive inflammatory response [42], vasculitis, renal vein thrombosis and renal artery dissection are the main vascular causes that can result in intrinsic acute kidney injury in elderly patients. In several studies it has been suggested that rapidly progressive glomerulonephritis is more common in the elderly and has a poorer prognosis [43].

Postrenal

Postrenal or obstructive causes in the elderly account for 9–30% of the AKI cases [44]. Depending on whether the obstruction is proximal or distal to the bladder, obstructive causes are subdivided into upper and lower. Upper urinary tract related causes include previous radiation therapy, nephrolithiasis, and malignancy and may result in unilateral hydronephrosis, which leads to AKI only if the contralateral kidney cannot compensate, whereas lower can usually cause bilateral hydronephrosis and include prostatic hypertrophy or malignancy in men and pelvic malignancy in women. Other causes in both sexes are neurogenic causes, previous trauma with subsequent urethral stricture or blood clots causing a bladder outlet obstruction.

Diagnosis of AKI

Despite the recent advances in defining AKI with RIFLE [45] and AKIN criteria [46], they are predominantly based on changes in serum creatinine concentration, which has multiple limitations and poor accuracy to its use as a marker of kidney function, especially in the non-steady states that accompany AKI. This can explain the previous lack of consensus and the existence of more than 30 different definitions of AKI. Furthermore, it is even more difficult to use serum creatinine as a marker for GFR evaluation as its values are depended on various factors that are altered in the elderly population. Elevations in creatinine are often delayed in relation to the onset of AKI and serum creatinine levels are influenced by factors other than kidney function including muscle mass, volume of distribution, catabolic state, and medications [47, 48]. As per the KDIGO criteria, monitoring relative (and not absolute) changes in the serum creatinine level, may be a better marker of AKI in the elderly patient [49]. Recent studies have proposed novel biomarkers for the early diagnosis of AKI in critically ill elderly patients, such as urinary interleukin 18, cystatin C, and neutrophil gelatinase-associated lipocalin (NGAL) [50]. However, none of them have been adequately validated, and therefore their use in routine clinical practice cannot be recommended. The features of prerenal AKI like low urine sodium concentration (UNa <20 meq/L), low fractional excretion of sodium (FENa <1%), low fractional excretion of urea (FEUrea <35%), high urine osmolality (UOsm >500 mosm/kg), and an elevated blood urea nitrogen (BUN)/serum creatinine ratio (>20:1) can be less useful in the elderly due to age-associated defects in sodium and water conservation [51]. A kidney biopsy is a low-risk procedure that is well tolerated by patients, even among the elderly. Approximately 30% of diagnoses were altered in one case series of kidney biopsies for AKI in older adults (age >60 years) [52].

Outcome of AKI

Many studies have shown that the elderly suffer from higher AKI-associated morbidity and mortality. A meta-analysis has shown that 31% of elderly patients did not show recovery of their renal function after an episode of AKI compared with 26% of younger patients [20], whereas in another study the risk of end-stage renal disease (ESRD) was 13 times higher in hospitalized elderly patients with AKI than in elderly patients without AKI [17]. In rapid onset ESRD (SORO-ESRD) which is an accelerated progression to ESRD from a priory stable CKD after an AKI event, age appeared to be a significant contributing pathogenetic factor [53–55]. Of the 15 patients with SORO-ESRD first described in 2010, mean age was 68 years, 9 of the 15 (60%) patients were aged 65 years and older and 6 of the 15 (40%) patients were aged 80 years or older [56]. These observations suggested that this syndrome was more common in the older adult CKD patient and that such acute yet irreversible ESRD may be related to the changes that occur concurrently in the aging kidney, otherwise described as renal senescence [2, 55]. There is also an absolute 2-year mortality risk increase of 29% for elderly patients with AKI compared with their elderly counterparts without AKI [18]. In the BEST Kidney study, 5.7% of 29,269 critically ill patients had ARF during their ICU stay and the overall hospital mortality was 60.3% whereas among survivors with a median age 67 years, dialysis dependence at discharge was 13.8%.

Conclusion

Age-related changes in the kidney make the elderly more prone to develop AKI and the AKI more severe. Furthermore, age-related changes in body composition and functioning require special assessment and care in this population.

References

1. Van Den Noortgate N, Mouton V, Lamot C, et al. Outcome in a post-cardiac surgery population with acute renal failure requiring dialysis: does age make a difference? Nephrol Dial Transplant. 2003;18:732–6.
2. Musso CG, Oreopoulos DG. Aging and physiological changes of the kidneys including changes in glomerular filtration rate. Nephron Physiol. 2011;119(Suppl 1):p1–5.
3. Castellani S, Ungar A, Cantini C, et al. Excessive vasoconstriction after stress by the aging kidney: inadequate prostaglandin modulation of increased endothelin activity. J Lab Clin Med. 1998;132:186–94.
4. Crane MG, Harris JJ. Effect of aging on renin activity and aldosterone excretion. J Lab Clin Med. 1976;87:947–59.
5. Silva FG. The ageing kidney: a review I. Int Urol Nephrol. 2005;37:185–205.
6. Silva FG. The ageing kidney: a review II. Int Urol Nephrol. 2005;37:419–32.
7. Glassock RJ, Rule AD. The implications of anatomical and functional changes of the aging kidney: with an emphasis on the glomeruli. Kidney Int. 2012;82:270–7.
8. Abdel-Kader K, Palevsky PM. Acute kidney injury in the elderly. Clin Geriatr Med. 2009;25:331–58.
9. Del Giudice A, Piemontese M, Valente G, et al. Acute kidney injury in the elderly: epidemiology, risk factors and outcomes. J Nephrol Ther. 2012;2:129.
10. Lindeman RD. Overview: renal physiology and pathophysiology of aging. Am J Kidney Dis. 1990;16:275–82.
11. Musso CG, Liakopoulos V, Ioannidis I, et al. Acute renal failure in the elderly: particular characteristics. Int Urol Nephrol. 2006;38:787–93.
12. Baylis C, Corman B. The aging kidney: insights from experimental studies. J Am Soc Nephrol. 1998;9:699–709.
13. Pascual J, Liano F, Ortuno J, et al. The elderly patient with acute renal failure. J Am Soc Nephrol. 1995;6:144–53.
14. Musso C, Liakopoulos V, Pangre N, et al. Renal physiology in elderly persons with severe immobility syndrome. Int Urol Nephrol. 2009;41:437–41.
15. Musso CG. Geriatric nephrology and the 'nephrogeriatric giants'. Int Urol Nephrol. 2002;34:255–6.
16. Ali T, Khan I, Simpson W, et al. Incidence and outcomes in acute kidney injury: a comprehensive population-based study. J Am Soc Nephrol. 2007;18:1292–8.
17. Wen J, Cheng Q, Zhao J, Ma Q, Song T, et al. Hospital-acquired acute kidney injury in Chinese very elderly persons. J Nephrol. 2013;26:572–9.
18. Ishani A, Xue JL, Himmelfarb J, et al. Acute kidney injury increases risk of ESRD among elderly. J Am Soc Nephrol. 2009;20:223–8.
19. Groeneveld AB, Tran DD, van der Meulen J, et al. Acute renal failure in the intensive care unit: predisposing, complicating factors affecting outcome. Nephron. 1991;59:602–10.
20. Schmitt R, Coca S, Kanbay M, et al. Recovery of kidney function after acute kidney injury in the elderly: a systematic review and meta-analysis. Am J Kidney Dis. 2008;52:262–71.
21. Hsu CY, Ordonez JD, Chertow GM, et al. The risk of acute renal failure in patients with chronic kidney disease. Kidney Int. 2008;74:101–7.

22. Huang TM, Wu VC, Young GH, et al. National Taiwan University Hospital Study Group of Acute Renal Failure. Preoperative proteinuria predicts adverse renal outcomes after coronary artery bypass grafting. J Am Soc Nephrol. 2011;22:156–63.
23. Coca SG, Cho KC, Hsu CY. Acute kidney injury in the elderly: predisposition to chronic kidney disease and vice versa. Nephron Clin Pract. 2011;119(Suppl 1):c19–24.
24. Musso CG, Belloso WH, Scibona P, et al. Impact of renal aging on drug therapy. Postgrad Med. 2015;127:623–9.
25. Westhoff JH, Schildhorn C, Jacobi C, et al. Telomere shortening reduces regenerative capacity after acute kidney injury. J Am Soc Nephrol. 2010;21:327–36.
26. Bolisetty S, Traylor AM, Kim J, et al. Heme oxygenase-1 inhibits renal tubular macroautophagy in acute kidney injury. J Am Soc Nephrol. 2010;21:1702–12.
27. Hu MC, Kuro-o M, Moe OW. The emerging role of Klotho in clinical nephrology. Nephrol Dial Transplant. 2012;27:2650–7.
28. Anderson S, Eldadah B, Halter JB, et al. Acute kidney injury in older adults. J Am Soc Nephrol. 2011;22:28–38.
29. Coca SG. Acute kidney injury in elderly persons. Am J Kidney Dis. 2010;56:122–31.
30. van Kraaij DJ, Jansen RW, Gribnau FW, et al. Diuretic therapy in elderly heart failure patients with and without left ventricular systolic dysfunction. Drugs Aging. 2000;16:289–300.
31. Pilotto A, Franceschi M, Leandro G, et al. NSAID and aspirin use by the elderly in general practice: effect on gastrointestinal symptoms and therapies. Drugs Aging. 2003;20:701–10.
32. Gurwitz JH, Avorn J, Ross-Degnan D, et al. Nonsteroidal anti-inflammatory drug associated azotemia in the very old. JAMA. 1990;264:471–5.
33. Jerkic M, Vojvodic S, Lopez-Novoa JM. The mechanism of increased renal susceptibility to toxic substances in the elderly. Part I. The role of increased vasoconstriction. Int Urol Nephrol. 2001;32:539–47.
34. Macias-Nunez JF, Lopez-Novoa JM, Martinez-Maldonado M. Acute renal failure in the aged. Semin Nephrol. 1996;16:330–8.
35. Chawla LS, Abell L, Mazhari R, et al. Identifying critically ill patients at high risk for developing acute renal failure: a pilot study. Kidney Int. 2005;68:2274–80.
36. Mehran R, Aymong ED, Nikolsky E, et al. A simple risk score for prediction of contrast-induced nephropathy after percutaneous coronary intervention: development and initial validation. J Am Coll Cardiol. 2004;44:1393–9.
37. Rosner MH, Okusa MD. Acute kidney injury associated with cardiac surgery. Clin J Am Soc Nephrol. 2006;1:19–32.
38. Song W, Zhang T, Pu J, et al. Incidence and risk of developing contrast-induced acute kidney injury following intravascular contrast administration in elderly patients. Clin Interv Aging. 2014;9:85–93.
39. Brenner BM, Rector FC. Brenner & Rector's the kidney. 8th ed. Philadelphia: Saunders Elsevier; 2008.
40. Davison AM, Jones CH. Acute interstitial nephritis in the elderly: a report from the UK MRC Glomerulonephritis Register and a review of the literature. Nephrol Dial Transplant. 1998;13:12–6.
41. Moore RD, Smith CR, Lipsky JJ, et al. Risk factors for nephrotoxicity in patients treated with aminoglycosides. Ann Intern Med. 1984;100:352–7.
42. Scolari F, Ravani P, Pola A, et al. Predictors of renal and patient outcomes in atheroembolic renal disease: a prospective study. J Am Soc Nephrol. 2003;14:1584–90.
43. de Lind van Wijngaarden RA, Hauer HA, Wolterbeek R, et al. Clinical and histologic determinants of renal outcome in ANCA-associated vasculitis: a prospective analysis of 100 patients with severe renal involvement. J Am Soc Nephrol. 2006;17:2264–74.
44. Feest TJ, Round A, Hamad S. Incidence of severe acute renal failure in adults: results of a community-based study. BMJ. 1993;306:481–3.
45. Bellomo R, Ronco C, Kellum JA, et al. Acute renal failure – definition, outcome measures, animal models, fluid therapy and information technology needs: the Second International

Consensus Conference of the Acute Dialysis Quality Initiative (ADQI) Group. Crit Care. 2004;8:R204–12.

46. Bagshaw SM, George C, Bellomo R, ANZICS Database Management Committe. A comparison of the RIFLE and AKIN criteria for acute kidney injury in critically ill patients. Nephrol Dial Transplant. 2008;23:1569–74.
47. Perrone RD, Madias NE, Levey AS. Serum creatinine as an index of renal function: new insights into old concepts. Clin Chem. 1992;38:1933–53.
48. Cheung CM, Ponnusamy A, Anderton JG. Management of acute renal failure in the elderly patient: a clinician's guide. Drugs Aging. 2008;25:455–76.
49. Palevsky PM, Liu KD, Brophy PD, et al. KDOQI US commentary on the 2012 KDIGO clinical practice guideline for acute kidney injury. Am J Kidney Dis. 2012;61:649–72.
50. Joannidis M, Druml W, Forni LG, et al. Critical Care Nephrology Working Group of the European Society of Intensive Care Medicine. Prevention of acute kidney injury and protection of renal function in the intensive care unit. Expert opinion of the Working Group for Nephrology ESICM. Intensive Care Med. 2010;36:392–411.
51. Lash JP, Gardner C. Effects of aging and drugs on normal renal function. Coron Artery Dis. 1997;8:489–94.
52. Haas M, Spargo BH, Wit EJ, et al. Etiologies and outcome of acute renal insufficiency in older adults: a renal biopsy study of 259 cases. Am J Kidney Dis. 2000;35:433–47.
53. Onuigbo MA, Onuigbo NT. The syndrome of rapid onset end-stage renal disease – a new mayo clinic dialysis services experience, January 2010-February 2011. In: Di Iorio B, Heidland A, Onuigbo M, Ronco C, editors. Hemodialysis: how, when and why. Hauppauge: NOVA Science Publishers; 2012. p. 443–85.
54. Onuigbo MAC, Onuigbo NT, Musso CG. Syndrome of rapid onset end stage renal disease in incident Mayo Clinic chronic hemodialysis patient. Indian J Nephrol. 2014;24:75–81.
55. Musso CG, Reynaldi J, Martinez B, et al. Renal reserve in the oldest old. Int Urol Nephrol. 2011;43:253–6.
56. Uchino S, Kellum JA, Bellomo R, et al. Acute renal failure in critically ill patients: a multinational, multicenter study. JAMA. 2005;94:813–8.

Nephroprevention in the Elderly

9

Maria Mercedes Capotondo and Carlos Guido Musso

Introduction

The nephroprevention strategies are practically the same to young and old individuals except for those applied to very old (≥80 years) or frail elderly patients, where it has to be evaluated if they should be modified based on the following fundamental geriatric principles [2, 3]:

1. Individualized therapy (always an ideal objective in medicine) is crucial in the elderly, since people age at different rhythms (aging is a heterogeneous process); consequently, at the age, for instance, 80 years, they can present different clinical status, even if they suffer from the same stage of chronic kidney disease.
2. Frailty phenotype consists of the decline in multiple physiological systems and the coordination among them (reduced homeostasis), while sarcopenia consists of a generalized decline in muscle mass and strength secondary to aging. Both conditions are tightly related and they can lead old individuals to diminish their physiological reserve and to increase their vulnerability to stressors, making them prone to lose their autonomy and increase their mortality risk. The appearance of frailty and sarcopenia reduce the homeostatic capability in the elderly, causing aging to become senescence. Thus, the

M. M. Capotondo
Nephrology Division, Hospital Italiano de Buenos Aires, Buenos Aires, Argentina

C. G. Musso (✉)
Nephrology Division, Hospital Italiano de Buenos Aires, Buenos Aires, Argentina

Physiology Department, Instituto Universitario del Hospital Italiano de Buenos Aires, Buenos Aires, Argentina

Ageing Biology Unit, Hospital Italiano de Buenos Aires,
Buenos Aires, Argentina
e-mail: carlos.musso@hospitalitaliano.org.ar

C. G. Musso et al. (eds.), *Clinical Nephrogeriatrics*,
https://doi.org/10.1007/978-3-030-18711-8_9

presence of frailty phenotype and sarcopenia should be evaluated in CKD elderly patients in order to adequate the nephroprevention strategies to their status of dependency.

3. In the oldest old patients, and particularly in frail ones, quality of life is much more important than quantity of life since the time of life is already short in this group. Thus, some therapies usually prescribed for the young patients could become harmful or futile in the very old frail patients, therefore they should be avoided for this population.

Dietary Salt

The KDIGO clinical practice guidelines (2012) for managing CKD in young adults recommend the consumption of <2.3 g of sodium per day (corresponding to 5 g of sodium chloride), unless it would be contraindicated (e.g., hypotension, etc.) [4].

The Dietary Guidelines for Americans (2015–2020) also recommends consuming <2.3 g of sodium per day as a healthy diet [5].

However, since there is an increased urine sodium loss in the elderly due to their reduced sodium reabsorption capability at the thick ascending limb of the loop of Henle and collecting tubules (nephrogeriatric giants) [4], it should be taken into account that when old patients become salt restricted, they could develop hyponatremia (senile sodium leakage hyponatremia), volume depletion (ortostatism, hypotension), and/or even prerenal acute renal failure, particularly those who are very old or frail individuals. Thus, low sodium diet prescription in the very old and/or frail patients should be followed by monitoring blood pressure, serum sodium level, and renal function in order to rule out any of the abovementioned complications, and if these complications are detected, a normal salt diet (e.g., 5 g/day) instead of a low sodium diet should be prescribed [6–8].

Serum Hemoglobin (Hb) and Anemia Management

The KDIGO clinical practice guidelines (2012) for managing CKD in young adult define anemia as a hemoglobin (Hb) <13.0 g/dl in males and <12.0 g/dl in females [9, 10]. However, these guidelines recommend that nondialysis CKD young adult patients who have Hb <10.0 g/dl should have to initiate erythropoiesis-stimulating agent (ESA) therapy, since higher Hb values increase the risk of suffering from hypertension and stroke [9].

In addition, ESA therapy has to be individualized depending on the Hb fall rate, response to iron therapy, need of blood transfusion, ESA adverse effects, and presence of symptomatic anemia [10, 11].

Anemia is associated with disability, poorer physical performance, and lower muscle strength, particularly in the elderly; and treating anemia has a beneficial effect on the functional status in elderly patients [9]. Moreover, anemia can exacerbate the geriatric syndromes (delirium, gait disorders, falls, immobility, incontinence), as well as the neurocognitive dysfunction in the elderly [12–15]. Therefore, it should be taken into account that very old and/or frail elderly patients often require higher Hb target (e.g., 11.5–12 g/dL) compared to recommended Hb target in the young, in order to avoid cognitive and gait disorders [8, 14–16].

Blood Pressure (BP) Targets

The KDIGO clinical practice guidelines (2012) for managing CKD in young adult recommend that diabetic and nondiabetic patients with CKD and urinary albumin excretion <30 mg/day whose office BP is >140 mm Hg systolic or >90 mm Hg diastolic should be treated with medications that lower BP to maintain it a <140 mm Hg systolic and <90 mm Hg diastolic levels. Regarding the diabetic and nondiabetic CKD young adult patients with urine albumin excretion > 30 mg/day, and office BP systematically >130 mm Hg systolic or >80 mm Hg diastolic, these guidelines recommend treating these patients with antihypertensive drugs to maintain BP <130 mm Hg systolic and <80 mm Hg diastolic. The guidelines recommend to treat diabetic CKD patients who have microalbuminuria (urine albumin: 30–300 mg/day) and CKD patients (diabetic or not) who have macroalbuminuria (urine albumin: >300 mg/day) with angiotensin converting enzyme inhibitors (ACEI) or angiotensin II receptor antagonists (ARA) [4].

Meta-analysis of observational studies indicate that the incidence of stroke, myocardial infarction, and overall mortality increased with increasing blood pressure in old and very old patients, although the relative risk decreased with increasing age. Additionally, the INVEST study highlighted a J-shaped relationship between systolic and diastolic BP and outcomes in hypertensive old individuals suffering from coronary arterial disease [17].

In this study, the mortality risk in the oldest old patients (≥80 years) increased when systolic BP was <140 mmHg or blood pressure was <70 mmHg. Even though, it has been documented that antihypertensive treatment in the oldest old was associated with a reduction in the frequency of strokes and major cardiac events, it showed no benefit in cardiovascular nor in general mortality [18]. Furthermore, the evidence provided by several studies (INVEST, STONE, HYVET) reassures to target a relatively higher BP level in the very old patient (BP <150–80 mmHg), although these aforementioned studies did not specifically address CKD patients [17]. Nonetheless, it has been recommended that target BP in the oldest old with CKD should be <150/90 mmHg and <140/80 mmHg in non-albuminuric and albuminuric patients, respectively. It is worth mentioning that these BP targets should be reached gradually, taking into account the patient's comorbidities to avoid the interactions between these conditions and the prescribed medication. For instance, antihypertensive drugs can induce, particularly in the oldest old and frail elderly, orthostatic hypotension, falls and bone fractures, and/or higher glomerular filtration rate (GFR) decline. In this sense, a clinical entity called "normotensive acute renal failure "has been reported, which consists of an acute GFR deterioration in CKD elderly patients whose blood pressure has been reduced to "normal range" [19, 20]. This phenomenon has been attributed to reduced kidney perfusion secondary to senile renal dysautonomy (nephrogeriatric giants) [21]. Moreover, it is worth noting that concomitant sodium sensitivity and endothelial dysfunction are increased in the very elderly people; therefore, low sodium diet (used with caution) and exogenous nitric oxide donors are often useful for treating resistant hypertension in this group [22]. Other antihypertensive drugs, such as thiazides, ACEI, ARA, and aldosterone antagonists should be used with caution in this population, specially with GFR <30 mL/min/1.73 m^2 due to the possibility of inducing a further GFR reduction, precipitating an acute renal injury, and/or water, electrolytes and acid-base disorders. In this sense, even though a recent meta-analysis did not find evidence that the use of RAAS blocking agent expedited the need for renal replacement therapy in patients with CKD stages 3–5, it has been described the *syndrome of rapid onset end stage renal disease* (SORO-ESRD), unanticipated acute and irreversible end-stage renal disease, more prevalent in CKD elderly patients on potential kidney damaging agents, such as ACEIs and ARBs [8, 23–26].

KDIGO clinical practice guideline for the management of BP in CKD also recommends a healthy weight (body mass index: 20–25), a low sodium diet, an exercise program compatible with the patient's cardiovascular health and tolerance (at least 30 minutes five times per week), low alcohol intake (no more than two standard drinks per day for men and no more than one standard drink per day for women), and no smoking [26].

In addition, the European Renal Best Practice (ERBP) guidelines on management of patients suffering from diabetes mellitus and 3b or higher CKD (eGFR <45 mL/min/1.73 m^2) recommends adjusting the BP to a target <140 mmHg of systolic BP, while monitoring tolerance and avoiding side effects. This population could suffer from autonomic dysfunction and consequently they are more prone to complications associated with sudden hypotension. Moreover, if diastolic BP is too low (˂60 mmHg), it can jeopardize coronary perfusion [27].

Hemoglobin A1C

Elderly people are at high risk of developing diabetes mellitus because of the presence of insulin resistance and pancreatic islet senile dysfunction [28, 29]. Since aging alters the counter-regulatory response to hypoglycemia, hypoglycemic episodes may present practically without previous symptoms in the elderly since these symptoms are mild and appear at lower levels of glycemia. Moreover, psychomotor coordination is more affected in hypoglycemic old individuals.

The KDIGO clinical practice guidelines (2012) for managing CKD in young adults recommends hemoglobin A1c (HbA1c) target <7.0% in order to prevent or delay the progression of microvascular complications of diabetes mellitus, including diabetic nephropathy [4]. However, it has been suggested that this HbA1c target can induce hypoglycemia in individuals with limited life expectancy, such as very old and/or frail elderly patients. Therefore, therapeutic strategies with less stringent HbA1c levels are recommended in the oldest old or frail diabetic patients since this subgroup visits the hospital twice as much due to hypoglycemia episodes than the general diabetic patients, and it has also been documented that hypoglycemia is related to cognitive impairment in the elderly. Thus, the consensus recommendation is a hemoglobin HbA1c target <8% for very elderly patients or for those who suffer from major clinical complications and/or comorbid conditions. Finally, a hemoglobin HbA1c target of 8–9% has been recommended for patients with low life expectancy (≤5 years) [8]. Additionally, diabetes mellitus is usually associated with high comorbidity in old people, and this subgroup cannot obtain cardiovascular benefit from strict glycemia control. Thus, glycemic control should be part of a complex therapeutic strategy in CKD diabetic patients, which addresses the BP and cardiovascular risk control, promoting the use of ACEI, ARA, statins, and platelet antiaggregant, of course if they are indicated [2, 28, 29].

Regarding glycemic control recommendations in diabetic advanced CKD older and/or frail individuals, the European Renal Best Practice (ERBP) says that intensive glycemic control is not appropriate for many or even most of this population; and if more intensive treatment is needed, it should be implemented with a medication that has a good safety profile and lower risk of hypoglycemia [30].The HbA1C targets in diabetic stage 3b-5 CKD patients should be 8.5% in those who have high risk of hypoglycemia, decreased general life expectancy, cardiovascular disease, and/or presence of microvascular complications.

In those who do not belong to the previously mentioned group and who receive treatment with drugs of low risk of hypoglycemia, the target of HbA1C should be <6.5%. Finally, those patients who do not belong to any of the aforementioned groups, the HbA1C target depends on the diabetes duration, being <7.2% if diabetes duration <10 years or <7.9% if diabetes duration >10 years [27].

Lipid Metabolism

The major determinants of the appearance of dyslipidemia in CKD patients are glomerular filtration rate (GFR) reduction, severe proteinuria, use of immunosuppressive agents, renal replacement modality, some comorbidities (e.g., diabetes mellitus, etc.), and nutritional status. An initial lipid profile evaluation mainly serves to establish the diagnosis of severe hypercholesterolemia (LDL >190 mg/dl), and/or severe hypertriglyceridemia (TG >1000 mg/dl), and potentially rule out secondary causes of dyslipidemia [31, 32].

In nondialysis CKD adults older than 50 years with GFR >60 ml/min/1.73 m^2, the recommended treatment is statins, while if their GFR < 60 ml/min/1.73 m^2, the recommended treatment is a combination of statins or statins/ezetimibe. Regarding nondialysis CKD adult patients (aged 18–49 years), treatment with statins is recommended in those who suffer from the following conditions: coronary disease, diabetes mellitus, ischemic stroke, estimated 10-year incidence of coronary death, or nonfatal myocardial infarction >10% [32]. Prior guidelines emphasized to achieve the specific LDL cholesterol targets by increasing the statin dose and/or combined therapy progressively [1, 7]. However, this approach is no longer recommended in CKD patients because of the lack of evidence to support this approach, the substantial personal variability in measured LDL cholesterol values, and the potential hypolipemiant toxicity [7, 8].

Since high cardiovascular risk in CKD patients who have nonelevated LDL cholesterol is currently the primary indication to initiate or adjust lipid-lowering treatment, further monitoring of LDL cholesterol may not be required for many patients, since normal LDL cholesterol variability over time reduces the clinical utility of its follow-up [29].

Regarding lipid lowering therapy in this population, an interesting study in very elderly patients documented a 15% reduction in coronary events in those treated with pravastatin. This suggests that this drug can be prescribed in the oldest old suffering from diabetes mellitus except in those with very poor life expectancy [8, 33].

Protein Diet and Physical Exercise

The KDIGO clinical practice guidelines (2012) for the evaluation and management of the young adult suffering from CKD recommend to lower the protein intake to 0.8 g/kg/day in patients with or without diabetes mellitus who have GFR <30 ml/min/1.73 m^2.

They recommend avoiding high protein intake (>1.3 g/kg/day) in young adult patients at risk of CKD progression. Additionally, these guidelines recommend that individuals suffering from CKD be encouraged to undertake physical activity compatible with cardiovascular health and tolerance (aiming for at least 30 minutes five times per week), and to achieve a healthy weight (BMI: 20–25) and to avoid smoking [4].

Although energy needs decline with age, very elderly people can be exposed to malnutrition because of anorexia, impaired taste and smell, chewing and swallowing problems, geriatric syndromes, and senile prevalent comorbidities which lead to difficulties in cooking and eating. Because of the above exposed reasons, a low protein (0.8/g/kg/day) diet should be prescribed with caution in very old and/or frail elderly patients in order to avoid their malnutrition. In these cases a normal protein diet (1/g/kg/day) could be a more appropriate prescription for this population [8].

The nutritional intervention in order to improve the nutritional status in the oldest old patients consists of using smaller but more frequent and fortified portions of food and/or adding nutrition supplements between meals. Moreover, sarcopenia is a prevalent entity in the elderly which may worsen when old individuals are on a low protein diet or suffer from conditions usually associated with aging, such as diabetes mellitus, heart failure, etc. Conversely, physical activity adequate to each patient's clinical situation can further improve functional status, even in those who have poor health status [8, 16, 28, 32].

Senescent Nephropathy in Nephroprevention

Frailty is a construct originally coined by gerontologists to describe cumulative declines across multiple physiological systems that occur with aging and lead individuals to a state of diminished physiological reserve and increased vulnerability to stressors (senescence) [33, 34]. Fried et al. coined the concept of "frailty phenotype," which is based on the evaluation of five clinical domains: shrinking, weakness, poor endurance and energy, slowness, and low physical activity, aiming to identify old people who are at risk of disability, falls, institutionalization, hospitalization, and premature death [35]. Some authors consider the presence of sarcopenia as part of the "shrinking domain" of the frailty phenotype [35–39]. This phenomenon could explain why the frailty phenotype is more prevalent in women than in men in all age categories [40–43].

Sarcopenia diagnosis is based on muscle mass assessment by body imaging techniques (computed tomography or magnetic resonance imaging), bioimpedance analysis (lean body mass), and muscle strength evaluated by measuring handgrip strength (hand-held dynamometer), and clinical scores (clinical sarcopenia stages) [32]. Sarcopenia explains why when kidney function is assessed in elderly people using estimating glomerular filtrate rate equation based on serum creatinine levels (eGFR-Cr), those patients with the lowest and highest eGFR values were associated with the highest mortality. This U-shape is more prominent in octogenarians, probably because higher eGFR-Cr partly reflects those with lower muscle mass and malnutrition [44].

From this concept of the frailty phenotype, those patients with three or more of the five domains are judged to have a frail phenotype, those with one or two domains as vulnerable individuals (pre-frail), and those with no domain as fit or robust elderly people [35–38]. Besides, it should be taken into account that the frailty phenotype is often exacerbated by three additional and prevalent problems in the elderly, such as the social isolation, depression, and cognitive impairment, which usually reinforce the frailty status [16, 37]. The frailty phenotype has been documented in 7% of elderly population and 14% of nondialysis CKD elderly patients, who are at a higher risk of hospitalization and mortality [39].

The Clinical Frailty Scale is the simplest and clinically useful and validated tool for evaluating a frailty phenotype, while the diagnosis of sarcopenia is based on muscle mass assessment by body imaging techniques, bioimpedance analysis, and muscle strength evaluated with a handheld dynamometer. Frailty treatment can be based on different strategies, such as exercise, nutritional interventions, drugs, vitamins, and antioxidant agents. Additionally, ACEI may improve the structure and biochemical function of skeletal muscle, and they may halt or slow senile decline in muscle strength. These interventions may slow patient's functional decline, reducing their need for hospitalization and risk of death [41–47].

Normal aging should be distinguished from pathological aging (senescence) as they occur through different mechanisms, and the latter characteristically reduced the homeostatic capability which makes the elderly frail [48].

CKD is usually associated with several conditions such as malnutrition, chronic inflammation, increased oxidative stress, protein-energy wasting, acidemia, impaired hormonal changes, anemia, accumulation of advanced glycation end-products, insulin resistance, vessels calcification, and reduction in bone mass, altered regulation of body methionine transmethylation reactions by the kidney and low physical activity, all of which contribute to the acceleration and worsening of the aging process (senescence), and consequently to induce the frailty phenotype [48]. Additionally, sarcopenia increases progressively along with the loss of renal function in CKD patients, and this phenomenon seems to be primarily due to type II fiber atrophy influenced by altered protein turnover rates, mitochondrial depletion, and low protein diet associated to CKD [37]. Moreover, coexistence of CKD and frailty has been shown to further increase risks of falls, fractures, hospitalization, and mortality [49].

Thus, there is a deteriorating interdependence between CKD and aging where CKD makes aging accelerate and worsen (senescence), while senescence makes CKD accelerate its deterioration (senescent nephropathy), being frailty status the common path which catalyzes this spiral of damage. This particular subgroup of CKD frail elderly patients suffers from a condition which has been called *senescent nephropathy*, since it usually has different clinical complications, therapeutic needs, and worse overall prognosis compared to CKD fit elderly patients (chronic nephropathy) (Table 9.1). Consequently, CKD elderly patients should be evaluated in order to discard the presence of the frailty phenotype. If the presence of the frailty phenotype is documented, rehabilitation therapy should be added to the CKD treatment, and standard nephroprevention targets should be adequate to the senescent nephropathy condition. In this sense, a practical algorithm for achieving this purpose, which should be validated, is proposed in Fig. 9.1 [48–58].

Finally, the dialytic treatment seems to prolong longevity in elders compared to conservative treatment, but not in the sickest elderly patients. Some authors have reported a loss of independence in very old CKD who started dialysis treatment, observing that many patients deteriorate their functional state at 3 months from the beginning of dialysis with a negative impact on their daily activities. Moreover, they can become more frail and sarcopenic since they have fewer activities which are limited by the dialysis treatment (time on dialysis, post-dialysis fatigue, etc.). In these cases conservative treatment could be a better therapeutic alternative [4, 20].

Table 9.1 Differences between chronic kidney disease (CKD) in fit elderly from senescent nephropathy (SN) patients

	CKD	SN
CKD diagnosis	Positive	Positive
Frailty phenotype score	Negative	Positive
Treatment	Corresponding CKD therapy	Corresponding CKD therapy adjusted to frailty status + frail rehabilitation and home assistance
CKD follow-up	Standard control rate	Tighter
CKD prognosis	Standard	Worse

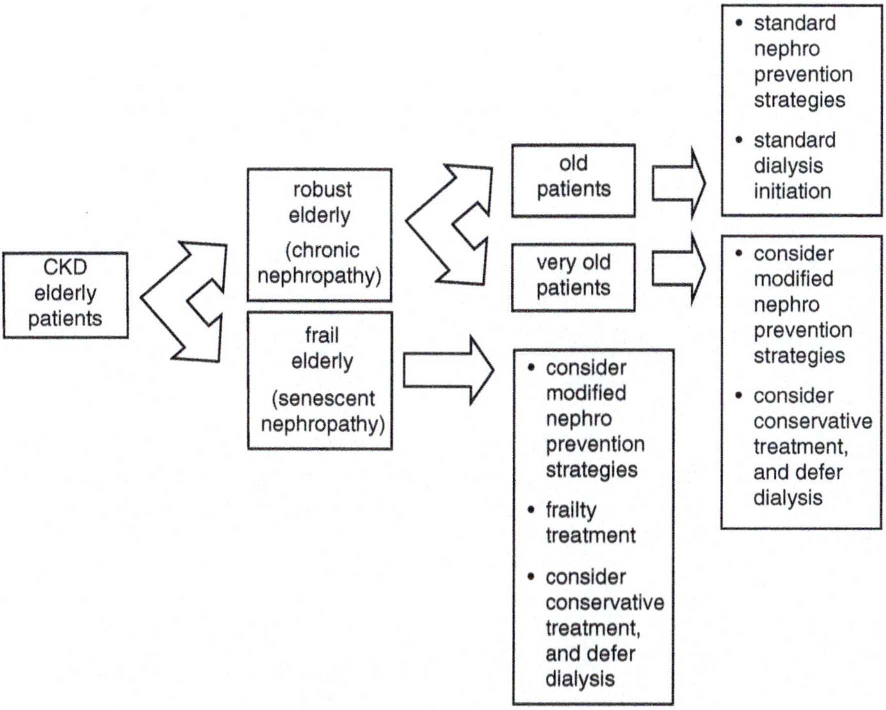

Fig. 9.1 Nephroprevention algorithm in chronic kidney disease (CKD) elderly patients

Interestingly, a study suggested an association between frailty and increased GFR at the start of dialysis, phenomenon which could be explained because the signs and symptoms of end-stage renal disease are not specific and it is possible that the presentation of frailty in these patients is assumed as a symptom of uremia and in this way leads to an earlier onset of dialysis. In addition, it is considered that GFR may be overestimated in these patients since their creatininemia is relatively lower because of their sarcopenia [18, 56–58]. Thus, in order to determine the best time to initiate dialysis, it would be important to consider factors other than the nephrological ones (GFR, electrolyte levels, etc.), and frailty status should also be included in this assessment [18].

The Guideline Development Group considers that it is important to identify those patients who would not benefit from closer nephrologic follow-up, and this evaluation can be based on the Bansal score, which is acceptable to determine the predicted mortality risk in older patients. As a consequence, the treatment for those patients who have a high predicted mortality risk should be focused on planning advanced care, while nephroprevention measures should be installed, as far as they do not interfere with their quality of life.

Since Bansal score was obtained and validated in a cohort with few frail patients, a low predicted mortality risk can be inaccurate in frail patients. Thus, in these frail patients an additional assessment of frailty should be performed, using a

Table 9.2 Differences nephroprevention targets (estimative) between chronic kidney disease (CKD) and senescent nephropathy (SN) patients

Nephroprevention treatment	CKD conventional targets	SN modified targets
Diet	Low sodium Low protein	Normal sodium Normal protein
Hemoglobin (g/dl)	11	11.5–12
Glycated hemoglobin (HbA_{1C}) (%)	<7	7.5–8.5
Blood pressure (mmHg)	≤130–80	≤140/150–80 Diastolic higher 60
Proteinuria (g/day)	<0.5	<1

well-validated tool, and if the frailty risk is high, the patient should be considered to have a high mortality risk, regardless of the Bansal score, and he/she should be managed accordingly [59].

Finally, the prescribed therapy should be individualized and based on a shared decision-making process which would be ideally initiated when the elderly patient is healthy enough to participate and share their goals and priorities (autonomy principle) [48, 53] (Table 9.2).

Conclusion

Even though, the nephroprevention strategies are similar between young adult and senior chronic kidney disease patients, standard targets should be adequate to very old and/or frail elderly individuals. Additionally, the diagnosis of senescent nephropathy in this population implies the need of prescribing anti-frailty interventions in order to slow patient's functional decline, hospitalization, and mortality.

References

1. Musso CG. Geriatric nephrology and the «nephrogeriatric giants. Int Urol Nephrol. 2002;34(2):255–6. Musso CG, Macías-Núñez J-F. Renal Handling of Water and Electrolytes in the Old and Old-Old Healthy Aged. In: Macías Núñez JF, Cameron S, Oreopoulos D, editors. Renal ageing: health and disease. New York: Springer;2008. p. 141–54. https://link.springer.com/chapter/10.1007/978-0-387-72659-5_8
2. Suzman R, Willis D, Manton K. The oldest old. Oxford: Oxford University Press; 1992.
3. Kidney Disease: Improving Global Outcomes (KDIGO) CKD Work Group. KDIGO 2012 clinical practice guideline for the evaluation and management of chronic kidney disease. Chapter 3: management of progression and complications of CKD. Kidney Int Suppl. 2013;3(1):73–90.
4. De Salvo KB, Olson R, Casavale KO. Dietary guidelines for Americans. JAMA. 2016;315(5):457–8.
5. Musso CG, Oreopoulos DG. Renal changes in the elderly. In: Katlic MR, editor. Cardiothoracic surgery in the elderly. New York: Springer; 2011. p. 293–9. https://link.springer.com/chapter/10.1007/978-1-4419-0892-6_22.
6. De Santo NG, Cirillo M. The impact of salt restriction on the effectiveness of antihypertensive therapy. In: Onuigbo M, editor. ACE Inhib Med Uses Mech Action Potential Adverse Eff Relat Top. 2013;2:135–58.

7. Musso CG, Vilas M, Onuigbo M. Nephroprevention in the oldest old with chronic kidney disease: special considerations. World J Nephrol. 2015;4(1):1–5.
8. Penninx BWJH, Pahor M, Cesari M, Corsi AM, Woodman RC, Bandinelli S, et al. Anemia is associated with disability and decreased physical performance and muscle strength in the elderly. J Am Geriatr Soc. 2004;52(5):719–24.
9. Kidney Disease: Improving Global Outcomes (KDIGO) Anemia Work Group. KDIGO Clinical Practice Guideline for Anemia in Chronic Kidney Disease. Chapter 1: Diagnosis and evaluation of anemia in CKD. Kidney Int Suppl. 2012;2(4):288–91.
10. Kidney Disease: Improving Global Outcomes (KDIGO) Anemia Work Group. KDIGO Clinical Practice Guideline for Anemia in Chronic Kidney Disease. Chapter 3: Use of ESAs and other agents to treat anemia in CKD. Kidney Int Suppl. 2012;2(4):299–310.
11. Kidney Disease: Improving Global Outcomes (KDIGO) Anemia Work Group. KDIGO clinical practice guideline for anemia in chronic kidney disease. Kidney Int, Suppl. 2012;2:279–335.
12. Lipschitz D. Medical and functional consequences of anemia in the elderly. J Am Geriatr Soc. marzo de. 2003;51(3 Suppl):S10–3.
13. Zamboni V, Cesari M, Zuccalà G, Onder G, Woodman RC, Maraldi C, Ranzini M, Volpato S, Pahor M, Bernabei R. Anemia and cognitive performance in hospitalized older patients: results from the GIFA study. Int J Geriatr Psychiatry. 2006;21(6):529–34.
14. Musso CG, Vilas M. Nephroprevention in the very elderly patient. Rev Colomb Nefrol. 2015;2(2):129–34.
15. Martin-Lester M. Cognitive function in dialysis patients. Case study of the anemic patient. ANNA J. 1997;24(3):359–65.
16. Forciea M, Lavizzo-Mourey R, Schwab E. Geriatric secrets. Philadelphia: Hanley Belfus; 2000.
17. Kidney Disease: Improving Global Outcomes (KDIGO) Blood Pressure Work Group. KDIGO Clinical Practice Guideline for the Management of Blood Pressure in Chronic Kidney Disease. Chapter 7: Blood pressure management in elderly persons with CKD ND. Kidney Int Suppl. 2012;2(5):377–81.
18. Onuigbo MAC, Onuigbo NTC. Late onset azotemia from RAAS blockade in CKD patients with normal renal arteries and no precipitating risk factors. Ren Fail. 2008;30(1):73–80.
19. Bowling CB, O'Hare AM. Managing older adults with CKD: individualized versus disease-based approaches. Am J Kidney Dis Off J Natl Kidney Found. 2012;59(2):293–302.
20. Musso GC, Alfie J. In: Onuigbo M, editor. ACEIs as Antihypertensives in the elderly (> 65 years old): a south American perspective. New York: NOVA Publishers; 2013. p. 129–34.
21. Somma C, Trillini M, Kasa M, Gentile G. Managing end-stage renal disease in the elderly: state-of-the-art, challenges and opportunities. Aging Health. 2013;9(5):539–52.
22. Musso CG, Macías-Núñez JF. Dysfunction of the thick loop of Henle and senescence: from molecular biology to clinical geriatrics. Int Urol Nephrol. marzo de. 2011;43(1):249–52.
23. Onuigbo MAC. Syndrome of rapid-onset end-stage renal disease: a new unrecognized pattern of CKD progression to ESRD. Ren Fail. 2010;32(8):954–8.
24. Nistor I, De Sutter J, Drechsler C, Goldsmith D, Soler MJ, Tomson C, Wiecek A, Donciu MD, Bolignano D, Van Biesen W, Covic A. Effect of renin–angiotensin–aldosterone system blockade in adults with diabetes mellitus and advanced chronic kidney disease not on dialysis: a systematic review and meta-analysis. Nephrol Dial Transplant. 2018.. 1;33(1):12–22.
25. Onuigbo MAC, Onuigbo NT, Musso CG. Syndrome of rapid onset end stage renal disease in incident Mayo Clinic chronic hemodialysis patient. Indian J Nephrol. 2014;24(2):75–81.
26. Onuigbo MA, Achebe NJ, Musso CG. The syndrome of rapid onset ESRD in the last 100 consecutive incident Northwestern Wisconsin Mayo Clinic chronic hemodialysis patients, 2010–2011. In: Onuigbo M, editor. ACE Inhib Med Uses Mech Action Potential Adverse Eff Relat Top. 2013;1:109–25.
27. Guideline development group, Bilo H, Coentrão L, Couchoud C, Covic A, De Sutter J, Drechsler C, Gnudi L, Goldsmith D, Heaf J. Clinical practice guideline on management of patients with diabetes and chronic kidney disease stage 3b or higher (eGFR <45 mL/min). Nephrol Dial Trans. 2015;30(suppl 2):1.. ii1–ii142

28. Kidney Disease: Improving Global Outcomes (KDIGO) Blood Pressure Work Group. KDIGO Clinical Practice Guideline for the Management of Blood Pressure in Chronic Kidney Disease. Summary of recommendation statements. Kidney Int Suppl. 2012;2(5):341–2.
29. Abaterusso C, Lupo A, Ortalda V, De Biase V, Pani A, Muggeo M, Gambaro G. Treating elderly people with diabetes and stages 3 and 4 chronic kidney disease. Clin J Am Soc Nephrol. 2008;3(4):1185–94. https://doi.org/10.2215/CJN.00410108.
30. Panduru NM, Nistor I, Groop PH, Van Biesen W, Farrington K, Covic A. Considerations on glycaemic control in older and/or frail individuals with diabetes and advanced kidney disease. Nephrol Dial Trans. 2017;32(4):1.. 591–59
31. Kirkman MS, Briscoe VJ, Clark N, Florez H, Haas LB, Halter JB, Huang ES, Korytkowski MT, Munshi MN, Odegard PS, Pratley RE, Swift CS. Diabetes in older adults. Diabetes Care. 2012;35(12):2650–64. https://doi.org/10.2337/dc12-1801.
32. Kidney Disease: Improving Global Outcomes (KDIGO) Lipid Work Group. KDIGO Clinical Practice Guideline for Lipid Management in Chronic Kidney Disease. Chapter 1: Assessment of lipid status in adults with CKD. Kidney Int Suppl. 2013;3(3):268–70.
33. Cruz-Jentoft AJ, Baeyens JP, Bauer JM, Boirie Y, Cederholm T, Landi F, Martin FC, Michel JP, Rolland Y, Schneider SM, Topinková E, Vandewoude M, Zamboni M. European working group on sarcopenia in older people. Sarcopenia: European consensus on definition and diagnosis: report of the European working group on sarcopenia in older people. Age Ageing. 2010;39(4):412–23. https://doi.org/10.1093/ageing/afq034.
34. Roshanravan B, Khatri M, Robinson-Cohen C, Levin G, Patel KV, de Boer IH, Seliger S, Ruzinski J, Himmelfarb J, Kestenbaum B. A prospective study of frailty in nephrology-referred patients with CKD. Am J Kidney Dis. 2012;60(6):912–21. https://doi.org/10.1053/j.ajkd.2012.05.017.
35. Johansen KL, Delgado C, Bao Y, Kurella Tamura M. Frailty and dialysis initiation. Semin Dial. 2013;26(6):690–6.
36. Fried LP, Tangen CM, Walston J, Newman AB, Hirsch C, Gottdiener J, Seeman T, Tracy R, Kop WJ, Burke G, McBurnie MA. Cardiovascular health study collaborative research group. Frailty in older adults: evidence for a phenotype. J Gerontol A Biol Sci Med Sci. 2001;56(3):M146–56.
37. Walker SR, Gill K, Macdonald K, Komenda P, Rigatto C, Sood MM, Bohm CJ, Storsley LJ, Tangri N. Association of frailty and physical function in patients with non-dialysis CKD: a systematic review. BMC Nephrol. 2013;14:228. https://doi.org/10.1186/1471-2369-14-228.
38. Ayaz T, Sahin SB, Sahin OZ, Bilir O, Rakıcı H. Factors affecting mortality in elderly patients hospitalized for nonmalignant reasons. J Aging Res. 2014;2014:584315. https://doi.org/10.1155/2014/584315.
39. Studenski S, Perera S, Patel K, Rosano C, Faulkner K, Inzitari M, et al. Gait speed and survival in older adults. JAMA. 2011;305(1):50–8.
40. Musso CG, Jauregui JR, Macías Núñez JF. Frailty phenotype and chronic kidney disease: a review of the literature. Int Urol Nephrol. 2015;47(11):1801–7.
41. Johansen KL, Chertow GM, Jin C, Kutner NG. Significance of frailty among dialysis patients. J Am Soc Nephrol JASN. 2007;18(11):2960–7.
42. Morley JE, Vellas B, van Kan GA, Anker SD, Bauer JM, Bernabei R, et al. Frailty consensus: a call to action. J Am Med Dir Assoc. 2013;14(6):392–7.
43. Roderick PJ. Chronic kidney disease in older people: a cause for concern? Nephrol Dial Transplant Off Publ Eur Dial Transpl Assoc – Eur Ren Assoc. 2011;26(10):3083–6.
44. Musso CG, Trigka K, Dousdampanis P, Jauregui J. Therapeutic alternatives and palliative care for advanced renal disease in the very elderly: a review of the literature. Int Urol Nephrol abril de. 2015;47(4):647–54.
45. Shastri S, Katz R, Rifkin DE, Fried LF, Odden MC, Peralta CA, Chonchol M, Siscovick D, Shlipak MG, Newman AB, Sarnak MJ. Kidney function and mortality in octogenarians: cardiovascular health study all stars. J Am Geriatr Soc. 2012;60(7):1201–7. https://doi.org/10.1111/j.1532-5415.2012.04046.x.

46. Bonanni A, Mannucci I, Verzola D, Sofia A, Saffioti S, Gianetta E, et al. Protein-energy wasting and mortality in chronic kidney disease. Int J Environ Res Public Health. 2011;8(5):1631–54.
47. Clegg A, Young J, Iliffe S, Rikkert MO, Rockwood K. Frailty in elderly people. Lancet Lond Engl. 2 de marzo de. 2013;381(9868):752–62.
48. Aiello F, Dueñas EP, Musso CG. Senescent nephropathy: the new renal syndrome. Healthcare (Basel). 2017;5(4):E81. https://doi.org/10.3390/healthcare5040081.
49. Latos DL. Chronic dialysis in patients over age 65. J Am Soc Nephrol. 1996;7(5):637–46.
50. Lindsay RM, Spanner E. Adequacy of haemodialysis in the elderly. Geriatr Nephrol Urol. 1997;7(3):147–56.
51. Kurella Tamura M, Covinsky KE, Chertow GM, Yaffe K, Landefeld CS, McCulloch CE. Functional status of elderly adults before and after initiation of dialysis. N Engl J Med. 2009;361(16):1539–47. https://doi.org/10.1056/NEJMoa0904655.
52. Arnold RM, Zeidel ML. Dialysis in frail elders – a role for palliative care. N Engl J Med. 2009;361(16):1597–8. https://doi.org/10.1056/NEJMe0907698.
53. Burns A, Davenport A. Functional status of elderly adults receiving dialysis. N Engl J Med. 2010;362(5):468; author reply 469. https://doi.org/10.1056/NEJMc0911236.
54. Farrington K, Covic A, Nistor I, Aucella F, Clyne N, De Vos L, Findlay A, Fouque D, Grodzicki T, Iyasere O, Jager KJ, Joosten H, Macias JF, Mooney A, Nagler E, Nitsch D, Taal M, Tattersall J, Stryckers M, van Asselt D, Van den Noortgate N, van der Veer S, van Biesen W. Clinical practice guideline on management of older patients with chronic kidney disease stage 3b or higher (eGFR < 45 mL/min/1.73 m^2): a summary document from the European Renal Best Practice Group. Nephrol Dial Transplant. 2017;32(1):9–16. https://doi.org/10.1093/ndt/gfw411.
55. Park JY, Yoo KD, Kim YC, Kim DK, Joo KW, Kang SW, Yang CW, Kim NH, Kim YL, Lim CS, Kim YS, Lee JP. Early dialysis initiation does not improve clinical outcomes in elderly end-stage renal disease patients: a multicenter prospective cohort study. PLoS One. 2017;12(4):e0175830. https://doi.org/10.1371/journal.pone.0175830.
56. Rosansky SJ, Schell J, Shega J, Scherer J, Jacobs L, Couchoud C, Crews D, McNabney M. Treatment decisions for older adults with advanced chronic kidney disease. BMC Nephrol. 2017;18(1):200. https://doi.org/10.1186/s12882-017-0617-3.
57. Swidler M. Dialysis decisions in the elderly patient with advanced CKD and the role of non-dialytic therapy. Am Soc Nephrol. 2009;1–8.
58. Fassett RG. Current and emerging treatment options for the elderly patient with chronic kidney disease. Clin Interv Aging. 2014;9:191–9.
59. Farrington K, Covic A, Aucella F, Clyne N, de Vos L, Findlay A, Fouque D, Grodzicki T, Iyasere O, Jager K. Clinical practice guideline on management of older patients with chronic kidney disease stage 3b or higher (eGFR <45 mL/min/1.73 m2). Nephrol Dial Transplant. 2016;31(suppl 2):ii1–ii66.

Hemodialysis in the Elderly

10

Luminita Voroneanu and Adrian Covic

The global population is aging. In 2017, there are an estimated 962 million people aged 60 or over in the world, comprising 13% of the global population [1, 2]. The number of older is expected to more than double by 2050 and to more than triple by 2100, rising to 2.1 billion in 2050 and 3.1 billion in 2100 [3]. Simultaneously, the number of elderly patients with ESRD has increased. For this category of patients, some essential question should be addressed:

1. Renal replacement therapy or conservative care?
2. What renal replacement therapy (RRT) modality is more appropriate for our elderly patients?
3. When to start dialysis?
4. What type of vascular access is proper for our patient?
5. Which is the adequate prescription of dialysis in the elderly?

Epidemiology

Data provided by the ERA-EDTA registry (2015) showed that 44% of the prevalent dialysis patients were aged ≥65 years [4]. Almost 52% of the incident dialysis patients were aged ≥65 years. The mean age of the patients commencing RRT in all countries and regions combined was 64.6 years. However, data provided by a large and comprehensive cohort from the 29 European registries showed a significant difference between the incidence of RRT among the elderly across European countries and regions; the

L. Voroneanu (✉)
University of Medicine "Grigore T. Popa" and University Hospital "C. I. Parhon", Iasi, Romania

A. Covic
University of Medicine "Grigore T. Popa" and University Hospital "C. I. Parhon", AOSR, Iasi, Romania

C. G. Musso et al. (eds.), *Clinical Nephrogeriatrics*,
https://doi.org/10.1007/978-3-030-18711-8_10

difference between the highest and the lowest incidence is almost sixfold (from 157 to 924 per million age-related population, whereas among patients 20–74 years of age the difference was only twofold) [5]. These differences could be partly explained by: (1) diverse usage of conservative management in the care of patients with ESRD; (2) Information provided to patients by nephrologists and other renal unit staff plays an important role when older adults are choosing between dialysis and conservative management; (3) different management of patients during the progression of CKD; a better management could reduce the number of comorbidities and increase the number of elderly patients who benefit from dialysis [5]. In Canada, the proportion of incident dialysis patients who are 65 years or older has increased from 41.8% in 1994 to 53.5% in 2013 [6]. In United States, nearly half of incident dialysis patients are senior citizens, with the median age at dialysis initiation over 64 years [7, 8].

Renal Replacement Therapy or Conservative Care in the Elderly? (Survival and Quality of Life)

Elderly undergoing dialysis are at an amplified risk for poor outcomes, including death, with a mortality rate of up to 37.0 deaths/100 person-years within the first 6 months of dialysis therapy initiation [9]. The median survival for elderly in dialysis is almost 4 years for patients who start dialysis over the age of 70 [7]. Because elderly patients with ESRD could be associated with multiple comorbid conditions, frailty, or cognitive and functional decline, a decision regarding dialysis initiation is frequently difficult. It has been doubted if these categories of patients are expected to benefit from dialysis. The option of a conservative care as an alternative to dialysis had produced increased interest for this category of patients. However, adequate survival data, particularly in elderly patients, are limited. A number of studies have showed survival in elderly dialysis patients compared with conservative care [10–13]. However, in these studies, the numbers of enrolled patients are usually small, the studies are performed in heterogeneous study populations, and there is significant variability in starting points used in survival analyses. In the largest cohort analysis that has been published so far, Chadna et al. studied 844 patients, 689 (82%) of whom had been treated by dialysis and 155 (18%) with conservative care. Median survival was less in conservative management than in dialysis (21.2 vs. 67.1 months; $p < 0.001$) [12]. However, in patients aged >75 years when corrected for age, high comorbidity and diabetes, the survival advantage from dialysis was only 4 months, which was not statistically significant [12]. In a retrospective survival analysis performed in a single-center cohort in the Netherlands, 311 patients with ESRD ages ≥70 years old opted for conservative care or dialysis. In total, 107 patients chose conservative management, and 204 chose dialysis. Median survival was higher in the dialysis group (median; 75th to 25th percentiles: 3.1, 1.5–6.9 versus 1.5, 0.7–3.0 years; log-rank test: $p < 0.001$). However, the survival advantage of these patients was no longer noticed in patients aged ≥80 years old (median; 75th–25th percentiles: 2.1, 1.5–3.4 versus 1.4, 0.7–3.0 years; log-rank test: $p = 0.08$) and in patients aged ≥70 years old with Davies comorbidity scores of ≥3, particularly with cardiovascular comorbidity [13, 14]. Similar data were reported by Hussain et al. The survival benefit of dialysis was also lost in patients >80 years, with a poor performance status and high comorbidity score [15].

In a prospective observational study, including 273 predialysis patients who had usual nephrology care and 122 nondialysis pathway patients who also attended a renal supportive care clinic adding the skills of a palliative medicine team and further 72 patients commenced dialysis during this period without attending, Brawn et al. found that elderly patients managed via a nondialysis pathway that includes renal supportive survived a median of 16 months [13]. These patients had a lower survival than (younger) patients attending the predialysis clinic but there was no substantially difference in their adjusted survival compared with dialysis patients who had not attended the predialysis clinic. During this time, the majority of patients had improvement in their symptoms by utilizing the skills of a palliative care team [13].

In a recent systematic review and meta-analysis of cohort studies (12 studies, 11.515 patients) the authors founded that elderly who chose dialysis therapy were younger (mean age: 72 years), were able to care for themselves, and had an average Karnofsky performance score of 73; in contrast, patients who opted for conservative care were elderly (mean age: 80 years old), required occasional assistance, and had an average Karnofsky performance score of 63 [16]. In multivariate analysis, patients preferring dialysis had a pooled adjusted hazard ratio for mortality of 0.53 (95% CI 0.30–0.91, $p = 0.02$) relative to those deciding for conservative management; however, significant heterogeneity precluded definitive conclusions [16].

As an intermediary conclusion, all these studies seem to suggest that dialysis may extend life among elderly patients without comorbidities; there is no significant survival advantage in patients >80 years old and with important comorbidities. However, the decision is often very difficult.

In this context, clinical risk prediction tools may help patients and providers in this decision-making process by comparing their risk for mortality to that of other similar patient. There are several scores developed in the last 10 years. Couchoud et al. derived a clinical score to predict *6-month mortality* based on a national end-stage renal disease registry of adults 75 years and older initiating dialysis therapy in France; the Couchoud score consisted of nine predictors, body mass index <18.5 kg/m^2 (2 points), diabetes (1), congestive heart failure stages III–IV (2), peripheral vascular disease stages III–IV (2), dysrhythmia (1), active malignancy (1), severe behavioral disorder (2), total dependency for transfers (3), and unplanned dialysis (2) [17]. Mortality rates ranged from 8% in the lowest risk group (0 point) to 70% in the highest risk group (≥9 points) and 17% in the median group (2 points) [17]. Thamer et al. did a comparable score with US-based Medicare and Medicaid patients 67 years and older initiating dialysis therapy in 2009–2010. The simple risk score (total score: 0–9) included age (0–3 points), low albumin level, assistance with daily living, nursing home residence, cancer, heart failure, and hospitalization (1 point each) [18]. A median score of 3 indicating 12% risk in 3 months and 20% in 6 months, and the highest scores (≥8) indicating 39% risk in 3 months and 55% in 6 months [18]. A third prediction score was published last year. This is the first score developed using population-level data—a cohort of 2199 older adults (aged >65 years) in Alberta, Canada; it is a 19-point risk score for 6-month mortality that included age 80 years or older (2 points), glomerular filtration rate of 10–14.9 mL/min/ 1.73 m2 (1 point) or >15 mL/min/1.73 m2 (3 points), atrial fibrillation (2 points), lymphoma (5 points), congestive heart failure (2 points), hospitalization in the prior 6 months (2 points), and metastatic cancer (3 points) [19]. A score <5 equated to <25% of individuals dying in 6 months, whereas a score >12 predicted that more than half the individuals would die in the first 6 months [19].

Another important issue is the impact of dialysis on the quality of life in elderly patients. It was already demonstrated 10 years ago a marked decline in functional status during the period surrounding the initiation of dialysis; these functional decline continues despite the initiation of dialysis; at 1 year after the start of dialysis *only one* by eight U.S. nursing home residents had functional capacity that was maintained at the predialysis level [20]. The lowest level of physical functioning was seen in patients aged over 75 years old. In contrast, emotional health is well preserved in patients over 75 years old; the relatively good emotional health in elderly patients may reflect lower expectations and a higher level of satisfaction with being alive despite functional disabilities [20].

In this context (moderate survival benefit, decline in functional status), several elderly patients may regret their initial decision. In a cross-sectional study including 103 elderly dialysis patients from Singapore, 81% reported no decision regret about choosing dialysis over conservative management; 11% reported ambivalence ("Neither agree nor disagree") and 8% reported clear regret [21]. Additionally, 16% indicated they would not undergo dialysis if they had to do it over again and 19% felt that dialysis had led to harm [21]. One possible explanation for this perception is the significant healthcare-related burden reported by participants, in terms of the number of daily medications they needed to take, their number of comorbidities, monthly medical costs, and past year hospitalization days.

What RRT Modality Is More Appropriate for Our Elderly Patients? (Mortality, Quality of Life)

Elderly patients on dialysis typically receive in center hemodialysis, and only a small proportion are on peritoneal dialysis. The principal benefit of PD is the avoidance of the disturbance and discomfort of visits to hospital in all types of weather and regardless of how the patient is feeling. Some other advantages are as follows: no need for vascular access, less surgical procedures required, no use of central venous catheter and reduced risk of related infection, better hemodynamic tolerance, no need for transportation, and better residual renal function preservation. Realistically, although some elderly patients are able to perform their own PD, for many it is impossible. Family members could help, but typically, when this is not possible, patients are included in HD with all its difficulties, or on conservative care or in best cases, on assisted PD.

A recent meta-analysis of observational studies (15 studies involving >631,421 elderly patients) suggested a higher risk for death in elderly patients receiving PD than in those receiving HD was noticed (HR with PD was 1.10 (95% CI, 1.01 to

1.20)) [22]. When the subgroup analysis was stratified by possible confounding factors, the decreased survival of the PD group was more prominent in the presence of diabetes mellitus and long dialysis durations [22]. However, there was significant heterogeneity among the included observational studies. Also, because the incorporated studies are observational and mainly from registry databases, it is likely that crucial confounders may not have been corrected for (for example frailty), limiting the validity of the study [22].

There are several observational studies which particularly compared QoL outcomes in elderly patients on HD or PD. The North Thames Dialysis study explicitly examined outcomes and quality of life in dialysis patients older than 70 years of age who were starting dialysis [23]. The 1-year survival of 71% was influenced by age but not by dialysis modality. There was no difference in survival, hospitalization rate, or quality of life at 6 and 12 months [23]. The Broadening Options for Long-term Dialysis in the Elderly (BOLDE) study is a cross-sectional, multicenter study which assessed quality of life, depression, symptoms, and illness intrusion in 140 (aged 65 years or older) on PD and HD patients from 3 large hospitals in South East England [24]. Although HD and PD patients did not differ in the quality of life, in physical component scores, PD patients had marginally but significantly better mental component scores. PD patients also had a lower number of symptoms, significantly less possible depression and lower illness intrusion (caused by greater intrusion of HD in the domain of health and diet, with no significant difference in the other 11 intrusion scales) [24].

Most of the elderly could not choose PD because of functional impairment and cognitive dysfunction. In several countries, assisted PD is used in elderly ESRD patients. Assisted PD program is available in French, Danish, Italy, Belgium, The Netherlands, Norway, Sweden, Canary Islands, UK, Canada, Brazil, and China. Data from the French Peritoneal Dialysis Registry for 1615 patients older than 75 years of age (1232 on assisted PD) showed that the median survival is 27.1 months; median pure technique survival was 21.4 months and the median survival free of peritonitis was 32.1 months [25]. Assisted PD seems to be a safe alternative to in-center HD also in terms of hospitalization risk. Oliver et al. in a recent paper publication analyzed the hospitalization rate in 203 assisted PD patients and 872 in-center HD patients and reported similar findings in both groups, i.e., 11.1 versus 12.9 days/year, which corresponds to 0.8 versus 0.7 hospital/admissions per year [26]. Patients on assisted peritoneal dialysis were more likely to be hospitalized for dialysis-related complications (admitted for 2.4 day/year) compared with 1.6 day/year in the hemodialysis group; $p = 0.04$). This difference was partly explained by more hospital days because of peritonitis. The assisted PD seems to be also cost effective. Additional assistance from normal PD could increase the cost to the same level as HD. In an observational study including 251 patients (129 assisted PD and 122 HD), there were no differences in measures of QoL and physical function, except for treatment satisfaction, which is higher in patients on PD [27]. Assisted PD should be considered as an alternative to HD for older patients, allowing them to make their preferred choices [27].

When to Start Dialysis?

The optimal timing for dialysis initiation in the elderly is unknown. The IDEAL study found no advantage when dialysis was started with a higher (10–14 mL/min per 1.73 m^2) versus lower eGFR; however, these finding could not be adequately extrapolated in elderly population, because elderly, particularly with frailty or serious comorbidities were underrepresented in this trial [28]. O'Hare et al. reviewed the medical records of a random sample of patients who initiated maintenance dialysis in the Department of Veterans Affairs (n = 1691) and showed that the mean eGFR at initiation increased from 9.8±5.8 to 11.0±5.5 mL/min per 1.73 m^2 ($p < 0.001$) between fiscal years 2000 and 2009 [29]. This trend was not elucidated by variations in clinical presentation over time: neither the percentage of patients presenting with an acute illness or the distribution of different types of clinical signs and/or symptoms at the time of dialysis initiation different substantially during this time period [29].

In a contemporary cohort of United States veterans with advanced CKD (n = 73,349), Tamura et al. founded that the eGFR at which survival with dialysis exceeded survival with medical management varied by age; an apparent benefit of dialysis was evident at higher eGFRs for older patients [30]. At the same time, the potential gain in life expectancy associated with dialysis was diminished for older patients and at higher eGFRs [30]. Provision of dialysis at higher levels of kidney function may extend survival for some older patients, but the corresponding increase in life expectancy may not outweigh the burden of therapy.

Vascular Access in Elderly

The optimal vascular access in elderly hemodialysis patients remains controversial. Many national clinical guidelines recommended arteriovenous fistulae (AVFs) as the optimal vascular access in HD patients, based on several justifications: better longevity, less intervention to maintain long-term patency, lower mortality and infection risk for this category of patients, and less access-related costs [31].

However, in elderly HD patients, there are some suggestions that AVFs are not always the right choice [32]. There are some possible explanations for this particular situation: (1) many elderly patients have a heavy burden of comorbidities and an increased risk of death before dialysis initiation in this group or if they are already on hemodialysis they may not live long enough to see the benefits of prolonged AVF survival; (2) many elderly patients have inadequate vasculature for fistula maturation, resulting in a reduced rate of AVF patency [33]; in a systematic review and meta-analysis including 13 relevant studies a statistically significantly higher rate of radial-cephalic arteriovenous fistula failure in elderly patients compared with non-elderly adults at 12 (odds ratio [OR], 1.525; $p = 0.001$) and 24 months (OR, 1.357, $p = 0.019$) was reported [34].

The selection of a site for AV access must be individualized for each elderly patient. Guidelines advise performing distal limb AVF procedures first as an approach to preserve more proximal venous anatomy [35]. But in the elderly, the mortality rates are higher, so the preservation of the vein in proximal sites is of smaller importance. Additionally, peripheral vascular disease (frequently founded in the elderly) can prejudice the inflow of blood to the AVF and consequently affect its maturation. This has led to a surgical preference for creating a brachiocephalic AVF rather than a radio cephalic AVF in elderly [36]. In a systematic review and meta-analysis, McGrogan et al. described the pooled 12-month AVF patency rates in elderly patients and compared the primary and secondary AVF patencies at 12 months for radio cephalic versus brachiocephalic AVFs [37]. This meta-analysis showed that adequate 12-month primary and secondary AVF patency rates can be achieved in elderly patients (the pooled 12-month primary AVF patency rates were 53.6% and secondary AVF patency was 71.6%). Brachiocephalic AVFs have both superior primary and secondary patency rates at 12 months compared with radio cephalic AVFs (primary (OR, 0.72; 95% CI, 0.55–0.93; and secondary (OR, 0.76; 95% CI, 0.58–1.00; patency rates) [37].

What about the optimal time for AVF placement in the elderly? The Fistula First Breakthrough Initiative and 2006 KDOQI9 recommend that "a fistula should be created at least 6 months or with sufficient lead time before the anticipated start of haemodialysis treatments for fistula maturation [38–40]." This allows for adequate time for an AVF to mature and necessary interventions to be performed to ensure successful AVF use at dialysis initiation. If the access is created too late, the patient is more likely to initiate dialysis with a catheter and to experience sepsis. However, if dialysis access is created too early, it may not be necessary, especially in the elderly, because it is more likely to die before the start of dialysis. Additionally, the progression rate of CKD is slowly in the elderly; moreover, the rate of clotting and stenosis necessitating invasive procedures may be also augmented [40].

Using data from the US Renal Data System with Medicare claims data (17,511 patients ≥67 years old on incident HD, with an AVF placed as the first predialysis access), Hod et al. founded that placing an AVF >6–9 months before first HD did not improve the success rate at HD initiation but was associated with an increased number of interventional procedures [41]. The subgroup analysis revealed that the trends were more pronounced in patients with chronic heart failure and with diabetes [41]. One potential explanation is that, in patients with comorbidities, it may lead to endothelial dysfunction and vascular wall abnormalities, and the hemodynamic shear stress of an AVF might cause increased neointimal hyperplasia with a lack of vascular dilation [41]. In this context, placing an AVF too early may increase the exposure time to neointimal hyperplasia and AVFs failure [41]. Similar data were reported by Richardson et al. [42]. Among patient's ≥70 years old undergoing AVF creation, only 39% of AVFs were patent at 1 year, and only 50% of patients were alive at 18 months. As a consequence, only 35% of patients who died ever used their AVF [42]. Comparable results were reported also in a large nationally representative cohort of 3418 elderly patients with predialysis CKD undergoing preemptive AVFs or AVG. Sixty-seven percent of the patients initiate dialysis during a 2-year follow-up [40]. Two recent Canadian studies found analogues results. Similar data were also reported in two canadian cohorts; 70% of patients (in the first study) and 81%

(in the second) initiated dialysis within 2 years of access placement [43, 44]. Moreover, as a consequence of maturation failure almost one half of patients receiving AVFS initiated dialysis with a catheter.

In this context, some authors suggest that elderly patients should be referred later to decrease the risk of creating an AVF that will never be used. In this interest, the AVG converts into a valid option form of vascular access if no appropriate anatomy for AVF creation and slow renal progression are present. In this context, the use of early stick graft might be proper. It was already demonstrated that almost half of those with AVF placement-initiated dialysis using a central venous catheter (CVC); in contrast, among patients that received a graft as first access only 25.4% started dialysis with a CVC; in other words, patients who obtain a graft are less probable to necessitate a catheter at first HD treatment compared to those who receive a fistula [45].

But do not forget that a substantial number of elderly have poor vasculature, leading to poor fistula or graft function or arterial steal syndromes; also, other number of patients have short predicted survival times, fistula arm swelling, or prolonged bleeding periods after each dialysis, which compromise their quality of life. In this context, CVC prevalence in the elderly dialysis population remains high. In 14,966 elderly, incident HD patients from the MUNDO initiative, CVC prevalence ranged from 32 to 69% and significantly decreased in all regions in the first year on dialysis [46]. North America had the highest prevalence of CVC by the end of the 1st year, while Asia Pacific showed the largest decrease in CVC prevalence at the end of year 1. Younger (70–79 years) patients were more likely to convert to a non-CVC access as compared to those ≥80 years old [46]. Similar data were showed in the DOPPS cohort; the prevalence of permanent, as the dialysis access was highest among those older than 75 years [47]. Permanent central venous catheters were used more frequently in the elderly versus younger patients in Europe, ANZ, and North America but were very rarely used in Japan. These data indicate that the elderly is less probable to start dialysis with an AV fistula and predominantly elderly women have a higher percentage of catheters than men [47].

That about vascular access and main outcomes? In reported comparisons, patients initiating hemodialysis with a catheter have greater mortality rates of more than 70% than those starting with an AVF, encouraging a strong emphasis on the fistula first, catheter last initiative. In the first large population-based study in the elderly evaluating survival outcomes with the vascular access placed in the predialysis period, *fistula first is not the clearly superior strategy in the elderly population, particularly for octogenarians and nonagenarians*. The patients with a catheter as the first predialysis access placed had significantly inferior survival compared with those patients with a fistula (HR = 1.77; 95% CI = 1.73 to 1.81; $p < 0.001$) [45]. However, no significant mortality difference was found between those patients with a graft as the first access placed and those patients with a fistula (HR = 1.05; 95% CI = 1.00 to 1.11; $p = 0.06$). Moreover, analyzing mortality stratified by age groups, grafts as the first predialysis access placed had inferior mortality outcomes compared with fistulas for the 67 to ≤ 79 years' age group (HR = 1.10; 95% CI = 1.02–1.17; $p = 0.007$) [45, 48].

In a cohort of 115,425 patients on incident hemodialysis ≥67 years old from the US Renal Data System with linked Medicare, Brawn et al. compared mortality outcomes in patients initiating hemodialysis with a fistula placed first (9794 patients), a catheter after a fistula placed first failed (8230), or a catheter placed first (n = 90,517)—the reference group (47). The patients receiving an AVF first were younger, men, whites, those who were normal or overweight by body mass index rather than underweight or obese, and those who had more predialysis nephrology care than those in the CVC group. The fistula group had the lowest mortality over 58 months (HR, 0.50; 95% CI 0.48–0.52; $p < 0.001$). However, the group initiating hemodialysis with a catheter after fistula placement failed also had significantly lower mortality rates than the catheter group had over 58 months (hazard ratio, 0.66; 95% confidence interval, 0.64–0.68; $p < 0.001$). The authors concluded that patient factors affecting fistula placement, even when patients are hemodialyzed with a catheter instead, may explain at least two thirds of the mortality benefit observed in patients with a fistula [49].

Conversion from a CVC to a non-CVC access within the first 6 months does result in a significantly lower risk of death in all age groups, particularly beneficial in those older than 80 years. Furthermore, patients who were maintained on CVC as their primary vascular access had a higher risk of death compared to those who converted from CVC to arteriovenous graft (AVG) or AVF. In conclusion, it seems that elderly patients who started HD with a CVC should be changed to a non-CVC access as soon as possible [50].

Economically speaking, AVFs have been found to be the most cost-effective form of hemodialysis access; however, in elderly HD patients, the cost-effectiveness is critically dependent on life expectancy [51]. Using a Markov model to estimate the cost-effectiveness of placing an AVF or AVG or continued CVC use in a hypothetical cohort of elderly (age ≥65 years old) patients initiating hemodialysis with a CVC, Hall et al. founded that placement of an AVF was more cost-effective than continued CVC use for all age and life expectancy groups except 85- to 89-year-olds in the lowest life expectancy quartile. AVFs were more cost effective than AVGs for all quartiles of life expectancy among the 65- to 69-year-old age group [52]. AVFs are no more cost effective than AVGs for those with a life expectancy of <2 years, and neither form of vascular access is more cost effective than catheters for patients with a life expectancy of <6 months. These results support continued CVC use after dialysis initiation as reasonable vascular access options for older adults with limited life expectancy [52, 53].

Probably the best decision regarding the optimal vascular access in the elderly should be based on life expectancy in addition to age. A definitive answer about the relative benefits of AVFs and AVGs in terms of pattern survival, mortality, hospitalization, and costs would necessitate large, multicenter, randomized clinical trials (RCTs), in which patients are randomized to receive one of these vascular access types.

Until then, the optimal choice depends on the clinical judgment of nephrologists and surgeons caring for these patients. Probably the best decision regarding the optimal vascular access should be based on (1) life expectancy in addition to age;

(2) the possibility of efficacious AVF maturation; (3) the outcomes of a preceding vascular access.

Which Is the Adequate Prescription of Dialysis in the Elderly?

The current European guidelines as well as American guidelines recommend a minimum of three dialysis sessions per week, with a Kt/V of at least 1.2 for each session (this target generally requires 4 h of treatment) [2]. The guidelines accept for modification to take account of renal function. This recommendation is independent of patient's age, frailty, or comorbidities [54].

Kt/V is defined as the dialyzer clearance of urea (K) multiplied by the duration of the dialysis treatment (t, in minutes) divided by the volume of distribution of urea in the body (V, in mL), which is approximately equal to the total body water, corrected for volume lost during ultrafiltration. In the elderly, some important changes are founded on these parameters [55]:

- Body water volume (TBW) has a major influence on Kt/V. In elderly, a relatively lower total body water volume has been described, changing from around 65% in young people to around 50% in male, and 40% in female elderly people. Thus, old people have 10–20% lower TBW content compared to young people. Conversely, TBW is relative high (60%) in elderly patients suffering from immobility syndrome [56];
- Moreover, when Kt/V is considered using online clearance, V calculated using anthropometric data is often used. This is likely to be highly inaccurate in the elderly.
- Elderly patients associate a reduced metabolic rate and a reduced protein intake; in this context, these patients have lower levels of uremic toxins [57].

The current guidelines recommend a hemodialysis dose of an eKt/V ≥1.2 (standard Kt/V ≥1.4) per session in a thrice-weekly program. The optimum dialysis dose in elderly patients with or without comorbidities is unknown. There is no study in the literature which had specifically determined hemodialysis characteristics in the elderly.

Elderly patients have also lower salt and water intake. The interdialytic weight gain is reduced. This has a tendency to decrease the necessity for ultrafiltration, permitting either a slower ultrafiltration rate at the same dialysis time or a shorter dialysis with the same ultrafiltration rate compared with younger patients. The DOPPS recent analysis confirms this theory. The mean ultrafiltration rate was lower in the elderly than in the younger age groups [47]. These selected elderly patients with lower generation of uremic toxins and lower interdialytic weight gain could also tolerate twice-weekly HD. The comparison of the outcomes between twice versus thrice weekly dialysis is needed.

Additionally, these patients associate important cardiovascular comorbidities; in this context, a decreased tolerance to ultrafiltration and an amplified risk of hypotension is present. Hypotension often causes premature cessation of dialysis and inadequate dialysis dose. Moreover, vascular problems may cause a poor vascular access and finally, insufficient/disrupted dialysis.

In this context, an ERBP paper recently published conclude that the prescription of dialysis in the elderly should be individualized, taking multiple factors into account [54].

Incremental dialysis uses the idea of adjusting dialysis dose according to residual renal function so that the dialysis dose is individualized [58]. The foundation is to provide enough dialysis to minimum removal of uremic solutes and control of hypervolemia and then escalating the dose of dialysis as residual renal function decline. There are only few observational studies that examined clinical outcomes in those incremental HD. A recent large one found that there was no difference in survival rates between patients treated by incremental versus standard HD. However, higher mortality rates are noticed in patients with inadequate baseline renal urea clearance ($\leq$3.0 mL/min/1.73 m^2; HR, 1.61; 95% CI, 1.07–2.44) or urine volume <600 mL/day. The advantages of this type of HD could be particularly important for the elderly. An RCT is required to compare the safety and efficacy of incremental dialysis with standard full-dose HD in elderly dialysis patients [59]. In a recent narrative review of 12 observational cohort studies of twice weekly compared with to thrice weekly HD, incremental HD was associated with several benefits including preservation of residual kidney function as well as extending the event-free life of arteriovenous fistulas and grafts. However, serious risks must also be considered, including increased hospitalization and mortality perhaps related to fluid and electrolyte shifts after a long interdialytic interval [60].

The recent ERBP paper on this subject recommends that the prescription of dialysis in the elderly should be individualized, taking multiple factors into account [54]. An individualized Kt/V may be useful in controlling dialysis dose and detecting problems in delivery. However, achievement of a specified Kt/V may not result in any benefit to an elderly patient and could be counterproductive.

Additional HD-Related Complications

Elderly patients are at increased risk of *accidental falls*; this risk is amplified in hemodialysis patients due to added risk of the kidney disease burden as well as the HD technique itself [61, 62]. Anemia and malnutrition, depression, cognitive impairment, sleep disorder, the fluid and electrolyte shift from HD session, the increased risk of hypotension, and arrhythmias are additional risk factors in the elderly hemodialysis patients [63]. In this context, a higher rate of falls compared with general elderly population was described (1.2–1.8 vs. 0.6–0.8 falls per patient-year, respectively) [62–64]. Falls are likely to occur annually among 25% or more of HD patients, even in a cohort that is not primarily elderly. Falls in the elderly population are related with increased hospitalization, need for long-term care, and mortality [65]. Other concerns include fear of falling, resulting in physical activity restriction, functional decline, and frailty [63]. Compared with non-fallers, HD elderly fallers had a 2.13-fold increase in risk of death, a 3.5-fold increase in risk of nursing home admission, and nearly a 2-fold increase in the number and duration of hospitalizations [65].

Given the increased incidence of seniors in an outpatient dialysis setting and the reported fall rate in these patients, clinical nephrologists and other health care providers should consider fall risk when providing general care for these patients.

There is increasing evidence that HD procedure itself might contribute *to brain injury in the elderly* [66]. It was already reported an increased risk of stroke in first month on HD in the elderly; the stroke rate decreased in the months after dialysis initiation but remained approximately twice the baseline rate by 1 year [66]. This stabilization may signify partial recovery of cerebrovascular autoregulation in response to acute volume and electrolyte shifts after the first months of dialysis sessions. It may also be a survivor phenomenon, with dialysis functioning as a stress test [66]. Using [15O]H_2O positron-emission tomography-computed tomography to measure cerebral blood flow (CBF), Polinder-Bos et al. demonstrated a significant decline in global CBF by 10% ± 15% during hemodialysis session [67]. The decline in CBF was similar for the various individual brain regions that were studied and therefore, most likely, affected both the anterior (i.e., the internal carotid arteries) and posterior (i.e., the vertebral and basilar arteries) circulation. The decline in CBF was symptomatic in only one patient. HD treatment-related factors that might explain the intradialytic CBF decline were a higher tympanic temperature, a greater UF volume and UF rate, and a higher pH [67].

Cognitive impairment, including *dementia,* is a usual but poorly recognized complication among elderly dialysis affecting 16–38% of patients [68]. Dementia increases the risk for death, disability, hospitalization, and dialysis withdrawal and increases costs of care [68]. Additionally, may interfere with capacity for self-care and informed decision-making. Besides common traditional risk factors, like increasing age, diabetes, male gender, smoking, hypertension, or hypercholesterolemia, and CKD-related factors (inflammation, oxidative stress, vascular calcification, etc.), some other important factors, induced by hemodialysis session itself, like intradialytic hypotension, cerebral edema, and hyperviscosity, are significant in the development of dementia [68]. The risk of dementia is higher in elderly hemodialysis patients compared with PD. A recent analysis of a large national database (121.623 patients) demonstrated that persons whose initial dialysis modality is PD have a 25% lower risk of acquiring a dementia diagnosis than persons who initiated dialysis on HD, even adjusting for a comprehensive set of demographic and clinical characteristics in a well matched analysis [69].

Conclusion

1. Conservative care/dialysis modality choice should be a patient-centered, individual decision.
2. No survival advantage for elderly with comorbidities; functional decline after dialysis initiation.
3. No essential difference in survival on HD compared with PD, in mortality, quality of life in technique survival or peritonitis free period.

4. The optimal time for dialysis initiation is unknown. There are some data that facility of dialysis at higher levels of kidney function may extend survival for some older patients, but the corresponding increase in life expectancy may not outweigh the burden of therapy.
5. Fistula first could be a right choice for elderly patients with good chance of AVF maturation and a reasonable life expectancy; for elderly patients with little chance of successful maturation and reasonable life expectancy, an AVG is a reasonable alternative. However, for patients with extensive peripheral vascular disease, short life expectancy from other comorbidities, or chronic hypotension, a tunneled dialysis catheter is a judicious choice.
6. The optimum dialysis dose in elderly patients, with or without comorbidities is unknown. There is no study in the literature which had specifically determined hemodialysis characteristics in the elderly. Use of incremental dialysis or changes in hemodialysis frequency could be used as a substitute and can ameliorate quality of life in elderly patients.
7. Hemodialysis can be complicated by vascular access-related problems, decreased tolerance to ultrafiltration, and an amplified risk of hypotension, brain injury, dementia, and increased risk of accidental falls.

References

1. http://www.un.org/en/sections/issues-depth/ageing/.
2. National Kidney Foundation. KDOQI Clinical Practice Guideline for Hemodialysis Adequacy: 2015 update. Am J Kidney Dis. 2015;66(5):884–930.
3. https://www.un.org/development/desa/en/news/population/world-population-prospects-2017.html.
4. Pippias M, Kramer A, Noordzij M, Afentakis N, Alonso de la Torre R, Ambuhl PM, et al. The European renal association – European dialysis and transplant association registry annual report 2014: a summary. Clin Kidney J. 2017;10(2):154–69.
5. van den Brand J, Pippias M, Stel VS, Caskey FJ, Collart F, Finne P, et al. Lifetime risk of renal replacement therapy in Europe: a population-based study using data from the ERA-EDTA registry. Nephrol Dial Transplant. 2017;32(2):348–55.
6. Organ CIfHIC, End-Stage RRARTo, Canadian Institute for Health Information. Canadian Organ Replacement Register Annual Report: Treatment of End-Stage Organ Failure in Canada, 2003 to 2013. Accessed 8 Oct.
7. https://www.usrds.org/2017/view/v2_05.aspx.
8. Anand S, Kurella Tamura M, Chertow GM. The elderly patients on hemodialysis. Minerva Urolo Nefrol = Italian J Urol Nephrol. 2010;62(1):87–101.
9. Foley RN, Chen SC, Solid CA, Gilbertson DT, Collins AJ. Early mortality in patients starting dialysis appears to go unregistered. Kidney Int. 2014;86(2):392–8.
10. Reindl-Schwaighofer R, Kainz A, Kammer M, Dumfarth A, Oberbauer R. Survival analysis of conservative vs. dialysis treatment of elderly patients with CKD stage 5. PLoS One. 2017;12(7):e0181345.
11. Martinez Echevers Y, Toapanta Gaibor NG, Nava Perez N, Barbosa Martin F, Montes Delgado R, Guerrero Riscos MA. Survival of patients ≥70 years with advanced chronic kidney disease: Dialysis vs. conservative care. Nefrologia. 2016;36(3):283–91.

12. Chandna SM, Da Silva-Gane M, Marshall C, Warwicker P, Greenwood RN, Farrington K. Survival of elderly patients with stage 5 CKD: comparison of conservative management and renal replacement therapy. Nephrol Dial Transplant. 2011;26(5):1608–14.
13. Brown MA, Collett GK, Josland EA, Foote C, Li Q, Brennan FP. CKD in elderly patients managed without dialysis: survival, symptoms, and quality of life. Clin J Am Soc Nephrol: CJASN. 2015;10(2):260–8.
14. Verberne WR, Geers AB, Jellema WT, Vincent HH, van Delden JJ, Bos WJ. Comparative survival among older adults with advanced kidney disease managed conservatively versus with dialysis. Clin J Am Soc Nephrol: CJASN. 2016;11(4):633–40.
15. Hussain JA, Mooney A, Russon L. Comparison of survival analysis and palliative care involvement in patients aged over 70 years choosing conservative management or renal replacement therapy in advanced chronic kidney disease. Palliat Med. 2013;27(9):829–39.
16. Wongrakpanich S, Susantitaphong P, Isaranuwatchai S, Chenbhanich J, Eiam-Ong S, Jaber BL. Dialysis therapy and conservative management of advanced chronic kidney disease in the elderly: a systematic review. Nephron. 2017;137(3):178–89.
17. Couchoud C, Labeeuw M, Moranne O, Allot V, Esnault V, Frimat L, et al. A clinical score to predict 6-month prognosis in elderly patients starting dialysis for end-stage renal disease. Nephrol Dial Transplant. 2009;24(5):1553–61.
18. Thamer M, Kaufman JS, Zhang Y, Zhang Q, Cotter DJ, Bang H. Predicting early death among elderly dialysis patients: development and validation of a risk score to assist shared decision making for dialysis initiation. Am J Kidney Dis. 2015;66(6):1024–32.
19. Wick JP, Turin TC, Faris PD, MacRae JM, Weaver RG, Tonelli M, et al. A clinical risk prediction tool for 6-month mortality after dialysis initiation among older adults. Am J Kidney Dis. 2017;69(5):568–75.
20. Kurella Tamura M, Covinsky KE, Chertow GM, Yaffe K, Landefeld CS, McCulloch CE. Functional status of elderly adults before and after initiation of dialysis. N Engl J Med. 2009;361(16):1539–47.
21. Tan EGF, Teo I, Finkelstein EA, Chan CM. Determinants of regret in elderly dialysis patients. Nephrology (Carlton). 2018.
22. Han SS, Park JY, Kang S, Kim KH, Ryu DR, Kim H, et al. Dialysis modality and mortality in the elderly: a meta-analysis. Clin J Am Soc Nephrol: CJASN. 2015;10(6):983–93.
23. Harris SA, Lamping DL, Brown EA, Constantinovici N. Clinical outcomes and quality of life in elderly patients on peritoneal dialysis versus hemodialysis. Perit Dial Int: J Int Soc Perit Dial. 2002;22(4):463–70.
24. Brown EA, Johansson L, Farrington K, Gallagher H, Sensky T, Gordon F, et al. Broadening Options for Long-term Dialysis in the Elderly (BOLDE): differences in quality of life on peritoneal dialysis compared to haemodialysis for older patients. Nephrol Dial Transplant. 2010;25(11):3755–63.
25. Castrale C, Evans D, Verger C, Fabre E, Aguilera D, Ryckelynck JP, et al. Peritoneal dialysis in elderly patients: report from the French Peritoneal Dialysis Registry (RDPLF). Nephrol Dial Transplant. 2010;25(1):255–62.
26. Oliver MJ, Al-Jaishi AA, Dixon SN, Perl J, Jain AK, Lavoie SD, et al. Hospitalization rates for patients on assisted peritoneal dialysis compared with in-center hemodialysis. Clin J Am Soc Nephrol: CJASN. 2016;11(9):1606–14.
27. Iyasere OU, Brown EA, Johansson L, Huson L, Smee J, Maxwell AP, et al. Quality of life and physical function in older patients on dialysis: a comparison of assisted peritoneal dialysis with hemodialysis. Clin J Am Soc of Nephrol: CJASN. 2016;11(3):423–30.
28. Harris A, Cooper BA, Li JJ, Bulfone L, Branley P, Collins JF, et al. Cost-effectiveness of initiating dialysis early: a randomized controlled trial. Am J Kidney Dis. 2011;57(5):707–15.
29. O'Hare AM, Wong SP, Yu MK, Wynar B, Perkins M, Liu CF, et al. Trends in the timing and clinical context of maintenance dialysis initiation. J Am Soc Nephrol. 2015;26(8):1975–81.
30. Kurella Tamura M, Desai M, Kapphahn KI, Thomas IC, Asch SM, Chertow GM. Dialysis versus medical management at different ages and levels of kidney function in veterans with advanced CKD. J Am Soc Nephrol. 2018.

31. Leake AE, Yuo TH, Wu T, Fish L, Dillavou ED, Chaer RA, et al. Arteriovenous grafts are associated with earlier catheter removal and fewer catheter days in the United States Renal Data System population. J Vasc Surg. 2015;62(1):123–7.
32. Lomonte C, Forneris G, Gallieni M, Tazza L, Meola M, Lodi M, et al. Erratum to: the vascular access in the elderly: a position statement of the vascular access working group of the Italian society of nephrology. J Nephrol. 2017;30(4):617.
33. Saggi SJ, Allon M, Bernardini J, Kalantar-Zadeh K, Shaffer R, Mehrotra R. Considerations in the optimal preparation of patients for dialysis. Nat Rev Nephrol. 2012;8(7):381–9.
34. Lazarides MK, Georgiadis GS, Antoniou GA, Staramos DN. A meta-analysis of dialysis access outcome in elderly patients. J Vasc Surg. 2007;45(2):420–6.
35. Sidawy AN, Spergel LM, Besarab A, Allon M, Jennings WC, Padberg FT Jr, et al. The society for vascular surgery: clinical practice guidelines for the surgical placement and maintenance of arteriovenous hemodialysis access. J Vasc Surg. 2008;48(5 Suppl):2s–25s.
36. Misskey J, Faulds J, Sidhu R, Baxter K, Gagnon J, Hsiang Y. An age-based comparison of fistula location, patency, and maturation for elderly renal failure patients. J Vasc Surg. 2018;67(5):1491–500.
37. McGrogan D, Al Shakarchi J, Khawaja A, Nath J, Hodson J, Maxwell AP, et al. Arteriovenous fistula outcomes in the elderly. J Vasc Surg. 2015;62(6):1652–7.
38. Fistula first breakthrough initiative: fistula first national access improvements initiative. Available at: http://esrdncc.org/ffcl/. Accessed 3 June.
39. Clinical practice guidelines for vascular access. Am J Kidney Dis. 2006;48 Suppl 1:S176–247.
40. Lee T, Thamer M, Zhang Y, Zhang Q, Allon M. Outcomes of elderly patients after predialysis vascular access creation. J Am Soc Nephrol. 2015;26(12):3133–40.
41. Hod T, Patibandla BK, Vin Y, Brown RS, Goldfarb-Rumyantzev AS. Arteriovenous fistula placement in the elderly: when is the optimal time? J Am Soc Nephrol. 2015;26(2):448–56.
42. Richardson AI 2nd, Leake A, Schmieder GC, Biuckians A, Stokes GK, Panneton JM, et al. Should fistulas really be first in the elderly patient? J Vasc Access. 2009;10(3):199–202.
43. Oliver MJ, Quinn RR, Garg AX, Kim SJ, Wald R, Paterson JM. Likelihood of starting dialysis after incident fistula creation. Clin J Am Soc Nephrol. 2012;7(3):466–71. https://doi.org/10.2215/CJN.08920811.
44. Weber CL, Djurdjev O, Levin A, Kiaii M. Outcomes of vascular access creation prior to dialysis: building the case for early referral. ASAIO J. 2009;55(4):355–60. https://doi.org/10.1097/MAT.0b013e31819f635c.
45. DeSilva RN, Patibandla BK, Vin Y, Narra A, Chawla V, Brown RS, et al. Fistula first is not always the best strategy for the elderly. J Am Soc Nephrol. 2013;24(8):1297–304.
46. Raimann JG, Barth C, Usvyat LA, Preciado P, Canaud B, Etter M, et al. Dialysis access as an area of improvement in elderly incident hemodialysis patients: results from a cohort study from the international monitoring dialysis outcomes initiative. Am J Nephrol. 2017;45(6): 486–96.
47. Canaud B, Tong L, Tentori F, Akiba T, Karaboyas A, Gillespie B, et al. Clinical practices and outcomes in elderly hemodialysis patients: results from the Dialysis Outcomes and Practice Patterns Study (DOPPS). Clin J Am Soc Nephrol: CJASN. 2011;6(7):1651–62.
48. O'Hare AM. Vascular access for hemodialysis in older adults: a "patient first" approach. J Am Soc Nephrol. 2013;24(8):1187–90.
49. Brown RS, Patibandla BK, Goldfarb-Rumyantzev AS. The survival benefit of "fistula first, catheter last" in hemodialysis is primarily due to patient factors. J Am Soc Nephrol. 2017;28(2):645–52.
50. Dhruve MJ, Chan CT. Vascular access in the elderly: does one size fit all? Am J Nephrol. 2017;45(6):484–5.
51. Leermakers JJ, Bode AS, Vaidya A, van der Sande FM, Evers SM, Tordoir JH. Cost-effectiveness of vascular access for haemodialysis: arteriovenous fistulas versus arteriovenous grafts. Eur J Vasc Endovasc Surg. 2013;45(1):84–92.
52. Hall RK, Myers ER, Rosas SE, O'Hare AM, Colon-Emeric CS. Choice of hemodialysis access in older adults: a cost-effectiveness analysis. Clin J Ame Soc Nephrol: CJASN. 2017;12(6):947–54.

53. Lee T, Allon M. Reassessing recommendations for choice of vascular access. Clin J Am Soc Nephrol: CJASN. 2017;12(6):865–7.
54. Tattersall J, Farrington K, Gentile G, Kooman J, Macias Nunez JF, Nistor I, et al. Is Kt/V useful in elderly dialysis patients? Pro and con arguments. Nephrol Dial Transplant. 2018;33(5):742–50.
55. Daugirdas JT, Depner TA, Greene T, Levin NW, Chertow GM, Rocco MV. Standard Kt/Vurea: a method of calculation that includes effects of fluid removal and residual kidney clearance. Kidney Int. 2010;77(7):637–44.
56. Mean? WdaADditE, Usefulness of Kt/V FSaIDiEP.
57. Nowson C, O'Connell S. Protein requirements and recommendations for older people: a review. Nutrients. 2015;7(8):6874–99.
58. Wong J, Vilar E, Davenport A, Farrington K. Incremental haemodialysis. Nephrol Dial Transplant. 2015;30(10):1639–48.
59. Obi Y, Streja E, Rhee CM, Ravel V, Amin AN, Cupisti A, et al. Incremental hemodialysis, residual kidney function, and mortality risk in incident dialysis patients: a cohort study. Am J Kidney Dis. 2016;68(2):256–65.
60. Mathew AT, Obi Y, Rhee CM, Chou JA, Kalantar-Zadeh K. Incremental dialysis for preserving residual kidney function-does one size fit all when initiating dialysis? Semin Dial. 2018;31(4):343–52.
61. Tinetti ME, Williams CS. Falls, injuries due to falls, and the risk of admission to a nursing home. N Engl J Med. 1997;337(18):1279–84.
62. Kutner NG, Zhang R, Huang Y, Wasse H. Falls among hemodialysis patients: potential opportunities for prevention? Clin Kidney J. 2014;7(3):257–63.
63. Cook WL, Tomlinson G, Donaldson M, Markowitz SN, Naglie G, Sobolev B, et al. Falls and fall-related injuries in older dialysis patients. Clin J Am Soc Nephrol: CJASN. 2006;1(6):1197–204.
64. Farragher J, Rajan T, Chiu E, Ulutas O, Tomlinson G, Cook WL, et al. Equivalent fall risk in elderly patients on hemodialysis and peritoneal dialysis. Perit Dial Int:J Int Soc Perit Dialysis. 2016;36(1):67–70.
65. Abdel-Rahman EM, Yan G, Turgut F, Balogun RA. Long-term morbidity and mortality related to falls in hemodialysis patients: role of age and gender – a pilot study. Nephron Clin Pract. 2011;118(3):c278–84.
66. Murray AM, Seliger S, Lakshminarayan K, Herzog CA, Solid CA. Incidence of stroke before and after dialysis initiation in older patients. J Am Soc Nephrol. 2013;24(7):1166–73.
67. Polinder-Bos HA, Garcia DV. Hemodialysis induces an acute decline in cerebral blood flow in elderly patients. J Am Soc Nephrol. 2018;29(4):1317–25.
68. Kurella Tamura M, Yaffe K. Dementia and cognitive impairment in ESRD: diagnostic and therapeutic strategies. Kidney Int. 2011;79(1):14–22.
69. Wolfgram DF, Szabo A, Murray AM, Whittle J. Risk of dementia in peritoneal dialysis patients compared with hemodialysis patients. Perit Dialysis Int: J Int Soc Perit Dial. 2015;35(2):189–98.

Frailty Among Elderly Patients on Chronic Maintenance Hemodialysis for ESRD: Not Simply a Matter of Chronological Age

11

Macaulay Amechi Chukwukadibia Onuigbo and Nneoma Agbasi

Introduction: Definition of Frailty

Frailty is a medical syndrome that is characterized by diminished strength, endurance, and reduced physiologic function, and it increases an individual's vulnerability for loss of independence and death [1]. Frailty is a clinical state in which there is an increase in an individual's vulnerability for developing increased dependency and/or mortality when exposed to a stressor [1]. There are several measures of frailty in clinical medicine.

They include the Fried phenotype scale and the 7-point Clinical Frailty Scale (CFS) developed by The Canadian Society of Health and Aging [2, 3].

In the Fried phenotype scale, frailty was defined as a clinical syndrome in which three or more of the following criteria were present: unintentional weight loss (10 lbs in past year), self-reported exhaustion, weakness (grip strength), slow walking speed, and low physical activity (Table 11.1) [2]. For the Clinical Frailty Scale, the following were the 7-point categories of frailty: (1) very fit; (2) well without active disease; (3) well with treated comorbid disease; (4) apparently vulnerable; (5) mildly frail; (6) moderately frail; and (7) severely frail (Table 11.2) [3].

Besides, the prevalence of frailty is considerably higher among patients on hemodialysis than among community-dwelling elders: more than five times as high as community-dwelling older adults, at 30–42% [4, 5]. Furthermore, frail patients are at higher risk of hospitalization and mortality than nonfrail patients [5, 6]. Indeed, a higher severity of frailty as defined by the Clinical Frailty Scale (CFS) score at dialysis initiation has been demonstrated to be associated with higher

M. A. C. Onuigbo (✉)
The Robert Larner, M.D. College of Medicine, University of Vermont, Burlington, VT, USA

College of Business, University of Wisconsin MBA Consortium, Eau Claire, WI, USA

N. Agbasi
NELFT Quality Improvement Programme, NELFT NHS Foundation Trust, Basildon, Essex, UK

C. G. Musso et al. (eds.), *Clinical Nephrogeriatrics*,
https://doi.org/10.1007/978-3-030-18711-8_11

Table 11.1 Fried frailty phenotype criteria

Domains	Definition
Weight loss	≥10 lb (4.5 kg) of unintentional weight loss in last 12 months
Weakness	Grip strength in the lowest 20% at baseline, adjusted to gender and body mass index
Poor endurance and energy	Self-report exhaustion
Slowness	Walking time/15 ft (4.5 m)—slowest 20% The slowest 20%, adjusting to gender and standing height
Low physical activity level	Kilocalories expended per week—lowest 20%

Frail: 3 or more domains
Prefrail or intermediate: 1 or 2 domains
Robust: no domain

Table 11.2 Clinical frailty scale criteria

1. Very fit	People who are robust, active, energetic, and motivated. These people commonly exercise regularly. They are among the fittest for their age
2. Well fit	People who have no active disease, symptoms but are less fit than category one. Often they exercise or are very active occasionally
3. Managing well	People whose medical problems are well controlled, but are not regularly active beyond routine walking
4. Vulnerable	While not dependent on others for daily help, often symptoms limit activities. A common complaint is being "slowed up" and/or being tired during the day
5. Mildly frail	These people often have more evident slowing and need help in high orders (finances, medication, transportation, heavy housework)
6. Moderately frail	People need help with all outdoor activities. Indoors they need help with housekeeping, and often have problems with stairs. They also need help with bathing and might need minimal assistance with dressing
7. Severely frail	Completely dependent for personal care, from either cause (physical or cognitive). Even so, they seem stable and not at high risk of dying

If dementia is present, the degree of frailty usually corresponds to the degree of dementia

Mild dementia: includes forgetting the details of recent events though still remembering the event itself, repeating the same question/story and social withdrawal

Moderate dementia: recent memory is very impaired, even though they seemingly can remember their past life events well. They can do personal care with prompting

Severe dementia: they cannot do personal care without help

mortality [7]. Moreover, overall, there is a general tendency to associate frailty simply with aging. Indeed, de Labra in a recent published study, the VERISAÚDE study, introduced frailty as a multidimensional clinical geriatric syndrome [8].

In this chapter, without prejudice to the foregoing discussion about frailty, we would present evidence from the Mayo Clinic Health System, Wisconsin, Hemodialysis Program, that frailty sometimes could be very dissociated with age and that octogenarians can indeed present with minimal frailty scores and have a sustainable and good quality life on outpatient maintenance in-center hemodialysis. We shall present clinical summaries of three patients all aged >65 years who were in our hemodialysis program and who exhibited excellent quality of life outcomes while on maintenance hemodialysis.

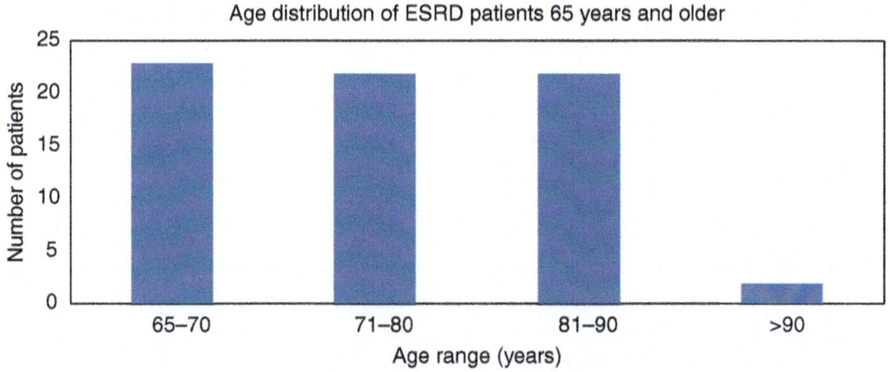

Fig. 11.1 Age distribution of the 69 ESRD patients aged ≥65 years in August 2017

Number of Patients Aged 65 Years and Older on Maintenance Outpatient In-Center Hemodialysis in August 2017 at the Mayo Clinic Health System Hemodialysis Units, in Wisconsin, USA

The first author was an attending nephrologist at the Mayo Clinic Health System Hemodialysis Program, Wisconsin (WI), USA, from September 2002 to January 2018.

We had completed a one-time cross-sectional assessment of all the end-stage renal disease (ESRD) patients on maintenance outpatient in-center hemodialysis in all four Hemodialysis Units in Eau Claire, WI (2), in Barron, WI (1), and in Menomonie, WI (1). Specifically, on August 27, 2017, of the 139 listed patients on maintenance outpatient hemodialysis in all four hemodialysis units, 69 (50%) were 65 years of age or older. They consisted of 43 males and 26 females; mean age 75.8 ± 7.8 (Standard Deviation, SD) years, range 65–92 years. They had been on hemodialysis for a mean of 45.8 ± 37.4 months (SD), range 1–162 months. Age at first hemodialysis treatment for these 69 patients was 71.9 ± 8.4 years (SD), range 53–87 years.

Figure 11.1 below shows the age distribution of the 69 patients who were aged 65 years and older in August 2017.

We shall now present three of these older ESRD patients aged 80 years and older as at August 2017 who despite the older age were still able to continue with outpatient maintenance in-center hemodialysis while maintaining a near-normal quality of life.

Case Reports

We present below brief synopses of three ESRD patients currently aged 80 years or older, as at January 2018 at the Mayo Clinic Dialysis Services in Northwestern Wisconsin, revealing the spectrum of quality of life/wellness associated with ongoing renal replacement therapy (RRT) for end-stage renal disease (ESRD) despite advanced age.

1. A is a Caucasian female patient, now aged 80 years as at January 2018, and had otherwise been on dialysis for nearly 10 years. She started hemodialysis in September 2010 for ESRD. She has a past medical history that included hypertension, obesity, type II diabetes, non-ST acute myocardial infarction in April 2011, coronary artery bypass graft (CABG) procedure in January 2005, redo sternotomy with one vessel CABG and aortic valve replacement for severe aortic stenosis in September 2011, against a background for a prior left nephrectomy over 40 years ago for recurrent urinary tract infection, recurrent kidney stones and a nonfunctional left kidney.

   She was switched to peritoneal dialysis in 2012 by choice. We note that sometime in September 2013, while on peritoneal dialysis (PD), she had experienced an unusual set of hypersensitivity reactions to Icodextrin that manifested as increasing lightheadedness, fatigue, exertional dyspnea, early-morning flu-like symptoms of the upper respiratory tract, dysgeusia, and hypotension [9]. She subsequently continued to do well on night-cycled PD without Icodextrin but was returned to outpatient in-center hemodialysis in June 2014 following repeated episodes of recurrent peritonitis.

   The patient, presently at age 80 years, remains otherwise cheerful, lives an active life, and in January 2018 was out shopping for a replacement new car, assisted by one of her grown daughters. She travels often to visit with her several grandchildren. More recently, the spouse was diagnosed with multiple myeloma and was started on chemotherapy and the patient is now a caregiver. She otherwise has an excellent quality of life as an octogenarian despite having been on maintenance RRT in the last 7 years for ESRD. She has remained very functional (Clinical Frailty Scale score of 3—well with treated comorbid disease), frailty phenotype 1, drives herself to and from dialysis, and has been the caretaker for the sick spouse in the last several months.
2. B is a Caucasian male patient, who encountered our Nephrology Service in July 2012 following a fall and a right hip fracture when he was shown to have experienced worsening renal failure with hyperkalemia and metabolic acidosis against a background of obstructive uropathy, hypertension, sleep apnea, chronic obstructive pulmonary disease (COPD), gout, previous kidney stones, anemia, and secondary hyperparathyroidism. The hip fracture was managed nonoperatively, and in mid-July 2012, he started hemodialysis initially via a tunneled dialysis catheter and subsequently via an arteriovenous (AV) fistula.

   He has now dialyzed for over 6 years and continues to have a good quality of life. He has always remained very functional (Clinical Frailty Scale score of 3—well with treated comorbid disease), and frailty phenotype 1. Now at 92 years, he remains very functional and still enjoys the great Wisconsin outdoors, and as at the last summer in 2017, he was still able to drive and take out his boat once a week sailing in the local waters and still carried out some fishing.

3. C is a Caucasian male patient who had been followed up in our Nephrology Clinic for nearly a decade [10]. He is an ex-smoker with a history of hypertension and had otherwise stable CKD V for about 8 years between 2005 and 2013, with a serum creatinine that ranged between 4.0 and 5.0 mg/dL (eGFR 8–14 mL/min per 1.73 m^2 BSA). During this period, he had remained asymptomatic from a renal point of view. Indeed, he had an AV fistula created in June 2004 and this AV fistula was revised in January 2006 due to poor maturation in anticipation of the need for renal replacement therapy. Nevertheless, he had become symptomatic in July 2013 with nausea, vomiting, and anorexia and has been on maintenance hemodialysis since August 2013 via his AV fistula. He was aged 85 years in August 2017, 4 years later, and was doing generally well. He lived with his spouse who at the time drove him back and forth for his hemodialysis treatments. He was still able to do some farm work at his farm between hemodialysis treatments.

Conclusions

Whereas frailty is significantly more common among the hemodialysis population and commonly associated with ageing, we have demonstrated in this report the reality that ageing alone is not the sine qua non lone determinant of frailty. Older patients, far into their 80s, could still live a near-normal life while on maintenance hemodialysis. The three patients described above, despite being 80 years or older, demonstrate evidence of mildly frail scores when subjected to either the Fried phenotype scale or the 7-point CFS developed by The Canadian Society of Health and Aging [2, 3].

Our message therefore is that frailty scores be utilized very early in the assessment of patients, both old and younger, who are about to transition to maintenance hemodialysis. Recently, there has been an increasing interest in the trauma of dialysis initiation which is addressed below.

Postscript: The Trauma of Dialysis Initiation

Recently, there has been an increasing interest in the trauma of dialysis initiation. Within nephrology, clinicians do not have a ready perspective, or even a language, with which to understand these turbulent transitions [11]. The evolution to dialysis therapy is a fragmenting experience, disturbing previously unexamined internal and external cohesions [11]. Externally, profound shifts in old and new interpersonal connections may distort one's sense of self [11]. The premises on which intimate relationships were built become warped [12]. Furthermore, the tensions introduced by altered roles and innate anxieties, which now place more demands on others, may lead to interpersonal discord [13].

From the foregoing, even for a younger nonfrail ESRD patient, the decision to initiate and continue hemodialysis must be a joint one between the medical team led by the nephrologist, the patient, and the patient's family. These exigencies of the trauma of dialysis initiation and maintenance are exaggerated and aggravated several-fold for the frail ESRD patient. We posit that frailty becomes a major consideration in the decision-making process to initiate dialysis for ESRD patients. But again, we must insist that frailty exists in both the old and the young and we conclude that frailty is not simply a matter of chronological age. Indeed, Alfaadhel et al. in a study of frailty and mortality among ESRD patients, published in 2015, showed that age at the start of dialysis did not modify the association between frailty and outcome; the mortality hazards ratio (HR) was comparable whether young or old [7].

We encourage the assessment of frailty scores as an additional clinical tool to help in the decision-making process of if and when to start or continue hemodialysis treatment, whether in the older or younger patients.

References

1. Morley JE, Vellas B, van Kan GA, Anker SD, Bauer JM, Bernabei R, et al. Frailty consensus: a call to action. J Am Med Dir Assoc. 2013;14(6):392–7. https://doi.org/10.1016/j.jamda.2013.03.022.
2. Fried LP, Tangen CM, Walston J, Newman AB, Hirsch C, Gottdiener J, Seeman T, Tracy R, Kop WJ, Burke G, McBurnie MA, Cardiovascular Health Study Collaborative Research Group. Frailty in older adults: evidence for a phenotype. J Gerontol A Biol Sci Med Sci. 2001;56:M146–56.
3. Rockwood K, Song X, MacKnight C, Bergman H, Hogan DB, McDowell I, Mitnitski A. A global clinical measure of fitness and frailty in elderly people. CMAJ. 2005;173: 489–95.
4. Johansen KL, Dalrymple LS, Delgado C, Kaysen GA, Kornak J, Grimes B, Chertow GM. Association between body composition and frailty among prevalent hemodialysis patients: a US Renal Data System special study. J Am Soc Nephrol. 2014;25:381–9.
5. McAdams-DeMarco MA, Law A, Salter ML, Boyarsky B, Gimenez L, Jaar BG, Walston JD, Segev DL. Frailty as a novel predictor of mortality and hospitalization in individuals of all ages undergoing hemodialysis. J Am Geriatr Soc. 2013;61:896–901.
6. Johansen KL, Dalrymple LS, Glidden D, Delgado C, Kaysen GA, Grimes B, Chertow GM. Association of performance-based and self-reported function-based definitions of frailty with mortality among patients receiving hemodialysis. Clin J Am Soc Nephrol. 2016;11:626–32.
7. Alfaadhel TA, Soroka SD, Kiberd BA, Landry D, Moorhouse P, Tennankore KK. Frailty and mortality in dialysis: evaluation of a clinical frailty scale. Clin J Am Soc Nephrol. 2015;10(5):832–40. https://doi.org/10.2215/CJN.07760814. Epub 2015 Mar 4
8. de Labra C, Maseda A, Lorenzo-López L, López-López R, Buján A, Rodríguez-Villamil JL, Millán-Calenti JC. Social factors and quality of life aspects on frailty syndrome in community-dwelling older adults: the VERISAÚDE study. BMC Geriatr. 2018;18(1):66. https://doi.org/10.1186/s12877-018-0757-8.
9. Onuigbo MA. Unexplained hypotension and exertional dyspnea in a night-cycled peritoneal dialysis patient – a rare form of icodextrin hypersensitivity. Adv Perit Dial. 2014;30:87–9.
10. Onuigbo MA, Agbasi N. Chronic kidney disease prediction is an inexact science: the concept of "progressors" and "nonprogressors". World J Nephrol. 2014;3(3):31–49. https://doi.org/10.5527/wjn.v3.i3.31.

11. Hercz G. The trauma of dialysis initiation. J Am Soc Nephrol. 2017;28(10):2835–7. https://doi.org/10.1681/ASN.2017020212. Epub 2017 Aug 28
12. White Y, Grenyer BF. The biopsychosocial impact of end-stage renal disease: the experience of dialysis patients and their partners. J Adv Nurs. 1999;30:1312–20.
13. Cukor D, Cohen SD, Peterson RA, Kimmel PL. Psychosocial aspects of chronic disease: ESRD as a paradigmatic illness. J Am Soc Nephrol. 2007;18:3042–55.

Peritoneal Dialysis in the Elderly Patient

12

Clare B. Jones and Joanne M. Bargman

Dialysis in the Elderly Population

The general population is getting older, and dialysis patients are ageing too. In the United States, end-stage renal disease (ESRD) prevalence per million is highest in the 65–74-year age group and the highest incidence rate is found in patients aged 75 and over [1] (Figs. 12.1 and 12.2). In short, the elderly are the largest group of patients on dialysis. This is a trend seen throughout the developed world. Indeed, in some European regions, the median age of the dialysis population is now over 70 [2].

The decision whether to commence renal replacement therapy (RRT) or to pursue a conservative nondialytic management path in elderly patients is complex. The

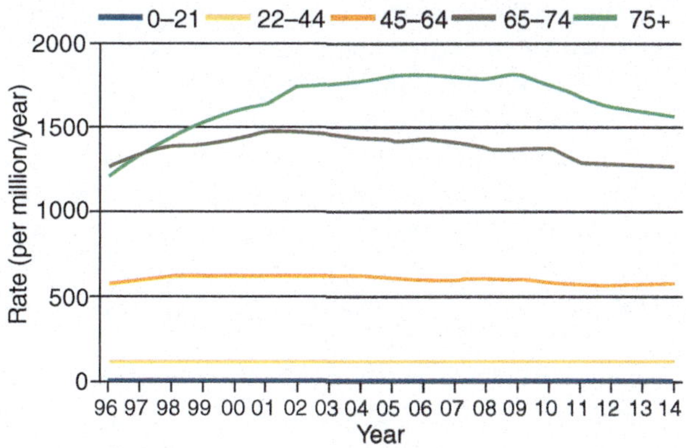

Fig. 12.1 Trends in adjusted ESRD incidence rate (per million/year, of ESRD, by age group, in the US population [1]

C. B. Jones · J. M. Bargman (✉)
University Health Network and University of Toronto, Toronto, ON, Canada
e-mail: joanne.bargman@uhn.ca

C. G. Musso et al. (eds.), *Clinical Nephrogeriatrics*,
https://doi.org/10.1007/978-3-030-18711-8_12

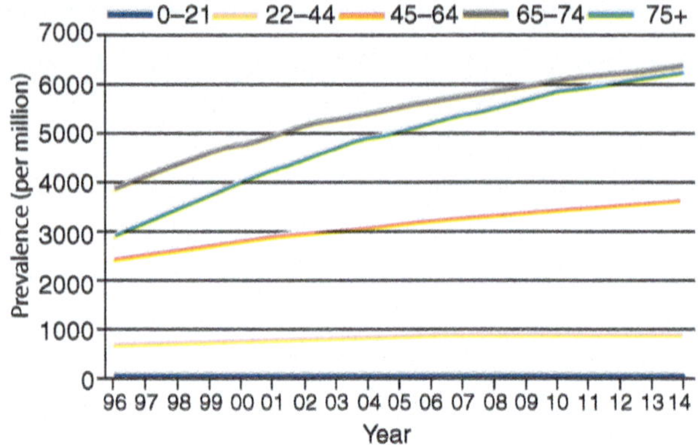

Fig. 12.2 Trends in the adjusted prevalence (per million) of ESRD, by age group, in the US population [1]

(often) competing factors of poor long-term prognosis coupled with the desire to control symptoms while maintaining quality of life can create a challenging discussion with the patient and family. As clinicians, we should always strive to maintain patient autonomy while being mindful of individual family dynamics and cultural backgrounds.

Where Are We Now?

A longitudinal study by Jain et al. reviewed data from 130 countries from 1996 to 2008 and reported that 11% of chronic dialysis patients around the world are treated with peritoneal dialysis, with increasing prevalence of utilization in developing countries [3]. However, the proportion of dialysis patients managed with PD is declining in the developed world. Health care financing and delivery play an important role in determining dialysis modality. Countries with private dialysis providers tend to use PD for a smaller proportion of patients compared to countries where publicly-funded providers predominate.

In most countries, elderly patients who commence RRT are much more likely to be commenced on hemodialysis (HD) than peritoneal dialysis (PD) [2]. This is despite PD offering comparable medical outcomes and potentially a better quality of life than hemodialysis, as will be discussed. In the United States, the prevalence of PD use is relatively low in the general dialysis population. However, this situation is further exacerbated in the elderly. USRDS data reveals that only 6.3% of the 65–74 age group and 5.6% of the over 75 age group are on PD as their mode of RRT [1].

In countries where PD is utilized more widely, such as in Canada, Australia, and parts of Europe, the trend of lower PD use in the elderly population persists. For example, in Denmark, Belgium, and Holland, 13–25% of dialysis patients aged 65–74 years and 9–13% of those aged over 75 start on PD compared to 20–41% of patients aged between 45 and 64 (Fig. 12.3) [4].

In contrast, France has a well-developed PD program for older patients where assisted peritoneal dialysis (usually CAPD) is frequently employed. Community

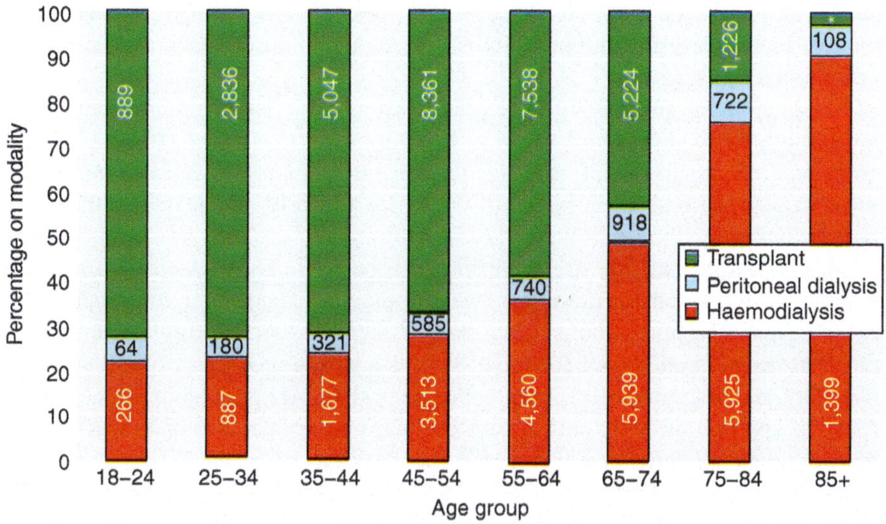

Fig. 12.3 Treatment modality distribution by age in prevalent RRT patients on 31/12/2014. (UK Renal Registry [5])

nurses utilize a "non-disconnect" UV flash system as it shortens the time needed for the nursing visit. The nurse can call the patient or relative to start the drain procedure so that on arrival, the nurse can remove the old bag and connect the new one leaving the fluid to drain in and the patient to fold up the bag [6]. In 2006, 54% of males and 59% of females on PD in France were over the age of 70. Other countries such as Hong Kong have adopted a "PD first" policy where PD is the default first-line RRT modality unless there is a contraindication or the patient wishes to pay for hemodialysis. As a consequence, PD is the modality used by 75.6% of the dialysis population. In Hong Kong, this policy has been in effect since 1985 and has proven to be cost-effective. Paradoxically, in other countries this *may* be the case from a payer's perspective but the use of PD may offer lower revenue or income margins for the provider [7].

Why Is PD Generally Underutilized in the Elderly?

PD has advantages for the elderly patient, not least the fact that it can be undertaken at home and is a gentle, continuous therapy. However, its relative low use compared to hemodialysis in this demographic is not congruent with these potential benefits.

How Are the Elderly Different?

The elderly patient with end-stage renal disease (ESRD) almost invariably has considerable co-morbidity—in part related to their renal disease and increased cardiovascular burden, but also secondary to the conditions affecting many older people, such as arthritic and mobility issues, cognitive impairment, and hearing or visual impairment [4].

The elderly are more likely to be prescribed multiple medications, often suffering the effects of polypharmacy, drug interactions, and adverse effects. To compound matters, psychosocial issues such as housing problems, financial compromise, social isolation, and depression are often particularly prevalent in the older population.

In addition, the elderly are more likely to be *frail*. The concept of frailty far exceeds its colloquial constraints of "weak and delicate" and is an important medical description which encompasses a state of increased vulnerability with reduced physical reserve and loss of function [8]. It is a strong predictor of morbidity and mortality and is known to be more common in the CKD population. Recognizing frailty is key to improving patient care and helps ensure patients and their families feel confident about the care their loved ones receive.

The NECOSAD study was a large prospective cohort study carried out in the Netherlands. The relationship between dialysis modality and health-related quality of life was explored. It reported that 50% of dialysis patients would choose PD if given a chance. However, patients over 70 were six times more likely to choose HD compared to patients aged 18–40. The factors that were associated with not choosing PD were older age, being female and living alone. The study also highlighted that patients who had received predialysis care were more likely to choose PD [9].

The use of PD in the elderly is likely limited by numerous factors. These include:

Health Policy

This varies among countries but greatly impacts dialysis trends. As previously discussed, high use of PD is found in countries such as Hong Kong where a "PD first policy" exists, whereas in the United States, peritoneal dialysis is reimbursed differently than hemodialysis [7].

Physician Bias

In many parts of the world, physicians have minimal experience with peritoneal dialysis which can significantly impact utilization. This factor is exemplified by the wide variation of PD uptake between different units even within the same country and payor system. Nephrologists with more training and experience with PD are more likely to effectively manage peritoneal catheter insertion and malfunction, volume status, infectious complications, and cardiovascular disease.

Patient Contraindications

Medical contraindications (although seldom absolute contraindications) include previous lower abdominal surgery, severe obesity, dexterity problems, and significant sensory impairment without a willing partner (although the latter could be overcome by the use of assisted PD) [10].

Psychosocial concerns include poor housing with limited storage space, anxiety regarding the ability to learn a new technique, the fear of undertaking dialysis at home and cognitive impairment.

There is some suggestion that the elderly are more likely to "crash land" onto dialysis. In other words, they present to a nephrologist late in the course of their disease affording minimal time for prognostic discussions and management planning. Roderick et al. conducted a retrospective study of 361 patients accepted for renal replacement therapy. Thirty-five percent were referred within 4 months of their needing to start dialysis and 23% within 1 month. These patients were found to be older and with more co-morbidity and had a high 6-month mortality rate [11]. Unfortunately, this group of patients is almost invariably commenced on hemodialysis and is likely to remain on this modality indefinitely.

Is Peritoneal Dialysis "Better"?

Over the past 30 years, numerous retrospective survival studies have been published comparing in-centre hemodialysis to peritoneal dialysis with variable and often conflicting results. Suffice to say; in the modern era survival is very comparable between the two modalities. However, we could, in this era of an ageing co-morbid population where prognosis in the elderly on ESRD is extremely poor, provocatively ask the question, who cares about length of survival [12]?

A large epidemiological study by Bloembergen et al. in 1995 paved the way for an overwhelming preference for hemodialysis as the dialysis modality of choice, particularly in the US population [13]. It was based on USRDS data and showed higher mortality rates in the PD population, particularly in older diabetics. Later work by Heaf et al. suggested that PD may confer an initial survival advantage which then resumes equality with hemodialysis after 2 years [14]. This has been explained by the preservation of residual renal function for longer in patients on peritoneal dialysis which in itself is known to confer survival benefits. Additional theories have stated that a "sicker" cohort of patients tend to be cordoned onto hemodialysis from the beginning. In other words, the initial survival advantage of PD is really the result of an accelerated early mortality on hemodialysis, especially in those starting with a venous catheter [15, 16].

These and other similar studies suffer from inherent methodological issues; conclusions are frequently based on complex statistics, subgroup analysis and are guilty of selection bias. It is considered impossible to conduct a randomized study on such an issue, and appropriately so. Patients value their autonomy and a decision regarding dialysis modality is clearly a personal and subjective one.

More recent work has focused specifically on elderly patients and attempts have been made to incorporate complex issues such as quality of life factors and examination of frailty. The North Thames dialysis study (NTDS) was the first prospective study looking at incident and prevalent elderly patients (over the age of 70) on dialysis. Mortality was not affected by dialysis modality and adjusted analyses also showed no significant differences in quality of life between PD and HD patients [17].

In the Broadening Options for Long-term Dialysis in the Elderly (BOLDE) study, 140 prevalent dialysis patients aged 65 and over were recruited with the intention of determining quality of life (amongst other variables) in patients on peritoneal dialysis compared to hemodialysis. Fifty percent of the cross-sectional cohort was on peritoneal dialysis. Illness intrusion rating scores (IIRS) were significantly *lower* in the peritoneal dialysis group. The IIRS assesses the impact of chronic illness on 13 life domains including health, diet, active recreation, relationship with partner and family relations [4].

How Important Is Survival?

As we have transitioned into the next millennium, our attitudes regarding medical care have, rightly, become more patient-focused. This ethos is particularly apt in the context of our ageing and co-morbid population. One could question why survival in terms of mortality rates on dialysis matters and it is becoming evident that patients themselves often do not care about this metric at all. If a survival advantage *does* exist for hemodialysis, any extended survival is likely to be spent in the hemodialysis unit.

Contrary to what may historically have been important to physicians with regard to their patients, a study by Manns et al. in Canada sought to identify concerns and unanswered questions important to patients nearing or on dialysis and to their families. The top 10 questions included issues such as access to transplantation and how intractable itch can be treated. There was only one question pertaining to survival in relation to modality but this only made it to the top 30 and was in the context of quality of life improvements [18].

Ahmed et al. demonstrated that independence is greatly valued in the elderly population. Patients are willing to initiate dialysis therapy as long as independence is sustained and symptoms are alleviated [19].

What Are the Benefits of PD in the Elderly?

Arguably PD is the superior dialysis therapy for both the "fit" and the "frail" elderly patient. At the fitter end of the spectrum, PD enables easier travel and encourages independence whereas for frailer patients, assistance is becoming increasingly available. As described above, PD appears to have, at least, comparable survival rates compared to hemodialysis and offers quality of life benefits. Other potential benefits are discussed below.

No Dependence on Vascular Access

Vascular access is the Achilles heel of hemodialysis. There is a high rate of fistula maturation failure in the elderly. Consequently, there is a higher rate of central venous catheter use which incurs issues with high infection risk and subsequent mortality [20]. A study by Perl et al. looked at mortality rates in hemodialysis versus peritoneal dialysis and found that mortality on hemodialysis was significantly worse in the 1st year when the patient had a central line as vascular access [15]. On the other hand, the frequently quoted mantra of "fistula first" may not always be appropriate in the elderly, and decisions regarding vascular access should be made on an individual patient basis.

Reduced Myocardial Stunning

Although cardiovascular related morbidity and mortality appear to be similar in hemodialysis and PD, there is evidence that PD is not associated with myocardial stunning [21]. In hemodialysis, hemodynamic changes can precipitate subclinical myocardial ischemia which negatively impacts morbidity. There is no evidence that this positively affects outcomes in PD as studies have been small and there are likely multiple conflicting and converging factors. However, at least in the elderly, the lack of regional wall motion abnormalities identified during PD may at least suggest that it is a more tolerable therapy for our frail elderly. The large swings in blood pressure and hemodynamic instability that are frequently experienced during a hemodialysis session are not usually an issue during the continuous and gentler nature of PD treatment.

This may also tie in to the evidence that "recovery time" after a conventional hemodialysis session (even for younger patients) may be as long as 6 h [22]. If travelling time to and from the hemodialysis unit 3 days a week is taken into consideration, it is understandable why conventional hemodialysis is associated with a greater degree of illness intrusion compared to PD.

Lower Incidence of De Novo Dementia

Similarly to cardiovascular disease, cerebrovascular disease and cognitive impairment is also more prevalent in the ESRD population compared to the general population. A large retrospective US cohort study by Wolfgram et al. evaluated the effect of initial dialysis modality on incidence of dementia. They found that patients who started RRT on PD had a 25% lower risk of acquiring a diagnosis of dementia compared to those on HD, despite adjusting for other risk factors/contributors such as age and diabetes [23]. Similarly to theories explaining myocardial stunning in hemodialysis, it has been postulated that the fluctuations in volume status and blood pressure that occur during HD can result in repeated episodes of cerebral ischemic injury.

There is also evidence that the incidence of subdural hematoma is higher in patients on hemodialysis which contributes to cerebrovascular morbidity and mortality [24].

Logistical Benefits

PD is a home-based therapy, meaning that there are few transportation costs. Additionally, for the elderly patient, travelling is frequently uncomfortable and time consuming.

Nutritional Benefits?

Nutrition is a vital component of a patient's well-being, particularly in the elderly dialysis patient. Malnutrition is common in dialysis patients and PD has some potential benefits with regard to this. Depending on the type of PD undertaken, the patient may absorb between 300 and 450 kcal per day via their dialysis. However, this may also be an undesirable effect for some resulting in unwanted weight gain [25].

A competing risk with the potential nutritional gain is the loss of protein that can occur via the dialysate. For example, APD has been shown to result in 10 g of protein loss each day [26]. Consequently, patients on PD are generally found to have lower serum albumin levels compared to patients on hemodialysis. Hypoalbuminemia has a striking correlation with mortality. However, a large cross-sectional study showed that the equivalent mortality risk in people on PD compared with HD occurred at different albumin thresholds; albumin levels were 0.2–0.3 g/dl lower in the PD patients [27].

PD solutions using amino acids instead of dextrose have been proposed as a treatment for protein malnutrition in PD patients. It is a 1.1% amino acid containing dialysate and has similar effective tonicity to a 1.5% glucose dialysis solution. It is most appropriately used for a 4–6 h dwell so could be used as part of a CAPD regimen or for the last fill/day dwell in APD. It has been shown to improve some nutritional markers but is most effective if the patient consumes calories whilst the fluid is indwelling. Since most malnutrition is the result of inflammation and not insufficient access to nutrients, the results have been disappointing. In addition, metabolic acidosis can supervene with potential catabolic effects [28].

Promoting PD in the Elderly

Many nephrology centres now pursue a multidisciplinary approach to patients who are predialysis but have progressively worsening renal function. This enables nonbiased information to be provided and patients given the opportunity to consider and decide upon dialysis versus nondialytic care and, if dialysis, home dialysis versus in-centre, and finally the dialysis modality. Peer support is also offered in some programs. The cognitive abilities of patients should be borne in mind during such discussions as well as the possible influence of uremia.

A retrospective study by Goovaerts et al. evaluated the influence of a predialysis education program on the mode of renal replacement therapy. This comprised talks from experienced nurses and the use of audiovisual tapes [29]. They found that a high percentage of patients opted for a self-care RRT modality following the education program [29].

Another study by Chanouzas et al. questioned 118 patients regarding the factors contributing to their choice of dialysis modality. It also highlighted that predialysis education encourages patients to choose self-care therapies. Furthermore, there was an overwhelming association of having a strong social support network and being functionally able, with choosing PD, emphasizing the need for assisted PD. The study helped to elucidate important factors for a dialysis education program including good quality information provision, written and easy to understand information, an education day and sufficient time for decision making. The study also focused on the importance of lifestyle preservation and coping skills [30].

As discussed previously, "crash-landers" are invariably commenced onto hemodialysis. However, in centres with willing surgeons or nephrologists capable of inserting PD catheters, initiating emergency PD in these circumstances should not be discounted.

Training and Assessment of Older Patients

Careful assessment of the potential PD candidate is essential and includes psychological, social and cognitive assessment in addition to consideration of medical issues. The utilization of the multidisciplinary team is key and may include the skills and knowledge of a social worker, geriatrician and psychiatrist.

Psychosocial Barriers

Accommodation issues including limited storage space, financial problems, transport limitations and functional impairment such as impaired dexterity can all significantly impact choice of modality. It is important to appreciate how involved families are likely to be in the care of the patient.

Cognitive Barriers

This is a particularly important as it may impact on an individual's ability to perform PD independently and safely, to comply with therapy and also whether they will even tolerate dialysis at all.

A MOCA (Montreal Cognitive Assessment) is a simple tool that can be performed in 10 minutes and can provide a quick initial screening method [31].

Medical Barriers

Have been discussed previously in "patient contraindications."

Training the elderly patient may take more time than for younger patients. Trainers should aim to be flexible; shorter more frequent training sessions may be appropriate. Educational materials may require adaptation such as the use of larger fonts or pictures to explain procedures. Aids such as clamp adaptors for those with dexterity problems can prove helpful.

MATCH-D

The Method to Assess Treatment Choices for Home Dialysis (MATCH-D) was developed by the Medical Education Institute, Inc., for Home Dialysis Central (www.HomeDialysis.org) to help nephrologists and dialysis staffs identify and assess candidates for home dialysis therapies. It is a useful "checklist" or aide memoire to refer to when assessing a predialysis patient.

Method to Assess Treatment Choices for Home Dialysis (MATCH-D)

This figure is reproduced with permission from the Medical Education Institute

Strongly encourage PD if a patient

- Is interested in doing dialysis at home
- Wants control of their health
- Is new to dialysis or has a failing renal transplant
- Is unhappy in the in-center environment
- Wants or needs a flexible schedule
- Wants or needs to travel
- Is a caregiver
- Lives far from the dialysis center and/or has ureliable transportation
- Has the manual dexterity to button a shirt
- Has the mental acumen to use an ATM
- I las hemodynamics that make in-center HD difficult (diabetic neuropathy, amyloidosis, severe ischemic cardiomyopathy, cirrhosis)
- Is no longer able to do HHD but would like to continue doing dialysis at home

Encourage PD after assessing & eliminating barriers

- Limited vision: consider using assist devices
- Hearing impairment: consider using light or vibrations for alarms
- Illiteracy: consider using pictures/videos
- Inability to understand language of intruction: use pictures/videos or an interpreter
- Cognitive impairment that inhibits short-term memory and ability to learn and/or make decisions related to treatment: assess availablity of assistance
- Angry or disruptive behavior: consider whether PD may help by providing increased control of their health
- Neuropathy in both hands or no use of hands: consider using assist devices
- Frailty: assess availability of assistance
- Poor personal hygiene: provide education
- Simple abdominal surgeries: consider laparoscopic PD catheter insertion
- Obese: consider using a presternal catheter, optimize dialysis prescription
- Colostomy: consider using a presternal catheter
- Large polycystic kidneys or back pain: consider night cycler with dry days or low volumes during daytime
- Unreliable electricity: consider CAPD
- Limited storage space at home: consider increased frequency of deliveries
- Pets at home: keep out of room during connections
- Lives in a nursing home: assess feasibility of training nursing home staff to do PD

May not be able to do PD

- Uncontrolled psychiatric symptoms (anxiety, psychosis)
- Active chemical dependency (alcohol, drugs) that impairs ability to asses health needs
- Inability to communicate (stroke or vegetative state), or significant cognitive impairment with no available helper
- Uncontrolled seizure disorder
- Homeless or hazardous home environment
- Inability to maintain personal hygiene (even after education)
- Absence of or unreliable electricity for CAPD and unable to do CAPD

PD Catheter Insertion

In recent times, the options for peritoneal dialysis catheter placement have broadened. Depending on the centre, open surgical, peritoneoscopic, laparoscopic, fluoroscopic, or the percutaneous Seldinger approach of peritoneal catheter insertion may be employed.

In the elderly patient, PD catheter insertion is not an insignificant undertaking. The patient may be on antiplatelet medications or anticoagulants and is less likely to tolerate the often heavy duty bowel preparation.

Percutaneous approaches obviate the use of general anesthesia and the risks that this entails, particularly for the elderly morbid patient. In some centres, nephrologists are undertaking these procedures at the bedside which can markedly reduce wait times for catheter insertion. Clearly, a percutaneous bedside approach may not be suitable for all patients. For example, those with a history of lower abdominal surgery or significant obesity would be better served with catheter insertion under direct visualization.

Laparoscopic surgery affords additional benefits. It permits the ability for simultaneous omentopexy, rectus sheath tunneling and adhesiolysis for those patients with prior abdominal surgery to maximize catheter function potential.

A meta-analysis by Boujelbane reviewed 13 peritoneal dialysis access studies comparing surgical and percutaneous placement of PD catheters and found no significant difference between rates of catheter dysfunction or in 1-year catheter survival rates [33].

Additionally, the concept of buried PD catheters may be appropriately utilized in the elderly. This is a concept whereby the PD catheter is inserted in advance of clinical need and the external tubing is embedded under the skin in the subcutaneous space. This helps to minimize the risk of a last-minute hemodialysis catheter being placed in the event of a sudden and unexpected change in renal function. It also means that the patient does not necessarily have to commence PD using low volumes as is often the case if the catheter has only just been inserted. However, especially in the elderly population, there may be a measurable number of futile placements, where the patient dies before ever needing dialysis [34].

Specific Considerations in the Elderly: Dialysis Modifications

Unfortunately, an elderly patient with ESRD on dialysis has a fairly dismal prognosis with USRDS data showing that the adjusted survival rate for patients greater than 75 years is 62.5% at 1 year and 17.1% at 5 years [1].

The Aim of PD in the Elderly Should Be Within the Remit of the Individual Patient's Goals of Care

Many of the dialysis guidelines and protocols we work towards in general may not be appropriate for the elderly patient. Parameters such as blood pressure recommendations and dialysis adequacy markers such as Kt/V_{urea} were formulated based on younger cohorts and their relevance and applicability for the elderly is questionable.

Dialysis modifications to consider in the elderly include:

Delayed Start of Dialysis Initiation

There is no good evidence to dictate the optimal dialysis initiation time in the elderly.

Anemia, volume overload and metabolic acidosis can be managed with erythropoietin stimulating agents (ESA's), judicious use of diuretics, salt restriction and sodium bicarbonate before dialysis is commenced.

A prospective study from the NECOSAD group looked at the association between the timing of dialysis initiation and the effect on survival [35]. Thirty-seven percent of the 253 patients started dialysis later than US guidelines advise. Timely starters had a small survival benefit after 3 years on dialysis; however, this was thought to be a reflection of lead time bias rather than a clear survival advantage.

Continuous Automated Peritoneal Dialysis (CAPD) v Automated Peritoneal Dialysis (APD)

The decision regarding whether to opt for CAPD or APD is ultimately patient preference. However, the decision may also be reliant on what assistance is available in the community (see Table 12.1).

Minimizing the Dialysis Prescription

The concept of incremental peritoneal dialysis is gaining momentum in the general dialysis population. It describes the gradual up titration of the dialysis prescription as residual kidney function (RKF) declines over time.

In a not dissimilar fashion, the elderly frail patient may often "get away" with a fairly minimal PD prescription. The elderly may be nutritionally challenged, of low muscle mass and have minimal energy expenditure. Their urea removal and ultrafiltration requirements may not be high and the patient can therefore achieve symptom benefit with fewer hours on dialysis and/or fewer exchanges but with some preservation of quality of life [36].

Table 12.1 Summary Table [32]

	PD advantages	PD disadvantages
Medical	Better preservation of residual kidney function Gentle treatment modality—avoids hemodynamic compromise → potentially less myocardial and cerebral stunning Vascular access not required	Risk of peritonitis, exit site infection, membrane failure Requires surgical procedure to insert PD catheter Inability to "fine tune" fluid removal, particularly in the anuric patient Risk of technique failure
Psychosocial	Performed at home—by patient, family member or nursing staff Less disruption to day-to-day life; particularly for frail patients with cognitive impairment Can continue to travel and engage in social activities Enables treatment flexibility—incremental dialysis, CAPD v APD, days off can be negotiated Avoids long, expensive, uncomfortable travel Fewer hospital visits	Reliance on family, caregivers or nurses to perform dialysis in many cases Treatment burden Less contact with medical staff Home storage space required May promote social isolation and dependence

Indeed as time goes by and the patient ages further, there may be the possibility of reducing dialysis complexity and hours further. The over-riding intention should be effective symptom control rather than a desire to achieve a certain Kt/V_{urea}.

For example, the elderly patient with cardio renal syndrome and resistance to large diuretic doses may benefit from CAPD with two exchanges of icodextrin over each 24 h period. There may also be a case for scheduling a "day off" intermittently in order to provide respite.

Assisted PD

Many older patients are simply not candidates for self-care or autonomous home-based dialysis and multiple studies have highlighted the benefits and successes of assisted peritoneal dialysis.

Assisted PD is available in parts of Europe, Canada and Australasia using health-care workers and also in the Middle East and Asian countries where help is provided by family members. In Canada, assisted APD or CCPD is generally offered and in France, the modality is usually CAPD. In the United States, assisted PD is not reimbursed.

In France, the elderly have been treated with assisted PD for more than a decade. The recent Frail Elderly Patient Outcomes on Dialysis (FEPOD) study suggested that quality of life is similar on assisted PD and in-centre hemodialysis although treatment satisfaction was higher on assisted PD [37]. The French experience also suggests that the cost of assisted PD is equal or even less expensive to that of in-centre hemodialysis. In France, registry data shows that in patients over the age of 75, the median survival for those requiring nursing assistance was 24 months which is similar to that in many parts of the world (the majority of whom would be on hemodialysis) [38].

APD is the most suited PD modality for the elderly requiring assistance as the home care nurse will need to attend the home just once or twice per day. Adequate training is clearly crucial and 24 h back-up from a medical centre is needed.

In France, private nurses provide care for those patients on assisted PD and they are seen by a nephrologist in a clinic every 8 weeks where the PD prescription is reviewed. The private nurses can send patients to the nephrologist on duty whenever necessary. Assisted CAPD is the norm but more places are beginning to offer assisted APD. In the 2010 report from the French Peritoneal Dialysis Registry (RDPLF), 76% of French PD patients over the age of 75 were on assisted PD. The median patient survival was 27.1 months, the median technique survival was 21.4 months and the median peritonitis free survival was 32.1 months [6].

Telemedicine is a growing area that could prove particularly useful in the management of elderly patients. More sophisticated systems including video conferencing and the ability to monitor patients' blood pressure, weight and ultrafiltration rate have been developed. Certain PD machines have programmable data cards—prescribed treatment details can be programmed onto this and data from each dialysis session can be captured. A health professional can access this remotely by modem/broadband; alternatively, the data can be accessed via a disc.

PD in the Nursing Home

PD is particularly appropriate for nursing home patients. The overnight cycler can be utilized and the patient then has time free in the day to partake in activities.

Potential Complications of PD

Peritonitis

Peritonitis is a serious complication of PD. However, it carries less morbidity compared to hemodialysis related central line infections. Studies regarding PD peritonitis in the elderly have revealed mixed findings. Overall, the risk of peritonitis does not appear to be increased in the elderly. For example, RDPLF data shows that the overall risk of peritonitis was not increased in the elderly and actually even lower in older patients compared to younger counterparts in those who have nursing assistance. However, there is evidence that elderly patients have higher short-term mortality rates and, in some cases, higher rates of relapsing peritonitis [39, 40].

Data was analyzed by Nessim et al. from the Baxter POET (Peritonitis Organism Exit Sites Tunnel Infections) database. Age was not associated with peritonitis among patients initiating PD between 2001 and 2005 [41].

Treatment should follow the International Society for Peritoneal Dialysis (ISPD) guidelines. However, antibiotic dosing may require specific attention particularly in frail elderly patients and a conscious observation for antibiotic-related side effects which may be more prevalent and more problematic in this population.

Of note, there is an association between peritonitis due to enteric organisms and severe constipation which is particularly common in older patients.

Exit Site Infections

This is another recognized complication that should be monitored and treated. However, a study by Szeto found that there appears to be a lower risk of exit site infections in the elderly than in younger patients. Whether this is related to fewer PD exchanges and therefore fewer connections and disconnections each day, or the result of reduced physical activity, is unclear [42].

Technique Survival

Observational studies vary in their assessment of this; some work has suggested an increased risk of transfer to hemodialysis in older adults whereas other studies found a reduced risk with increasing age [43]. On the one hand, one could theorize that the elderly are more likely to incur a change in health status necessitating a switch whereas on the other hand, arguably, the elderly are less likely to run into issues such as membrane failure due to their shorter expected duration on dialysis.

However, for patients who do require transfer to hemodialysis, there is evidence that this carries significant risk. The transfer may be due to modality related issues such as refractory peritonitis or patient factors such as change in health or social circumstance such as loss of housing. Additionally, transfer to HD as an emergency will likely involve hospitalization and central venous access and the risk that this entails.

Nutrition

Gastrointestinal symptoms are particularly prevalent in PD patients in comparison to age matched controls and also compared to patients on hemodialysis. This can further impact on the inability to reach nutrition targets. For example, they experience more dyspepsia, bloating and early satiety.

Contributing to the nutritional concerns for the elderly on PD are socioeconomic factors which may impede access to food and food preparation. However, in this scenario the absorbed calories from the PD solutions may be beneficial.

A significant proportion of the elderly on PD also have diabetes. The dextrose containing dialysis solutions frequently lead to increased blood glucose concentrations. To complicate this issue the action of hypoglycemic agents and insulin is likely to be prolonged in patients on dialysis [25].

Palliative Care in Peritoneal Dialysis

As expressed by Kidney Disease Improving Global Outcomes (KDIGO); (Controversies Conference on palliative care in Chronic Kidney Disease Populations): "the need for supportive care for kidney patients is equal to that for cancer patients and should be available based on need, not prognosis for patients at any stage of kidney disease" [44].

This statement is probably particularly pertinent for the elderly patient on dialysis who is more likely to experience multisymptom burden.

The BOLDE study showed that the median number of symptoms for patients on PD over the age of 65 was almost 9 [4]. Dialysis physicians should be particularly mindful of this and routinely enquire about symptoms [4].

Goals of care discussions and prognostication with patients and their families are critical to ensure optimal care for the elderly patient. This enables realistic and sensible decision making for the future. Prognostic scores are available to aid these frequently challenging consultations.

It is paramount for physicians to appreciate that one size does not fit all; each individual comes with their own collection of experiences, religious, and cultural beliefs. Much of the palliative care literature focuses on patient autonomy; shared decision making and honesty. There are many parts of the world where families take the burden of bad news, thus protecting their family member/patient from the grim reality. Empathy with these and other such ideals should be strived for. Many prognostication scores have been developed in the hemodialysis population but are likely to hold relevance in peritoneal dialysis too. However, studies have demonstrated that patients generally feel that advanced care planning is important [45, 46].

As the end of life approaches, decisions need to be made regarding continuation of dialysis. If dialysis is chosen to be continued, the focus should centre on symptom control as previously discussed. Other measures that can help alleviate burden for patients are to tolerate hypertension in order to avoid symptoms of low blood pressure and also to prevent the adverse effects of polypharmacy. Laboratory monitoring is not always necessary, particularly if it will not affect therapy and also a removal in dietary restrictions can enhance quality of life.

Conclusion

Our dialysis population is ageing. This fact has opened up new challenges for the nephrologist. In most countries, elderly people who start RRT are more likely to be commenced on hemodialysis rather than peritoneal dialysis. However, PD can offer unique benefits. Crucially, it is a home therapy permitting continued independence and can be "tailored" according to an individual's needs and treatment goals. Additionally, some countries such as France and Canada offer successful assisted PD programs to support even very frail patients at home.

Despite this, the number of elderly patients on PD in general remains low, which may be due to a combination of factors including health policy, physician bias, and perceived medical or psychosocial barriers. However, PD offers similar survival and quality of life benefits compared to HD with no dependence on vascular access. There may also be additional medical benefits such as less myocardial stunning compared to HD and potential nutritional advantages.

The use of multidisciplinary predialysis programs is vital to ensure that patients and their families receive balanced and relevant information in order to make informed choices about their care. It is also imperative that the necessary long-term support is available to enable elderly patients to pursue PD confidently.

References

1. USRDS: 2016 USRDS Annual Data Report (ADE). ESRD in the US http://www.usrds.org/adr.aspx. 10 Apr 2017, date last accessed.
2. ERA-EDTA: 2007 ERA-EDTA annual report. http://www.era-edta-reg.org/files/annualreports/pdf/Annrep2007.pdf. 10 Mar 2017, date last accessed.
3. Jain AK, Blake P, Cordy P, Garg AX. Global trends in rates of peritoneal dialysis. J Am Soc Nephrol. 2012;23(3):533–44.
4. Brown EA, Johansson L, Farrington K, et al. Broadening Options for Long-term Dialysis in the Elderly (BOLDE): differences in quality of life on peritoneal dialysis compared to hemodialysis for older patients. Nephrol Dial Transplant. 2010;25:3755–63.
5. Renal registry: UK Renal Registry 18th annual report: chapter 2 UK renal replacement therapy prevalence in 2014L national and centre-specific analyses. https://www.renalreg.org/wp-content/uploads/2015/01/02-Chap-02.pdf. 10 Mar 2017, date last accessed.
6. Castrale C, Evans D, Verger C, et al. Peritoneal dialysis in elderly patients: report from the French Peritoneal Dialysis Registry (RDPLF). Nephrol Dial Transplant. 2010;25(1):255–62.
7. Li PK, Chow KM. Peritoneal dialysis-first policy made successful: perspectives and actions. Am J Kidney Dis. 2013;62(5):993–1005.

8. Musso CG, Jauregui JR, Macias Nunez JF. Frailty phenotype and chronic kidney disease: a review of the literature. Int Urol Nephrol. 2014;47(11):18017.
9. Jager KJ, Korevaar JC, Dekker FW, et al. The effect of contraindications and patient preference on dialysis modality selection in ESRD patients in the Netherlands. Am J Kidney Dis. 2004;43:891–9.
10. Oliver MJ, Quinn RR. Selecting peritoneal dialysis in the older dialysis population. Perit Dial Int. 2015;35:618–21.
11. Roderick P, Jones C, Drey N, et al. Late referral for end-stage renal disease: a region-wide survey in the south west of England. Nephrol Dial Transplant. 2002;17(7):1252–9.
12. Lee MB, Bargman JB. Survival by dialysis modality – who cares? Clin J Am Soc Nephrol. 2016;11(6):1083–7.
13. Bloembergen WE, Port FK, Mauger EA, Wolfe RA. A comparison of mortality between patients treated with hemodialysis and peritoneal dialysis. J Am Soc Nephrol. 1995;6(2):177–83.
14. Heaf JG, Wehberg S. Relative survival of peritoneal dialysis and hemodialysis patients: effect of cohort and mode of dialysis initiation. PLoS One. 2014;9(3):e90119. https://doi.org/10.1371/journal.pone.0090119.
15. Perl J, Wald R, McFarlane P, et al. Hemodialysis vascular access modifies the association between dialysis modality and survival. J Am Soc Nephrol. 2011;22(6):1113–21.
16. Quinn RR, Hux JE, Oliver MJ, Austin PC, Tonelli M, Laupacis A. Selection bias explains apparent differential mortality between dialysis modality. J Am Soc Nephrol. 2011;22(8):1534–42.
17. Camping DL, Constantinovici N, Roderick P, et al. Clinical outcomes, quality of life and costs in the North Thames Dialysis Study of elderly people on dialysis: a prospective cohort study. Lancet. 2000;356(9241):1543–50.
18. Manns B, Hammelgarn B, Lillie E, et al. Setting research priorities for patients on or nearing dialysis. Clin Am J Soc Nephrol. 2014;9(10):1813–21.
19. Ahmed S, Addicott C, Qureshi M, Pendleton N, Clague JE, Horan MA. Opinions of elderly people on treatment for end-stage renal disease. Gerontology. 1999;45(3):156–9.
20. Woo K, Goldman DP, Romley JA. Early failure of dialysis access among the elderly in the ear of fistula first. Clin J Am Soc Nephrol. 2015;10(10):1791–8.
21. Selby NM, McIntyre CW. Peritoneal dialysis is not associated with myocardial stunning. Perit Dial Int. 2011;31:27–33.
22. Lindsay RM, Heidenheim PA, Nesrallah G, Garg AX, Suri R. Daily Hemodialysis Study Group London Health Sciences Centre. Clin J Am Soc Nephrol. 2006;1(5):952–9.
23. Wolfgram DF, Szabo A, Murray AM, Whittle J. Risk of dementia in peritoneal dialysis patients compared with hemodialysis patients. Perit Dial Int. 2015;35(2):189–98.
24. Wang IK, Cheng YK, Lin CL, et al. Comparison of subdural hematoma risk between hemodialysis and peritoneal dialysis patients with ESRD. Clin J Am Soc Nephrol. 2015;10(6):994–1001.
25. Johansson L. Nutrition in older adults on peritoneal dialysis. Perit Dial Int. 2015;35:655–8.
26. Westra WM, Kopple JD, Krediet RT, Appel M, Mehrotra R. Dietary protein requirements and sialysate protein losses in chronic peritoneal dialysis patients. Perit Dial Int. 2007;27:192–5.
27. Mehrotra R, Duong U, Jiwakanon S, et al. Serum albumin as a predictor of mortality in peritoneal dialysis comparisons with hemodialysis. Am J Kidney Dis. 2011;58(3):929–36.
28. Taylor GS, Patel V, Spencer S, Fluck RJ, McIntyre CW. Long term use of 1.1% amino acid dialysis solution in hypoalbuminemic continuous ambulatory peritoneal dialysis patients. Clin Nephrol. 2002;58:445–50.
29. Goovaerts T, Jadoul M, Goffin E. Influence of a pre-dialysis education programme (PDEP) on the mode of renal replacement therapy. Nephrol Dial Transplant. 2005;20(9):1842–7.
30. Chanouzas D, Ng KP, Fallouh B, Baharani J. What influences patient choice of treatment modality at the pre-dialysis stage? Nephrol Dial Transplant. 2012;27(4):1542–7.
31. Montreal cognitive assessment. http://www.mocatest.org. Accessed 24 Apr 2017.
32. Brown EA, Finkelstein FO, Iyasere OU, Kilger AS. Peritoneal or hemodialysis for the frail elderly patient, the choice of two evils? Kidney Int. 2017;91:294–303.
33. Boujelbane L, Fu N, Chapla K. Percutaneous versus surgical insertion of PD catheters in dialysis patients: a meta-analysis. J Vasc Access. 2015;16(6):498–505.

34. Crabtree JH, Burchette RJ. Peritoneal dialysis catheter embedment: surgical considerations, expectations, and complications. Am J Surg. 2013;206(4):464–71.
35. Korevaar JC, Jansen MA, Dekker FW, Jager KJ, Boeschoten EW, Krediet RT, et al. When to initiate dialyses: effect of proposed US guidelines on survival. Lancet. 2001;358:1046–50.
36. Hurst H, Figueiredo. The needs of older patients for peritoneal dialysis: training and support at home. Perit Dial Int. 2015;35:625–9.
37. Iyasere OU, Brown EA, Johansson L. Quality of life and physical function in older patients on dialysis: a comparison of assisted peritoneal dialysis with hemodialysis. Clin J Am Soc Nephrol. 2016;11:423–30.
38. Bechade C, Lobbedez T, Ivarsen P, Povlsen. Assisted peritoneal dialysis for older people with end-stage renal disease: the French and Danish experience. Perit Dial Int. 2015;35:663–6.
39. Duquennoy S, Bechade C, Verger C, Ficheux M, Ryckelynck JP, Lobbedez T. Is peritonitis risk increased in elderly patients on peritoneal dialysis? Report from the French Language Peritoneal Dialysis Registry (RDPLF). Perit Dial Int. 2016;36:291–6.
40. Lim WH, Dogra GK, McDonald SF, Brown FG, Johnson DW. Compared with younger peritoneal dialysis patients, elderly patients have similar peritonitis-free survival and lower risk of technique failure, but higher risk of peritonitis-related mortality. Perit Dial Int. 2011;31:663–71.
41. Nessim SJ, Bargman JM, Austin PC, Story K, Jassal SV. Impact of age on peritonitis risk in peritoneal dialysis patients: an era effect. Clin J Am Soc Nephrol. 2009;4(1):135–41.
42. Szeto CC. Peritoneal dialysis-related infection in the older population. Perit Dial Int. 2015;35:659–62.
43. Bieber SD, Mehrotra R. Patient and technique survival of older adults with ESRD treated with peritoneal dialysis. Perit Dial Int. 2015;35:612–7.
44. Davison SN, Levin A, Moss AH, et al. Executive summary of the KDIGO controversies conference on supportive care in chronic kidney disease: developing a roadmap to improving quality care. Kidney Int. 2015;88(3):447–59.
45. Grubbs V, Moss AH, Cohen LM. A palliative approach to dialysis care: a patient-centered transition to the end of life. Clin J Am Soc Nephrol. 2014;9(12):2203–9.
46. Meeus F, Brown EA. Caring for older patients on peritoneal dialysis at end of life. Perit Dial Int. 2015;35:667–70.

Kidney Transplant in Elderly

13

Lucas Petraglia and Kristian Heldal

Introduction

As survival rates improve, the prevalence of older patients with end-stage renal disease (ESRD) increases markedly. Both USA and European registries have shown a rise in the elderly population (≥60 years old) with renal replacement therapies (RRT) [1, 2]. In this scenario, kidney transplant is a relatively new discipline, and older adults have their own characteristics that determine organ availability, donor evaluation, and recipient outcomes including their clinical complications. Taking this into account we can make a comparison with their younger counterparts.

The Asymmetry in Transplant

The incidence and prevalence of ESRD patients in RRT over the last decades have shown a significant growth mostly due to an increased number of patients above 65 years of age. This pattern is seen in most western societies, including the USA, Europe, and the UK where the number of patients younger than 60 years old has been steady since the 1990s in contrast with the age group of 70 years and above that was substantially enlarged and reached a plateau just a few years ago [2–4].

L. Petraglia
Internal Medicine Department, Hospital Italiano de Buenos Aires, Buenos Aires, Argentina
e-mail: lucas.petraglia@hospitalitaliano.org.ar

K. Heldal (✉)
Clinic of Internal Medicine, Telemark Hospital Trust, Skien, Norway

Institute of Clinical Medicine, Faculty of Medicine, University of Oslo, Oslo, Norway

Department of Transplantation Medicine, Section of Nephrology, Oslo University Hospital, Oslo, Norway
e-mail: hkri@ous-hf.no

C. G. Musso et al. (eds.), *Clinical Nephrogeriatrics*,
https://doi.org/10.1007/978-3-030-18711-8_13

Table 13.1 Comparison between young (<65 years old) and old (≥65 years old) kidney transplant patients

Young patient	Old patient
Same incidence of ESRD in the last decades	Growing incidence of elderly with ESRD and RRT
Higher probability to receive an organ within the 1st year	Lower chance of being wait-listed or transplanted
Stable proportion of transplanted individuals in the last decades	Increasing proportion of elderly recipients
Survival benefit over dialysis	Survival benefit over dialysis
HRQoL benefit over dialysis	HRQoL benefit over dialysis
Higher risk of death-censored graft failure in <35 years old	Higher mortality in the early post-transplant and in the long term
Higher chronic allograft failure	Higher incidence of comorbidity and frailty
Higher risk of acute rejection with ECD organs	Higher risk of death-censored graft failure in >75 years old
Lower drug compliance	Higher death-censored graft survival than younger patients
	Decrease in the overall immune response and less acute rejection with aging
	Acute rejection is a strong predictor of premature death and graft loss
	Higher immunosuppressive drug levels and toxicity with a median lower dosage
	Higher drug compliance but lower adherence

ESRD end-stage renal disease, *ECD* extended criteria donor, *RRT* renal replacement treatment

Regarding the access to kidney transplant, data from the USA show an inverse relationship between percentage of patients wait-listed or transplanted and age. In 2012, 56% of US patients aging 0–17 years were waitlisted or transplanted within the first year after initiation of RRT compared to only 13% of patients aging 65–69 years [1].

Although there is a significant asymmetry in the total number of transplants in both age groups, the USRDS, the Eurotransplant, and the Scandiatransplant registries all show evidence that the proportion of organ recipients of 65 years and older have increased since 1992 while staying fairly constant for patients below 45 years [5] (Table 13.1).

Allocation Strategies

In 2002, the Organ Procurement Transplant Network (OPTN)/United Network for Organ Sharing (UNOS) adopted the extended criteria donor (ECD) allocation policy [6]. The intention was to use the marginal organs by allocating them to patients that otherwise would have low probability to receive a transplant. This resulted in more procurement and transplant, but the number of organs discharged did not change [7–9]. Those kidneys that were initially rejected in some centers proved no significant difference in 5-year patient survival and graft survival when allocated [10]. To optimize and guide the distribution, the Kidney Donor Risk Index (KDRI) was introduced as a refined version of the ECD score [11]. This was used in the "longevity matching program" that aims to pair kidneys expected to last the longest with people expected to live the longest [12]. In 1999, some years before the ECD was adopted, the Eurotransplant Senior Program was developed as an age matching policy in Europe. Organs from donors aged ≥65 years are allocated locally to recipients aged ≥65 years without HLA matching, ranked exclusively by waiting time. This led to shortened waiting and cold ischemia times for elderly but no significant change in graft or patient survival at the 1st and 5th year of follow-up, compared to the regular allocation strategy [13, 14].

Outcomes: Patient and Graft Survival

Most available evidence on recipients of ECD kidneys show worse outcomes including more delayed graft function (DGF) and lower glomerular filtration rate (GFR), more primary non-function and acute rejection when compared to "standard organs". Older transplant recipients also have higher mortality than the younger ones [15–24]. However, the benefit for this age group comes when comparing survival rates with their dialysis counterparts [23, 25].

Back in the 1990s, evidence describing the beneficial effect of renal transplant over staying wait-listed on the expected survival rates in patients older than 60 years (diabetic and non-diabetic) emerged [26, 27]. This was also described for patients 70 years and older in studies done in the following decade [28, 29]. Recently, favorable outcomes have been described even in octogenarians [30, 31]. Even for patients receiving marginal organs with high Kidney Donor Profile Index (KDPI), the cumulative survival at 5 years was better for transplantation than waiting for a more "favorable organ" [32]. Consequently, an absolute upper age limit for transplantation is not advocated.

Although the long-term outcomes are favorable for older recipients, it should be mentioned that a higher mortality is registered during the early post-transplant period, especially in the most comorbid individuals and high-KDPI organs [33, 34].

Using old to old allocation strategies, elderly patients will most probably receive organs from older donors that may be suboptimal. Although the survival after transplantation with organs from donors of advanced age has been described as acceptable and far better than expected for comparable patients on dialysis, there is evidence describing that recipients of kidneys from very advanced aged donors (70 years and over) have higher risk of graft loss and recipient mortality than recipients of ordinary ECD grafts [18].

The use of dual kidney transplants as a way to maximize the graft outcomes in recipients of margigal donors has been introduced in USA and Spain [35–38]. The incidence of DGF and graft loss at 1st year has been found to be similar to single transplants, but mortality results described were variable, showing in some cases a rise in 1st year mortality but a beneficial effect in the 5 year analysis [35–37, 39–43]. To our knowledge, most transplant centers do not use this dual kidney transplant strategy.

Recipient characteristics also have a fundamental role in the graft outcomes.

To this matter some pathological conditions of the elderly population, like cognitive impairment (although this is considered as a contraindication to transplantation by most centers), and comorbidities like diabetes mellitus and hypertension, have been described to be associated with morbidity and mortality after kidney transplantation [44–47]. In addition, increased dialysis vintage is found to be negatively associated with survival after transplantation [48].

There are two more elements that should be examined due to their impact on the transplant outcomes. The first of them is frailty, a syndrome characterized by diminished strength, endurance, and reduced physiologic function that increases an individual's vulnerability for developing increased dependency and/or death [49]. Frailty is more frequent with advanced age, particularly in combination with chronic kidney disease [50]. Frailty in the general population is associated with an increased mortality risk [51, 52]. Some studies of kidney transplant recipients have found a higher risk of delayed graft function and hospital readmission in frail patients [43, 53, 54]. There are several scores developed to determine frailty, but none of them is validated for elderly transplanted patients, and there are no existing guidelines that include frailty in the selection algorithm for kidney transplantation.

The second element of importance in older recipients is poor adherence to prescriptions. Seventy percent of nontransplanted patients older than 65 years showed nonadherence to medication after 3 months of hospital discharge, and compliance declines with the number of daily doses, which is of significant practical value considering the amount of medication used by this particular population [55, 56]. These observations may not be directly transferable to older transplant recipients since the recipients constitute a carefully selected group of patients eligible for transplantation. Interestingly, elderly transplant recipients tend to be more compliant to therapy than younger adults, but the rate of adherence is lower as a consequence of forgetting or confusing prescription and dosage [57]. This lack of adherence to medication and clinical visits has been related to late rejection episodes, graft failure, graft loss, and occurrence of infection, tumor, and cardiovascular disease [58–60].

Fortunately, there seems to be a trend over the past years toward even better outcomes after transplantation in older patients [61]. The most frequent cause of graft loss in older kidney transplant recipients is death with functioning graft and consequently patient survival has become the main factor that determines the organ survival [31, 62]. As a matter of fact, large cohorts show that the highest risk of death-censored allograft failure is found in young adults (18 ≤ 35 years old) and very old patients (≥75 years old). Compared with young adults, death-censored allograft failure risk was lower in patients aged 65 or older and decreased with every 5 years until the age of 75 [63, 64]. In older recipients, the incidence of death with a functioning organ due to cardiovascular disease, infection, or malignancy is higher than the incidence of chronic allograft failure [65].

Outcomes: Health-Related Quality of Life

It is not only the survival time that is important to evaluate as an outcome after an intervention. Also the quality of the remaining years is considered as important for the patients, especially in older patients for whom the expected life span is relatively short, regardless of any intervention. Up to recently, only limited data describing the effect of kidney transplantations was published [48, 66]. However, in a prospective, longitudinal study published in 2018, the authors describe that health-related quality of life (HRQoL) in recipients older than 65 years improves significantly for most dimensions 1 year post engraftment [67]. Time on dialysis was the most important variable associated with impaired HRQoL after transplantation. Data from the same study also describe that HRQoL decreases while the patients are waiting for a transplant [68].

Immunosuppression

As part of the physiological aging, metabolism, pharmacokinetics, and immune system experience noticeable changes that determine a decrease in the overall immune response. There is evidence in murine models supporting the reduction in memory T cell helper function, effector T-cell alloreactivity, production of interferon by CD4+ memory T cell, proliferative response of T cells, and a rise in oligoclonal expansion of a memory T-cell subpopulation with reduced CD28 expression and impaired intracellular signaling [69–76], as well as B cell alterations characterized by a decreased antibody response [77]. On the other hand, organs from older donors are suspected to be more "immunogenic" than organs from younger donors, and as a consequence, receiving an organ from an older donor is associated with increased risk of rejection [48, 68, 78].

In humans this is reflected in the fact that organs from older donors have higher risk of rejection when allocated to younger individuals, in contrast to elderly recipients where there seems to be a reduced activation of the immune system [64, 79, 80].

The presence of reduced gastric emptying, impaired gastrointestinal motor function, decreased splanchnic blood flow, decreased renal clearance, changes in cytochrome IIIA isoenzymes and P-glycoprotein, decreased protein binding, and decreased hepatic blood flow are particularities of this age group that could potentially interfere with immunosuppressant drug metabolism [81].

There are no protocols specially designed for old patients receiving ECD organs. Pharmacokinetics should also play a fundamental role when deciding immunosuppressive regimens. Older adults reach higher calcineurin inhibitor (CNI) levels with a median lower dosage [82]. This is important knowing that older recipients tend to have higher frequency of CNI-induced nephrotoxicity, infections, cardiovascular events, and malignancies. There is also a trend toward a higher proportion of infections as a cause of death in elderly recipients, especially among those who received rejection treatment [48, 83].

It has been proposed that older recipients should profit from less intense immunosuppressive regimens, and studies have been designed to find the balance between targeting lower blood levels of immunosuppressant drugs and the risk of acute rejection [84].

European studies have described fewer episodes for patients over 60 years in comparison to the younger patients [24]. The risk of acute rejection also seems to be reduced with increasing age. An analysis of Norwegian data made by Heldal et al. found that recipients older than 70 had acute rejection rates of 35% within the first 12 weeks of post-transplantation in contrast with the 44% in patients aged 60–69 years and 45% among the control group aged 40–54 years [24, 85]. Even though the incidence of acute rejection decreased with increasing age, it seems to be more detrimental once it occurs. Acute rejection episodes during the first 3 months post engraftment were a strong predictor of premature death and graft loss in the elderly (≥70 years) and in the senior (60–69 years) age groups [48]. A likely explanation for these findings could be that the older recipients do not tolerate the intense immunosuppression that is included in the treatment of an acute rejection. According to this theory, immunosuppression should not be reduced in older recipients unless they experience side effects or complications to the treatment.

As for induction agents in recipients older than 60 years, many centers will consider antithymocyte globulin (ATG) as the drug of choice in high-risk recipients with high-risk donors [86], but because of the increased risk of infections and the reduced survival described in patients receiving more than 6 mg/kg of ATG, it would be advisable to aim lower doses [87]. Interleukin-2 antagonist (IL2R) may also be an attractive alternative for older recipients due to better tolerability. In a Norwegian study comparing outcomes after transplantation with kidneys from donors older than 60 years, induction therapy with IL2R was, compared to no induction therapy, associated with reduction in incidence of acute rejection episodes as well as improved 2-year graft survival [48, 88]. A direct comparison of IL2R versus ATG in older recipients has however to our knowledge not been performed.

Aging Kidney Transplantation

It is worth mentioning that there are several immunological and nonimmunological factors related to kidney graft deterioration and histological lesions as is the case of interstitial fibrosis and tubular atrophy overlap with those observed in aging kidneys. Therefore, it has been proposed that renal transplant aging could contribute to graft loss. In this sense, the cell aging process displays characteristics such as an increased expression of specific aging suppressor genes, shortened telomeres, increased expression of negative regulators of the cell cycle, and mitochondrial changes [89].

Tubular frailty, which is one of the main aged-related renal changes, makes aged kidney graft susceptible to ischemia, reperfusion, toxic injury, and inflammation. Moreover, renal tissue injury not only predisposes the older graft to progressive deterioration due to glomerular hyperfiltration but also triggers acute rejection due to increased immunogenicity [89, 90].

Conclusion

Kidney transplantation is an attractive treatment option for ESRD patients that after a standard medical evaluation are found suitable for the surgery and the following medical treatment. Both survival and HRQoL are improved in transplanted patients compared to what should be expected if they were not transplanted, and consequently transplantation should be considered as the treatment of choice provided that there are organs available and no contraindications exist. There should be no absolute upper age limit for accepting patients for transplantation.

References

1. 2015 USRDS Annual Data Report [Internet]. [Cited 2018 Sep 29]. Report no.: volume 2 – ESRD in the United States. Chapter 1: incidence, prevalence, patient characteristics, and treatment modalities. 2015. Available from: https://www.usrds.org/2015/download/vol2_ 01_ IncidenceandPrevalence_15.pdf.
2. Amsterdam UMC, location AMC, Department of Medical Informatics, Amsterdam, the Netherlands. ERA-EDTA Registry: ERA-EDTA Registry Annual Report 2016. 2018.
3. The Renal Association. UK Renal Registry. The seventeenth annual report. 2014.
4. T. L. Annual report Norwegian renal registry 2016 2017. 2018. Available from: http://www.nephro.no/registry.html.
5. Scandiatransplant. Annual Scandiatransplant data report. 2017.
6. Port FK, Bragg-Gresham JL, Metzger RA, Dykstra DM, Gillespie BW, Young EW, et al. Donor characteristics associated with reduced graft survival: an approach to expanding the pool of kidney donors1. Transplantation. 2002;74(9):1281–6.
7. Sung RS, Guidinger MK, Lake CD, McBride MA, Greenstein SM, Delmonico FL, et al. Impact of the expanded criteria donor allocation system on the use of expanded criteria donor kidneys. Transplantation. 2005;79(9):1257–61.
8. Schold JD, Howard RJ, Scicchitano MJ, Meier-Kriesche H-U. The expanded criteria donor policy: an evaluation of program objectives and indirect ramifications. Am J Transplant. 2006;6(7):1689–95.
9. Sung RS, Guidinger MK, Leichtman AB, Lake C, Metzger RA, Port FK, et al. Impact of the expanded criteria donor allocation system on candidates for and recipients of expanded criteria donor kidneys. Transplantation. 2007;84(9):1138–44.
10. Dahmane D, Audard V, Hiesse C, Pessione F, Bentaarit B, Barrou B, et al. Retrospective follow-up of transplantation of kidneys from "marginal" donors. Kidney Int. 2006;69(3): 546–52.
11. Rao PS, Schaubel DE, Guidinger MK, Andreoni KA, Wolfe RA, Merion RM, et al. A comprehensive risk quantification score for deceased donor kidneys: the kidney donor risk index. Transplantation. 2009;88(2):231–6.
12. Israni AK, Salkowski N, Gustafson S, Snyder JJ, Friedewald JJ, Formica RN, et al. New national allocation policy for deceased donor kidneys in the United States and possible effect on patient outcomes. J Am Soc Nephrol. 2014;25(8):1842–8.
13. Cohen B, Smits JM, Haase B, Persijn G, Vanrenterghem Y, Frei U. Expanding the donor pool to increase renal transplantation. Nephrol Dial Transplant. 2005;20(1):34–41.
14. Frei U, Noeldeke J, Machold-Fabrizii V, Arbogast H, Margreiter R, Fricke L, et al. Prospective age-matching in elderly kidney transplant recipients—a 5-year analysis of the Eurotransplant Senior Program. Am J Transplant. 2008;8(1):50–7.

15. Collini A, De Bartolomeis C, Ruggieri G, Barni R, Bernini M, Carmellini M. Long-term outcome of renal transplantation from marginal donors. Transplant Proc. 2006;38(10):3398–9.
16. Cicciarelli J, Iwaki Y, Mendez R. The influence of donor age on kidney graft survival in the 1990s. Clin Transplant. 1999;13:335–40.
17. Gjertson DW. A multi-factor analysis of kidney regraft outcomes. Clin Transplant. 2002;2:335–49.
18. Chavalitdhamrong D, Gill J, Takemoto S, Madhira BR, Cho YW, Shah T, et al. Patient and graft outcomes from deceased kidney donors age 70 years and older: an analysis of the Organ Procurement Transplant Network/United Network of Organ Sharing database. Transplantation. 2008;85(11):1573–9.
19. Moers C, Kornmann NSS, Leuvenink HGD, Ploeg RJ. The influence of deceased donor age and old-for-old allocation on kidney transplant outcome. Transplantation. 2009;88(4):542–52.
20. Carrier M, Lizé JF, Québec-Transplant Programs. Impact of expanded criteria donors on outcomes of recipients after kidney transplantation. Transplant Proc. 2012;44(7):2227–30.
21. Schnitzler MA, Lentine KL, Gheorghian A, Axelrod D, Trivedi D, L'Italien G. Renal function following living, standard criteria deceased and expanded criteria deceased donor kidney transplantation: impact on graft failure and death. Transplant Int. 2011;25(2):179–91.
22. Aubert O, Kamar N, Vernerey D, Viglietti D, Martinez F, Duong-Van-Huyen J-P, et al. Long term outcomes of transplantation using kidneys from expanded criteria donors: prospective, population based cohort study. BMJ. 2015;351:h3557.
23. Goldberg RJ, Smits G, Wiseman AC. Long-term impact of donor-recipient size mismatching in deceased donor kidney transplantation and in expanded criteria donor recipients. Transplantation. 2010;90(8):867–74.
24. Mendonça HM, Dos Reis MA, de Castro de Cintra Sesso R, Câmara NOS, Pacheco-Silva A. Renal transplantation outcomes: a comparative analysis between elderly and younger recipients. Clin Transplant. 2007;21(6):755–60.
25. Hellemans R, Stel VS, Jager KJ, Bosmans JL, Abramowicz D. Do elderly recipients really benefit from kidney transplantation? Transplant Rev. 2015;29(4):197–201.
26. Wolfe RA, Ashby VB, Milford EL, Ojo AO, Ettenger RE, Agodoa LY, et al. Comparison of mortality in all patients on dialysis, patients on dialysis awaiting transplantation, and recipients of a first cadaveric transplant. N Engl J Med. 1999;341(23):1725–30.
27. Port FK, Wolfe RA, Mauger EA, Berling DP, Jiang K. Comparison of survival probabilities for dialysis patients vs cadaveric renal transplant recipients. JAMA. 1993;270(11):1339–43.
28. Heldal K, Hartmann A, Grootendorst DC, de Jager DJ, Leivestad T, Foss A, et al. Benefit of kidney transplantation beyond 70 years of age. Nephrol Dial Transplant. 2010;25(5):1680–7.
29. Gill JS, Tonelli M, Johnson N, Kiberd B, Landsberg D, Pereira BJG. The impact of waiting time and comorbid conditions on the survival benefit of kidney transplantation. Kidney Int. 2005;68(5):2345–51.
30. Lønning K, Midtvedt K, Leivestad T, Reisæter AV, Line P-D, Hartmann A, et al. Are octogenarians with end-stage renal disease candidates for renal transplantation? Transplantation. 2016;100(12):2705–9.
31. Huang E, Poommipanit N, Sampaio MS, Kuo H-T, Reddy P, Gritsch HA, et al. Intermediate-term outcomes associated with kidney transplantation in recipients 80 years and older: an analysis of the OPTN/UNOS database. Transplantation. 2010;90(9):974–9.
32. Massie AB, Luo X, Chow EKH, Alejo JL, Desai NM, Segev DL. Survival benefit of primary deceased donor transplantation with high-KDPI kidneys. Am J Transplant. 2014;14(10):2310–6.
33. Kauffman HM, McBride MA, Cors CS, Roza AM, Wynn JJ. Early mortality rates in older kidney recipients with comorbid risk factors. Transplantation. 2007;83(4):404–10.
34. Gill JS, Schaeffner E, Chadban S, Dong J, Rose C, Johnston O, et al. Quantification of the early risk of death in elderly kidney transplant recipients. Am J Transplant. 2013;13(2):427–32.
35. Gill J, Cho YW, Danovitch GM, Wilkinson A, Lipshutz G, Pham P-T, et al. Outcomes of dual adult kidney transplants in the United States: an analysis of the OPTN/UNOS database. Transplantation. 2008;85(1):62–8.

36. Tanriover B, Mohan S, Cohen DJ, Radhakrishnan J, Nickolas TL, Stone PW, et al. Kidneys at higher risk of discard: expanding the role of dual kidney transplantation. Am J Transplant. 2014;14(2):404–15.
37. Cruzado JM, Fernandez L, Riera L, Bestard O, Carrera M, Torras J, et al. Revisiting double kidney transplantation: two kidneys provide better graft survival than one. Transplant Proc. 2011;43(6):2165–7.
38. Andrés A, Morales JM, Herrero JC, Praga M, Morales E, Hernández E, et al. Double versus single renal allografts from aged donors. Transplantation. 2000;69(10):2060–6.
39. Frutos MA, Mansilla JJ, Cabello M, Soler J, Ruiz P, Lebrón M, et al. Optimization of expanded donors using dual kidney transplantation: case-control study. Transplant Proc. 2012;44(7):2060–2.
40. Snanoudj R, Rabant M, Timsit MO, Karras A, Savoye E, Tricot L, et al. Donor-estimated GFR as an appropriate criterion for allocation of ECD kidneys into single or dual kidney transplantation. Am J Transplant. 2009;9(11):2542–51.
41. Rigotti P, Capovilla G, Di Bella C, Silvestre C, Donato P, Baldan N, et al. A single-center experience with 200 dual kidney transplantations. Clin Transplant. 2014;28(12):1433–40.
42. Medina-Polo J, Pamplona-Casamayor M, Miranda-Utrera N, González-Monte E, Passas-Martínez JB, Andrés Belmonte A. Dual kidney transplantation involving organs from expanded criteria donors: a review of our series and an update on current indications. Transplant Proc. 2014;46(10):3412–5.
43. Ekser B, Furian L, Broggiato A, Silvestre C, Pierobon ES, Baldan N, et al. Technical aspects of unilateral dual kidney transplantation from expanded criteria donors: experience of 100 patients. Am J Transplant. 2010;10(9):2000–7.
44. Garonzik-Wang JM, Govindan P, Grinnan JW, Liu M, Ali HM, Chakraborty A, et al. Frailty and delayed graft function in kidney transplant recipients. Arch Surg. 2012;147(2):190–3.
45. McAdams-Demarco MA, Grams ME, Hall EC, Coresh J, Segev DL. Early hospital readmission after kidney transplantation: patient and center-level associations. Am J Transplant. 2012;12(12):3283–8.
46. Karim A, Farrugia D, Cheshire J, Mahboob S, Begaj I, Ray D, et al. Recipient age and risk for mortality after kidney transplantation in England. Transplantation. 2014;97(8):832–8.
47. Heldal K, Hartmann A, Leivestad T, Foss A, Midtvedt K. Risk variables associated with the outcome of kidney recipients >70 years of age in the new millennium. Nephrol Dial Transplant. 2011;26(8):2706–11.
48. Heldal K, Hartmann A, Leivestad T, Svendsen MV, Foss A, Lien B, et al. Clinical outcomes in elderly kidney transplant recipients are related to acute rejection episodes rather than pretransplant comorbidity. Transplantation. 2009;87(7):1045–51.
49. Morley JE, Vellas B, van Kan GA, Anker SD, Bauer JM, Bernabei R, et al. Frailty consensus: a call to action. J Am Med Dir Assoc. 2013;14(6):392–7.
50. Anand S, Johansen KL, Kurella-Tamura M. Aging and chronic kidney disease: the impact on physical function and cognition. J Gerontol A Biol Sci Med Sci. 2014;69(3):315–22.
51. Theou O, Brothers TD, Peña FG, Mitnitski A, Rockwood K. Identifying common characteristics of frailty across seven scales. J Am Geriatr Soc. 2014;62(5):901–6.
52. Musso CG, Jauregui JR, Macías Núñez JF. Frailty phenotype and chronic kidney disease: a review of the literature. Int Urol Nephrol. 2015;47(11):1801–7.
53. McAdams-DeMarco MA, Law A, Salter ML, Chow E, Grams M, Walston J, et al. Frailty and early hospital readmission after kidney transplantation. Am J Transplant. 2013;13(8):2091–5.
54. Exterkate L, Slegtenhorst BR, Kelm M, Seyda M, Schuitenmaker JM, Quante M, et al. Frailty and transplantation. Transplantation. 2016;100(4):727–33.
55. Pasina L, Brucato AL, Falcone C, Cucchi E, Bresciani A, Sottocorno M, et al. Medication non-adherence among elderly patients newly discharged and receiving polypharmacy. Drugs Aging. 2014;31(4):283–9.
56. Claxton AJ, Cramer J, Pierce C. A systematic review of the associations between dose regimens and medication compliance. Clin Ther. 2001;23(8):1296–310.

57. Chisholm-Burns MA, Kwong WJ, Mulloy LL, Spivey CA. Nonmodifiable characteristics associated with nonadherence to immunosuppressant therapy in renal transplant recipients. Am J Health Syst Pharm. 2008;65(13):1242–7.
58. Schmid-Mohler G, Thut MP, Wüthrich RP, Denhaerynck K, De Geest S. Non-adherence to immunosuppressive medication in renal transplant recipients within the scope of the integrative model of behavioral prediction: a cross-sectional study. Clin Transpl. 2009;24(2):213–22.
59. Denhaerynck K, Dobbels F, Cleemput I, Desmyttere A, Schäfer-Keller P, Schaub S, et al. Prevalence, consequences, and determinants of nonadherence in adult renal transplant patients: a literature review. Transpl Int. 2005;18(10):1121–33.
60. Djamali A, Samaniego M, Muth B, Muehrer R, Hofmann RM, Pirsch J, et al. Medical care of kidney transplant recipients after the first posttransplant year. Clin J Am Soc Nephrol. 2006;1(4):623–40.
61. McAdams-DeMarco MA, James N, Salter ML, Walston J, Segev DL. Trends in kidney transplant outcomes in older adults. J Am Geriatr Soc [Internet]. 2014. Available from: https://doi.org/10.1111/jgs.13130
62. Rose C, Schaeffner E, Frei U, Gill J, Gill JS. A lifetime of allograft function with kidneys from older donors. J Am Soc Nephrol. 2015;26(10):2483–93.
63. Molnar MZ, Streja E, Kovesdy CP, Shah A, Huang E, Bunnapradist S, et al. Age and the associations of living donor and expanded criteria donor kidneys with kidney transplant outcomes. Am J Kidney Dis. 2012;59(6):841–8.
64. Tullius SG, Tran H, Guleria I, Malek SK, Tilney NL, Milford E. The combination of donor and recipient age is critical in determining host immunoresponsiveness and renal transplant outcome. Ann Surg. 2010;252(4):662–74.
65. Schratzberger G, Mayer G. Age and renal transplantation: an interim analysis. Nephrol Dial Transplant. 2003;18(3):471–6.
66. Balogun SA, Balogun R, Philbrick J, Abdel-Rahman E. Quality of life, perceptions, and health satisfaction of older adults with end-stage renal disease: a systematic review. J Am Geriatr Soc. 2016;65(4):777–85.
67. Lønning K, Heldal K, Bernklev T, Brunborg C, Andersen MH, von der Lippe N, et al. Improved health-related quality of life in older kidney recipients 1 year after transplantation. Transplant Direct. 2018;4(4):e351.
68. Lønning K, Midtvedt K, Bernklev T, Brunborg C, Andersen MH, von der Lippe N, et al. Changes in health-related quality of life in older candidates waiting for kidney transplantation. Nephrology. 2018;23(10):948–56.
69. Murasko DM, Weiner P, Kaye D. Decline in mitogen induced proliferation of lymphocytes with increasing age. Clin Exp Immunol. 1987;70(2):440–8.
70. Suvas S. Advancing age and immune cell dysfunction: is it reversible or not? Expert Opin Biol Ther. 2008;8(5):657–68.
71. Haynes L, Eaton SM, Burns EM, Randall TD, Swain SL. CD4 T cell memory derived from young naive cells functions well into old age, but memory generated from aged naive cells functions poorly. Proc Natl Acad Sci U S A. 2003;100(25):15053–8.
72. Denecke C, Bedi DS, Ge X, Kim IK-E, Jurisch A, Weiland A, et al. Prolonged graft survival in older recipient mice is determined by impaired effector T-cell but intact regulatory T-cell responses. PLoS One. 2010;5(2):e9232.
73. Rosenberg AS, Sechler JM, Horvath JA, Maniero TG, Bloom ET. Assessment of alloreactive T cell subpopulations of aged mice in vivo. CD4+ but not CD8+ T cell-mediated rejection response declines with advanced age. Eur J Immunol. 1994;24(6):1312–6.
74. Linton PJ. Antigen-independent changes in naive CD4 T cells with aging. J Exp Med. 1996;184(5):1891–900.
75. Mu XY, Thoman ML. The age-dependent cytokine production by murine CD8 T cells as determined by four-color flow cytometry analysis. J Gerontol A Biol Sci Med Sci. 1999;54(3):B116–23.

76. Messaoudi I, Lemaoult J, Guevara-Patino JA, Metzner BM, Nikolich-Zugich J. Age-related CD8 T cell clonal expansions constrict CD8 T cell repertoire and have the potential to impair immune defense. J Exp Med. 2004;200(10):1347–58.
77. Frasca D, Blomberg BB. Effects of aging on B cell function. Curr Opin Immunol. 2009;21(4):425–30.
78. de Fijter JW, Mallat MJ, Doxiadis II, Ringers J, Rosendaal FR, Claas FH, et al. Increased immunogenicity and cause of graft loss of old donor kidneys. J Am Soc Nephrol. 2001;12(7):1538–46.
79. Arns W, Citterio F, Campistol JM. "Old-for-old"—new strategies for renal transplantation. Nephrol Dial Transplant. 2007;22(2):336–41.
80. Tullius SG, Milford E. Kidney allocation and the aging immune response. N Engl J Med. 2011;364(14):1369–70.
81. Danovitch GM, Gill J, Bunnapradist S. Immunosuppression of the elderly kidney transplant recipient. Transplantation. 2007;84(3):285–91.
82. Jacobson PA, Schladt D, Oetting WS, Leduc R, Guan W, Matas AJ, et al. Lower calcineurin inhibitor doses in older compared to younger kidney transplant recipients yield similar troughs. Am J Transplant. 2012;12(12):3326–36.
83. Meier-Kriesche HU, Ojo AO, Hanson JA, Kaplan B. Exponentially increased risk of infectious death in older renal transplant recipients. Kidney Int. 2001;59(4):1539–43.
84. Heldal K, Midtvedt K. Managing transplant rejection in the elderly: the benefits of less aggressive immunosuppressive regimens. Drugs Aging. 2013;30(7):459–66.
85. Heldal K, Leivestad T, Hartmann A, Svendsen MV, Lien BH, Midtvedt K. Kidney transplantation in the elderly—the Norwegian experience. Nephrol Dial Transplant. 2008;23(3):1026–31.
86. Gill J, Sampaio M, Gill JS, Dong J, Kuo H-T, Danovitch GM, et al. Induction immunosuppressive therapy in the elderly kidney transplant recipient in the United States. Clin J Am Soc Nephrol. 2011;6(5):1168–78.
87. Patel SJ, Knight RJ, Suki WN, Abdellatif A, Duhart BT Jr, Krauss AG, et al. Rabbit antithymocyte induction and dosing in deceased donor renal transplant recipients over 60 yr of age. Clin Transplant. 2011;25(3):E250–6.
88. Heldal K, Thorarinsdottir S, Hartmann A, Leivestad T, Reisæter AV, Foss AE, et al. Induction with interleukin-2 antagonist for transplantation of kidneys from older deceased donors: an observational study. Transplant Res. 2013;2(1):11.
89. Musso CG, Giordani MC, Imperiali N. Aging kidney transplantation. Rev Investig Clin. 2016;68(2):68–74.
90. Musso CG. Geriatric nephrology and the "nephrogeriatric giants". Int Urol Nephrol. 2002;34(2):255–6.

Nephrolithiasis in the Elderly

14

Neera K. Dahl and David S. Goldfarb

Introduction

Although kidney stones are famously painful, they are also often viewed merely as inconvenient and relatively minor on the list of common disorders affecting the world's populace. When they affect the elderly, however, there is a likelihood that they may lead to adverse effects that become more meaningful when experienced in the context of the comorbidities of the older population. As a disorder that is amenable to prevention, we are often struck that primary care practitioners, including geriatricians, apply their expertise in prevention to treatment of diabetes, metabolic syndrome, hypertension, and atrial fibrillation, without any regard for the possibility of preventing stone disease. In this review, we first offer some facts regarding stones in the general population and then consider how risk factors and treatment might be different in an older population.

General Considerations

Kidney stones are becoming more common and are associated with significant morbidity. The overall prevalence of kidney stones has increased in the United States from 3.8% of the population in 1976–1980 to 8.8% of the population in 2007–2010 based on NHANES data [1]. Non-Hispanic white men have the highest prevalence of stones, followed by Hispanic men, non-Hispanic white women, and Hispanic women.

N. K. Dahl (✉)
Section of Nephrology, Yale School of Medicine, New Haven, CT, USA
e-mail: neera.dahl@yale.edu

D. S. Goldfarb
Nephrology Section, New York Harbor VA Healthcare System and NYU Langone Health, New York, NY, USA
e-mail: david.goldfarb@va.gov

C. G. Musso et al. (eds.), *Clinical Nephrogeriatrics*,
https://doi.org/10.1007/978-3-030-18711-8_14

Non-Hispanic black men and women have the lowest prevalence of stones at 4.8% and 4.2% respectively [1]. The prevalence of kidney stones increases with age: 16% of men and 7% of women over the age of 70 had passed at least one stone in their lifetime. The prevalence of kidney stones increased in men until the age of 65, and in women until the age of 70 [2]. In a group of calcium oxalate stone formers, the prevalence of diabetes mellitus, hypertension, and increasing BMI, all risk factors for stone disease, increases from age 18 to 69 prior to declining in those aged 70 or more [3].

Risk Factors

Nutritional factors play a role in the development of kidney stones. Diets rich in magnesium, potassium, and calcium with good fluid intake decrease the risk of kidney stones, while diets high in fructose, sucrose, or sodium with low fluid intake increase risk of kidney stones [4]. Being overweight or obese increases the risk for a kidney stone in both men and women [1]. Lower household income also increased risk of developing a kidney stone [1]. Stones are more common in warmer climates [5].

Certain occupations may also increase risk of kidney stones. For example, taxi cab drivers [6], who have infrequent access to rest rooms, are at higher risk, as are those who work in hot environments or with infrequent access to fluids.

Risk factors for kidney stones which may disproportionately affect older individuals include diabetes mellitus, gout, obesity [1], and immobilization [7]. Institutionalized older patients may be at additional risk because of limited access to water and to an appropriate diet. Older individuals may be more likely to limit fluid intake due to concerns of worsening urinary incontinence or lower urinary tract symptoms (LUTS) and gastroesophageal reflux disease (GERD). Older individuals may have more lactose intolerance, or other dietary restrictions which further limit adherence to the dietary guidelines discussed below.

An initial evaluation of a kidney stone patient should include a detailed medical history. Bowel disease leading to chronic diarrhea or malabsorption increases risk of kidney stones. Bariatric surgery (Roux-en-Y gastric bypass), small bowel resection, and ileostomy will increase risk. Systemic diseases which increase urine or serum calcium will also increase risk and include primary hyperparathyroidism and sarcoidosis. Certain medications such as topiramate and other carbonic anhydrase inhibitors will increase risk. Hyperthyroidism [7] will increase risk of kidney stones. Renal anomalies leading to urinary stasis will also increase risk of recurrence.

Kidney stone composition varies with age and between men and women. Although calcium oxalate stones remain the most common type of stone, both men and women show an increased prevalence of uric acid and struvite stones with age. The percentage of uric acid stones shows significant increase after the age of 50. Young women have a higher prevalence of calcium phosphate stones. This decreases with age, as calcium oxalate becomes the predominant stone type [8]. Metabolic abnormalities noted by 24-hour urine measurements also vary with age and gender. Men are more likely to have hyperuricosuria, hyperoxaluria, and hypocitraturia [3].

Appropriate Diet and Dietary Guidelines

Dietary intake is a modifiable risk factor in the development of kidney stones. Maintaining a normal BMI, drinking an adequate amount of fluid (2 L or greater), eating a diet high in fruits and vegetables, and high in low-fat dairy products (such as the DASH diet), with adequate calcium intake (about 1000 mg per day), and low intake of sugar-sweetened beverages was associated with a significantly lower risk of incident kidney stones [9]. The only randomized clinical trial to demonstrate the ability of a diet to prevent stones was successful in Italian men with urine calcium excretion greater than 300 mg/day [10]. Compared with a low calcium, low oxalate diet, the higher calcium, low salt, oxalate, and animal protein diet was associated with nearly half as many recurrent stones after 5 years. Based on the findings of these population-based studies and review of existing clinical trials, both the American Urologic Association (AUA) [11] and the European Association of Urology (EAU) [12] recommend "normal" dietary calcium intake, limited sodium, and limited animal protein for patients with calcium-containing stones (Table 14.1). A recent Cochrane review

Table 14.1 AUA and EUA dietary guidelines for management of kidney stones

AUA guidelines	General preventative measures (EAU)
All stone formers should have fluid intake that will achieve a urine volume of 2.5 L daily	Fluid intake of 2.5–3.0 L/day
	Circadian drinking
	Neutral pH beverages
	Goal urine output of 2.0–2.5 L/daily
	Goal urine-specific gravity <1.010
Patients with calcium stones and high urinary calcium should limit sodium intake and consume 1000–1200 mg daily of dietary calcium	Nutritional advice: balanced diet
	Rich in vegetables and fiber
	Normal calcium content (1–1.2 g/day)
	Limited sodium chloride (4–5 g/day)
	Limited animal protein 0.8–1.0 g/kg/day
Patients with calcium oxalate stones and high urinary oxalate should limit intake of oxalate-rich foods and maintain normal calcium consumption	If a 24-hour urine shows hyperoxaluria, oxalate should be restricted
Patients with calcium stones and low urinary citrate should increase intake of fruits and vegetables, and limit non-dairy animal protein	If a 24-urine shows high sodium excretion, sodium should be restricted
Patients with uric acid stones or calcium stones with high urinary uric acid should limit non-dairy animal protein	If a 24-hour urine shows a small urine volume then fluid intake should be increased
Patients with cystine stones should limit sodium and protein intake	If a 24-hour urine shows high intake of animal protein, then excess animal protein intake should be avoided
	Lifestyle advice
	BMI for adults: 18–25 kg/m^2
	Stress limitation measures
	Adequate physical activity
	Balancing excessive fluid loss

AUA American Urologic Association, *EUA* European Association of Urology, *BMI* body mass index also found a benefit from a normal calcium, low protein, and low salt diet for stone patients with hypercalciuria [13]. The EAU recommends general preventative measures for all stone formers, including specific dietary management based on a 24-hour urine.

In contrast, the American College of Physicians (ACP), which limits its recommendations to those based on randomized clinical trials (RCTs), only has a single guideline for dietary management of kidney stones, promoting a goal of increased fluid intake, spread throughout the day to achieve a daily urine volume of at least 2 L. Beyond stating that sodas acidified with phosphoric acid should be avoided, there were no strong, evidence-based recommendations for additional dietary interventions [14].

The AUA and EAU note that high risk stone formers are likely to benefit from medical therapy and have issued guidelines regarding appropriate treatment based on stone composition or metabolic factors. The ACP also evaluated the role of medical therapy. None of the guidelines specifically address the most appropriate strategies in older adults, or ask whether such strategies might be different than those of younger people.

The mainstays of pharmacologic management of calcium kidney stones include thiazides, to lower urinary calcium excretion, potassium citrate to inhibit calcium oxalate precipitation, and allopurinol to reduce hyperuricosuria in those without higher urine calcium. Uric acid stones are best treated with alkali to achieve an increase in urine pH [11, 12, 14]. Each of these therapies may potentially pose greater risk in older patients. Use of thiazides may lead to hyponatremia (especially when patients are advised to increase their fluid intake), or orthostatic hypotension, increasing fall risk. Thiazides may also cause erectile dysfunction, fatigue, and muscle symptoms, further limiting use [15]. On the other hand, thiazides also have the potential for important benefits in older people. They are generally considered effective therapy for systolic hypertension, associated with better cardiovascular outcomes [16]. In addition, probably by lowering urine calcium, they are associated with increased bone mineral density and reduced fracture rates [17].

Potassium citrate may cause GI symptoms, especially in older patients. Careful monitoring is advised in patients with reductions in estimated glomerular filtration rate (eGFR), particularly those who are adherent to low salt diets (which will further limit potassium excretion), or those treated with medications which impair potassium excretion such as angiotensin-converting enzyme inhibitors, angiotensin receptor blockers, or mineralocorticoid antagonists. Sodium bicarbonate may worsen a tendency toward fluid retention and heart failure, though this risk is small compared with sodium chloride. Allopurinol can be used safely in patients with reduced eGFR if started at lower doses and titrated upwards gradually. Thus, the risks and benefits of medical treatment of kidney stones need to be carefully considered in older individuals. If medical therapy is initiated, more frequent monitoring for side effects and laboratory abnormalities would be prudent.

Are Older Patients at Risk of Recurrent Stones?

Usui and colleagues examined metabolic risk factors in stone patients over the age of 65 [18]. Most patients in stone clinic were younger than 65; those older than 65 comprised only 9.6% of the total patient population. Recurrent stones were noted in about 15% of those over the age of 65, with higher urinary calcium associated with recurrence. However, the probability of stone recurrence was the same in the older patients compared to the younger ones.

A unique calculator was developed to predict the risk of stone recurrence. The Recurrence of Kidney Stone (ROKS) nomogram [19] assigns a point score based on the sum of 11 predictors (age, male gender, white race, family history of kidney stones, gross hematuria with a symptomatic stone, uric acid stones, stone in the uretero-vesicular junction, stone in the renal pelvis, any concurrent asymptomatic stones, and history of a prior suspected stone event). The older the age of a first time stone former, the lower the risk of recurrence. Thus, a low-risk patient, for instance, a 65-year-old woman with an obstructing calcium oxalate stone, and no other risk factors, may have only a 10% risk of recurrence over 10 years and may therefore not benefit from either dietary or medical therapy to further reduce her risk of recurrence. Utilization of the ROKS nomogram may therefore be helpful in identifying low-risk patients. Unfortunately, the ROKS nomogram may underestimate those patients at higher risk, because it does not include known metabolic risk factors, such as hypertension, diabetes mellitus, presence of metabolic syndrome, or obesity, in the risk calculation. It also has not been validated in a population other than that seen at Mayo Clinic, and does not take into account the results of 24-hour urine collections.

How Do Metabolic Risk Factors for Kidney Stones Change with Age?

We examined differences in urine and serum chemistry in patients greater than 60 years compared to younger patients [20]. In the referral clinic at University of Chicago, 12.8% of women (97 out of 760) and 5% of men (81 of 1617) were older. Each patient had three baseline 24-hour urine collections and a corresponding serum chemistry sample drawn 12 hours after the last meal. Older patients (both men and women) had higher baseline creatinine and potassium values. Significant changes noted in the 24-hour urine collections are shown in Table 14.2.

Older men and women had lower urinary calcium, uric acid, creatinine, magnesium, and phosphorus compared to younger men and women. Lower urinary calcium led to a lower (better) supersaturation (SS) for calcium oxalate and calcium phosphate despite a decline in urine pH with age. In these older patients, other factors in addition to supersaturations may be determining the increased risk for stones. This could be due to a defect in inhibitors of crystallization (the decline in urinary magnesium, for instance). Alternatively, it may be that although the urinary

Table 14.2 A comparison of urinary risk factors in older (age >60) and younger (age <60) stone patients

	Males		Females	
Measurement	Younger	Older	Younger	Older
Calcium	240	204	197	171
Uric acid	708	613	534	485
Creatinine	1872	1608	1186	1006
Sodium	187	177	139	115
Potassium	63	67	48	53
Magnesium	108	102	88	80
Phosphorus	1032	920	745	668
Urine pH	6.00	5.85	6.18	6.00
SS CaOx	9.24	7.77	9.08	7.75
SS CaP	1.60	1.04	1.70	0.84

All comparisons were significantly different $p \leq 0.05$. Calcium, uric acid, creatinine, magnesium, and phosphorus are in mg/dL; sodium and potassium in mEq/L
SS supersaturation, *CaOx* calcium oxalate, and *CaP* calcium phosphate [20]

calcium is lower, it is still sufficient for stone formation. Walker et al. show that although urinary calcium and creatinine decline with age, calcium clearance as a percentage of creatinine clearance increases with age in male and female stone formers [21].

Perinpam et al. [22] also found that urinary calcium, magnesium, and uric acid decreased with age, while urinary oxalate remained relatively stable. Similar results were noted by Friedlander et al. [23], with a decline in urine pH, uric acid, creatinine, and SS of CaOx and CaP with age in adjusted multivariate analysis.

Otto et al. found a linear association with age and urinary oxalate, lower urinary pH, and lower urinary uric acid [3] in calcium oxalate stone formers. Urinary calcium peaked in the age 40 to 49-year-old age group. There was no association between age and calcium oxalate supersaturation, but older patients had a lower supersaturation of calcium phosphate.

Some of the differences in these studies may be explained by the high rates of patients who were overweight (30%) or obese (40%) in the Otto cohort, as a higher BMI was associated with hyperuricosuria, hyperoxaluria, hypocitraturia, a lower urine pH, and hypercalciuria. They found that age, gender, and BMI performed best in predicting urinary abnormalities and suggested that the risks for calcium oxalate stones change with age. Younger patients may have hypocitraturia, middle-aged patients may have more calcium excretion, and older patients may have more hyperoxaluria [3].

Managing Osteoporosis and Kidney Stone Disease

Kidney stones can be conceptualized as a chronic pathophysiologic process [24], impacted by prevalent chronic diseases of diabetes mellitus, hypertension, and obesity. Factors affecting bone health, and the development of osteopenia or osteoporosis may also affect stone disease and influence therapy.

Osteoporotic fractures are reported to occur more commonly in patients with stones than in the general population [17], with symptomatic kidney stone patients having fourfold higher incidence of a vertebral fracture than a non-stone-forming population. Nephrolithiasis was associated with an increased risk of wrist but not hip fractures [25] based on data from the Nurses' Health Study (NHS) and Health Professionals Follow-up Study (HPFS). In contrast to these results, analysis of over 150,000 women from the Women's Health Initiative (WHI) showed no association between urinary tract stones and osteoporosis in postmenopausal women [26]. However, a recent meta-analysis of 26 smaller studies found an association with lower bone mineral density (BMD) and nephrolithiasis [27].

Reduced bone mineral density (BMD) is common in stone formers with higher urine calcium excretion [28]. Multiple factors contribute to this association. High salt consumption may lead to increased renal calcium loss, reducing BMD. High protein consumption may lead to an increase in metabolic acidosis which decreases bone formation and increases bone reabsorption and inhibits tubular calcium reabsorption. Hyperparathyroidism, hyperthyroidism, or genetic causes of higher urine calcium excretion may lead to a net negative calcium balance if dietary calcium intake is not optimal. However, patients with fasting higher urine calcium excretion, who are at high risk of bone loss, had PTH-independent calcium efflux, presumably from mobilization of calcium stores from bone although markers for bone turnover were not increased [28]. Based on these unique risks for both risks of bone loss and kidney stones in patients with higher urine calcium excretion, Arrabal-Polo and colleagues proposed tailored strategies for treatment including evaluation of bone density, and thiazide for patients with higher urine calcium excretion, or citrate for patients with an elevated calcium/citrate ratio [29].

Appropriate treatment with thiazide or indapamide to lower urine calcium and potassium citrate to minimize stone formation resulted in a decrease in stone formation and an improvement in bone density [30].

25-OH vitamin D deficiency is common in stone formers (roughly 30%) and is associated with higher parathyroid hormone levels [31]. However, 25-OH vitamin D status (levels between 20 and 100 ng/ml) was not associated with kidney stone incidence [32], and 25-OH vitamin D levels were not associated with an increased risk of incident kidney stones [33]. Since 25-OH vitamin D deficiency may be more common in older patients, we and others [34] recommend repletion of vitamin D in patients with deficiency and appropriate dietary intake of vitamin D. Short-term repletion studies show no increase in urinary calcium excretion or supersaturation for calcium oxalate or calcium phosphate in known stone formers [35], and longer-term studies show no increase in stone prevalence [36].

Appropriate Calcium Intake for Elderly Stone Formers

The WHI examined the role of calcium and vitamin D supplementation for the prevention of fractures in healthy postmenopausal women. Daily calcium (1000 mg of calcium carbonate) and vitamin D (400 IU of D3) resulted in a small but significant improvement in hip bone density but did not reduce hip fracture. However, there was an increased incidence of kidney stones in the group receiving supplementation [37]. A subsequent analysis of these data showed a modest increase in the risk of cardiovascular events associated with use of calcium supplements [38]; however, this topic remains controversial [39]. The USPSTF recommends against 25-OH vitamin D supplementation for the prevention of fractures; however, calcium and vitamin D supplements are still important in the treatment of bone disease [40, 41]. Urinary calcium concentration, and therefore risk of kidney stone formation could be effectively mitigated in patients taking 500 mg/day in calcium supplements if the urine volume was >2 L daily [42].

Therefore, we recommend vitamin D3, and calcium in the form of calcium-rich foods, not supplements, along with fluid intake of 2–3 L daily, for our stone patients who are postmenopausal or have been diagnosed with osteopenia or osteoporosis. In those lactose-intolerant patients we recommend lactose-free dairy products and calcium-fortified orange juice. If calcium supplements are absolutely necessary, we prefer calcium citrate, which may have a slightly more favorable effect on urinary supersaturation [43]. In addition, calcium citrate should be taken with or shortly after meals in order to bind oxalate in the intestinal lumen and reduce its absorption.

Role of Additional Therapies for Osteoporosis in Managing Kidney Stones

Currently there are many therapies, in addition to appropriate calcium and vitamin D intake, and weight-bearing exercise, which may be used for treatment of osteoporosis or management of osteopenia. Whether the combined use of medications for treatment of stone disease and for treatment of osteoporosis will have an additive affect in preserving bone mass remains largely unknown.

A recent small study suggests that there may be a synergistic effect in the use of thiazides and aminobisphosphonates [29, 44]. Presumably by reducing osteoclast-mediated bone turnover, some studies show that urinary calcium excretion declines and may be expected to reduce stone recurrence [29, 44]. Patients with hypercalciuria and decreased bone mineral density were randomized to receive either 50 mg/day hydrochlorothiazide and 70 mg/week of alendronate or 70 mg/week of alendronate alone. Both groups were encouraged to have 1000–1200 mg of dietary calcium from food, with moderate oxalate intake. After 2 years of treatment, the group receiving both hydrochlorothiazide and aminobisphosphonates showed improved urinary calcium and improved bone mineral density of the hip and lumbar spine. Given the concern about the relatively minor effects of vitamin D and possible risks of calcium supplementation, bisphosphonates may be a preferred therapy for reduced BMD in stone formers. Potassium citrate, which acts as potential base to neutralize acid, is also associated with increased BMD in older postmenopausal women [45]. The benefits of the pharmacologic prevention of stones should be clear: treatment is associated with increased BMD and reduced fracture rates.

There are no data regarding use of newer agents such as teriparatide, abaloparatide, denosumab, or selective estrogen receptor modulators (SERMs) in the management of patients with bone loss and kidney stones.

Kidney Stones, Chronic Kidney Disease (CKD), and Coronary Artery Disease (CAD)

Nephrolithiasis is associated with a twofold increase risk of chronic kidney disease (CKD) and end-stage kidney disease independent of other known CKD risk factors [46]. Some of the explanations may be patient-specific. For example, patients with the metabolic syndrome, diabetes mellitus, or hypertension are predisposed to nephrolithiasis as well as CKD. Patients with anatomic urinary tract abnormalities that predispose to stone formation may also be predisposed to renal disease, and those with infection stones may develop renal scarring due to chronic infection.

Recently, a large cohort study demonstrated that patients with nephrolithiasis have an approximately 18% increased risk of CAD compared to non-stone formers [47]. The effect was more pronounced in women (HR of 1.18 (1.08–1.28) in NHS I and HR of 1.48 (1.23–1.78) in NHS II). There was no association found in a cohort of men (HPFS). Alexander et al. conducted a cohort study of over three million members of the Alberta, Canada universal health care system between 1997 and 2009. They found that compared to non-stone formers, stone formers had a higher risk of acute myocardial infarction, angioplasty, and coronary artery bypass surgery and a higher risk of stroke. The risk was more pronounced for younger people and for women [48].

The mechanisms underlying these associations, including lifestyle, genetics, or diet, for example, remain to be discovered. It will be interesting to see if new insights into the physiology of stone formation and its interaction with CKD or CAD can be determined.

Proactive Care of Older People Undergoing Surgery (POPS)

Older patients with kidney stones have more risk factors for complications of ureteroscopy [49]. The prevalence of hypertension, diabetes mellitus, and use of anticoagulants increased with age. Diabetes mellitus, use of anticoagulants, cardiovascular disease, and obesity all increased the complication rate; older patients were more likely to have complications [49]. Given this increased risk of surgical complications. It is important to remember that uric acid stones, even those which are quite large, may respond to medical dissolution therapy [50]. For patients with multiple comorbidities, and non-obstructing uric acid stones, characterized by lower Hounsfield units (<500), a trial of either citrate or bicarbonate therapy for urinary alkalinization may therefore be an appropriate initial choice.

Patients aged 65 or older are an increasing demographic for urologists [51]. Awareness of this changing demographic has led to the development of geriatric urology. This has led to the development of a novel ward-based geriatric liaison service for older urological surgical patients [52]. Geriatrics team members rounded with the urology team. Improved outcomes included decreased length of stay, fewer postoperative complications, and fewer readmissions 30 days after discharge. These single center results are encouraging, and hopefully will lead to development of more programs in the future.

Conclusion

Older patients with kidney stones may have similar but not identical risk factors as younger patients. The comorbidities associated with stones including diabetes mellitus, hypertension, metabolic syndrome, and coronary artery disease however are more common in the geriatric population. Attention to treatment of these conditions is likely to address stone disease risk factors as well. It is particularly important for geriatricians to recognize that pharmacologic therapy of stone disease can also address osteoporosis, a related disorder clearly associated with an increase in mortality. In the summary below, we offer some of the recommendations for addressing calcium stones in the older patient population.

Summary of Recommendations for Older Stone Formers with Calcium-Containing Stones

1. Encourage fluid intake with a goal of 2–3 L daily, spread throughout the day to achieve a consistently diluted urine. If 2–3 L daily intake is not possible, then strict adherence to a low salt, lower protein diet should be advocated.
2. Replete vitamin D deficiency if present.
3. Minimize use of calcium supplements, particularly in individuals incapable of achieving high fluid intake.
4. Encourage intake of 1000 mg (men) to 1200 mg (postmenopausal women) of calcium through dietary sources.
5. Limit further medical therapy (thiazides, urinary alkalinization, or acidification) to individuals at high risk of recurrence. Start with lowest possible treatment doses, and monitor for side effects regularly.

References

1. Scales CD Jr, et al. Prevalence of kidney stones in the United States. Eur Urol. 2012;62(1):160–5.
2. Soucie JM, et al. Demographic and geographic variability of kidney stones in the United States. Kidney Int. 1994;46(3):893–9.
3. Otto BJ, et al. Age, body mass index, and gender predict 24-hour urine parameters in recurrent idiopathic calcium oxalate stone formers. J Endourol. 2017;31(12):1335–41.
4. Taylor EN, Fung TT, Curhan GC. DASH-style diet associates with reduced risk for kidney stones. J Am Soc Nephrol. 2009;20(10):2253–9.
5. Fakheri RJ, Goldfarb DS. Association of nephrolithiasis prevalence rates with ambient temperature in the United States: a re-analysis. Kidney Int. 2009;76(7):798.

6. Mass AY, Goldfarb DS, Shah O. Taxi cab syndrome: a review of the extensive genitourinary pathology experienced by taxi cab drivers and what we can do to help. Rev Urol. 2014;16(3):99–104.
7. Worcester EM, Coe FL. Clinical practice. Calcium kidney stones. N Engl J Med. 2010;363(10):954–63.
8. Lieske JC, et al. Stone composition as a function of age and sex. Clin J Am Soc Nephrol. 2014;9(12):2141–6.
9. Ferraro PM, et al. Dietary and lifestyle risk factors associated with incident kidney stones in men and women. J Urol. 2017;198(4):858–63.
10. Borghi L, et al. Comparison of two diets for the prevention of recurrent stones in idiopathic hypercalciuria. N Engl J Med. 2002;346(2):77–84.
11. Pearle MS, et al. Medical management of kidney stones: AUA guideline. J Urol. 2014;192(2):316–24.
12. Skolarikos A, et al. Metabolic evaluation and recurrence prevention for urinary stone patients: EAU guidelines. Eur Urol. 2015;67(4):750–63.
13. Escribano J, et al. Dietary interventions for preventing complications in idiopathic hypercalciuria. Cochrane Database Syst Rev. 2014;(2):Cd006022.
14. Qaseem A, et al. Dietary and pharmacologic management to prevent recurrent nephrolithiasis in adults: a clinical practice guideline from the American College of Physicians. Ann Intern Med. 2014;161(9):659–67.
15. Huen SC, Goldfarb DS. Adverse metabolic side effects of thiazides: implications for patients with calcium nephrolithiasis. J Urol. 2007;177(4):1238–43.
16. Pannarale G. Optimal drug treatment of systolic hypertension in the elderly. Drugs Aging. 2008;25(1):1–8.
17. Sakhaee K, et al. Nephrolithiasis-associated bone disease: pathogenesis and treatment options. Kidney Int. 2011;79(4):393–403.
18. Usui Y, et al. Urolithiasis in geriatric patients. Tokai J Exp Clin Med. 2003;28(2):81–7.
19. Rule AD, et al. The ROKS nomogram for predicting a second symptomatic stone episode. J Am Soc Nephrol. 2014;25(12):2878–86.
20. Goldfarb DS, Parks JH, Coe FL. Renal stone disease in older adults. Clin Geriatr Med. 1998;14(2):367–81.
21. Walker V, Stansbridge EM, Griffin DG. Demography and biochemistry of 2800 patients from a renal stones clinic. Ann Clin Biochem. 2013;50(2):127–39.
22. Perinpam M, et al. Effect of demographics on excretion of key urinary factors related to kidney stone risk. Urology. 2015;86(4):690–6.
23. Friedlander JI, et al. Age-related changes in 24-hour urine composition must be considered in the medical management of nephrolithiasis. J Endourol. 2014;28(7):871–6.
24. Scales CD, et al. Urinary stone disease: advancing knowledge, patient care, and population health. Clin J Am Soc Nephrol. 2016;11(7):1305–12.
25. Taylor EN, et al. Nephrolithiasis and risk of incident bone fracture. J Urol. 2016;195(5):1482–6.
26. Carbone LD, et al. Urinary tract stones and osteoporosis: findings from the Women's Health Initiative. J Bone Miner Res. 2015;30(11):2096–102.
27. Lucato P, et al. Nephrolithiasis, bone mineral density, osteoporosis, and fractures: a systematic review and comparative meta-analysis. Osteoporos Int. 2016;27(11):3155–64.
28. Letavernier E, et al. Determinants of osteopenia in male renal-stone-disease patients with idiopathic hypercalciuria. Clin J Am Soc Nephrol. 2011;6(5):1149–54.
29. Arrabal-Polo MA, et al. Effects of aminobisphosphonates and thiazides in patients with osteopenia/osteoporosis, hypercalciuria, and recurring renal calcium lithiasis. Urology. 2013;81(4):731–7.
30. Pak CYC, et al. Prevention of stone formation and bone loss in absorptive hypercalciuria by combined dietary and pharmacological interventions. J Urol. 2003;169(2):465–9.
31. Pipili C, Oreopoulos DG. Vitamin D status in patients with recurrent kidney stones. Nephron Clin Pract. 2012;122(3–4):134–8.

32. Nguyen S, et al. 25-hydroxyvitamin D in the range of 20 to 100 ng/mL and incidence of kidney stones. Am J Public Health. 2014;104(9):1783–7.
33. Taylor EN, Hoofnagle AN, Curhan GC. Calcium and phosphorus regulatory hormones and risk of incident symptomatic kidney stones. Clin J Am Soc Nephrol. 2015;10(4):667–75.
34. Tang J, Chonchol MB. Vitamin D and kidney stone disease. Curr Opin Nephrol Hypertens. 2013;22(4):383–9.
35. Leaf DE, et al. Effect of vitamin D repletion on urinary calcium excretion among kidney stone formers. Clin J Am Soc Nephrol. 2012;7(5):829–34.
36. Ferroni MC, et al. Vitamin D repletion in kidney stone formers: a randomized controlled trial. J Urol. 2017;197(4):1079–83.
37. Jackson RD, et al. Calcium plus vitamin D supplementation and the risk of fractures. N Engl J Med. 2006;354(7):669–83.
38. Bolland MJ, et al. Calcium supplements with or without vitamin D and risk of cardiovascular events: reanalysis of the Women's Health Initiative limited access dataset and meta-analysis. BMJ. 2011;342:d2040.
39. Kopecky SL, et al. Lack of evidence linking calcium with or without vitamin D supplementation to cardiovascular disease in generally healthy adults: a clinical guideline from the National Osteoporosis Foundation and the American Society for Preventive Cardiology. Ann Intern Med. 2016;165(12):867–8.
40. Kuehn BM. Uspstf: taking vitamin d and calcium doesn't prevent fractures in older women. JAMA. 2012;308(3):225–6.
41. Moyer VA, U.S.P.S.T. Force*. Vitamin D and calcium supplementation to prevent fractures in adults: U.S. Preventive Services Task Force recommendation statement. Ann Intern Med. 2013;158(9):691–6.
42. Harris SS, Dawson-Hughes B. Effects of hydration and calcium supplementation on urine calcium concentration in healthy postmenopausal women. J Am Coll Nutr. 2015;34(4):340–6.
43. Levine BS, et al. Effect of calcium citrate supplementation on urinary calcium oxalate saturation in female stone formers: implications for prevention of osteoporosis. Am J Clin Nutr. 1994;60(4):592–6.
44. Arrabal-Martin M, et al. Treatment with hydrochlorothiazide and alendronate in patients with stones and bone mineral density loss. Evolution of bone metabolism and calciuria with medical treatment. Arch Esp Urol. 2016;69(1):9–18.
45. Jehle S, Hulter HN, Krapf R. Effect of potassium citrate on bone density, microarchitecture, and fracture risk in healthy older adults without osteoporosis: a randomized controlled trial. J Clin Endocrinol Metab. 2013;98(1):207–17.
46. Keddis MT, Rule AD. Nephrolithiasis and loss of kidney function. Curr Opin Nephrol Hypertens. 2013;22(4):390–6.
47. Ferraro PM, et al. History of kidney stones and the risk of coronary heart disease. JAMA. 2013;310(4):408–15.
48. Alexander RT, et al. Kidney stones and cardiovascular events: a cohort study. Clin J Am Soc Nephrol. 2014;9(3):506–12.
49. Daels FPJ, et al. Age-related prevalence of diabetes mellitus, cardiovascular disease and anticoagulation therapy use in a urolithiasis population and their effect on outcomes: the Clinical Research Office of the Endourological Society Ureteroscopy Global Study. World J Urol. 2015;33(6):859–64.
50. Trinchieri A, Esposito N, Castelnuovo C. Dissolution of radiolucent renal stones by oral alkalinization with potassium citrate/potassium bicarbonate. Arch Ital Urol Androl. 2009;81(3):188–91.
51. Drach GW, Griebling TL. Geriatric urology. J Am Geriatr Soc. 2003;51(7 Suppl):S355–8.
52. Braude P, et al. Evaluation and establishment of a ward-based geriatric liaison service for older urological surgical patients: Proactive care of Older People undergoing Surgery (POPS)-Urology. BJU Int. 2017;120(1):123–9.

Nutrition in the Elderly with Renal Disease

15

Vincenzo Bellizzi, Filippo Aucella, Patrizia Calella, Philippe Chauveau, Lina Johansson, and Daniel Teta

Who Is the *True* Elderly Renal Patient and Which Target for Treatment?

The level of kidney function of *healthy* elderly individuals differs from that of young people; from a clinical perspective, however, it is not well defined whether or when the lower kidney function in the elderly has to be considered as a

V. Bellizzi (✉)
Division of Nephrology, Dialysis and Transplantation, Nephrology Unit, University Hospital "San Giovanni di Dio e Ruggi d'Aragona", Salerno, Italy

European Renal Nutrition (ERN) Working Group at the European Renal Association – European Dialysis Transplant Association (ERA-EDTA), London, UK

F. Aucella
Department of Nephrology and Dialysis, Scientific Institute for Research and Health Care "Casa Sollievo della Sofferenza" IRCCS, San Giovanni Rotondo, Italy

P. Calella
Department of Movement Sciences and Wellbeing, Parthenope University, Naples, Italy

P. Chauveau
European Renal Nutrition (ERN) Working Group at the European Renal Association – European Dialysis Transplant Association (ERA-EDTA), London, UK

Aurad Aquitaine et Service de Néphrologie CHU de Bordeaux, Bordeaux, France

L. Johansson
European Renal Nutrition (ERN) Working Group at the European Renal Association – European Dialysis Transplant Association (ERA-EDTA), London, UK

Department of Nutrition and Dietetics, Imperial College Healthcare NHS Trust, London, UK

D. Teta
European Renal Nutrition (ERN) Working Group at the European Renal Association – European Dialysis Transplant Association (ERA-EDTA), London, UK

Service of Nephrology, Hospital of Sion and University of Lausanne, Lausanne, Switzerland

C. G. Musso et al. (eds.), *Clinical Nephrogeriatrics*,
https://doi.org/10.1007/978-3-030-18711-8_15

physiological or a pathological condition. The kidney function is multidimensional and includes either quantitative or qualitative elements; actually, the kidney dysfunction can result from impaired filtration or epithelial transport, which respectively represents glomerular or tubular failure, but also from vascular damage. In addition, the intrinsic renal aging has to be distinguished from the vascular aging which impacts on glomerular function and can simulate the renal aging [1]. Also, renal aging and chronic kidney disease (CKD) have several shared conditions; besides the lower glomerular filtration rate (GFR) levels, the maximum urine concentration and the dilution capability, such as the reduction of urea and sodium reabsorption or the renal functional reserve, are similarly impaired; in contrast, other conditions such as urine acidification, erythropoietin synthesis, and parathyroid (PTH) levels are quite normal in the elderly [2].

The prevalence of CKD, defined by estimated GFR (eGFR) <60 ml/min per 1.73 m^2 or albuminuria persisting for 3 months or more, increases in the adult population [3]. However, the prevalence by these markers of kidney disease is strikingly related to age, increasing from 4% in 20–39-year-old individuals to 47% in 70- and more year-old subjects. Nonetheless, in elderly the prevalence of reduced eGFR is much higher than the presence of albuminuria [4]. Overall, it seems the eGFR level alone is not truly representative of the renal function impairment in the elderly. In other words, the eGFR per se is not capable to discriminate among aging and disease (subclinical vascular disease or renal structural changes), which may also be both present at the same time in an elderly subject. Hence, in elderly the diagnosis of CKD by mean of eGFR should take into account potential sources of bias (e.g., sarcopenia or malnutrition). Since to identify patients who will benefit from closer renal follow-up is of paramount importance, the *European Best Practice Guidelines* suggested to base this decision on two factors: the risk prediction for survival and the risk prediction for progression of renal insufficiency [5]. The preferred tool for the risk prediction for survival in older patients is the Bansal score. High-risk patients should be admitted to an advanced care plan and nephroprotective measures which should not interfere with their quality of life. Nevertheless, a low predicted mortality risk can be misleading in frail patients, and additional assessment of frailty should be performed using a specific geriatric multidimensional assessment. It is worth mentioning that patients with high frailty risk should be considered like high mortality risk patients, regardless of the Bansal score, and be managed accordingly.

The current thresholds of eGFR to identify the CKD should not be modified in the elderly [6], mainly because in the elderly the reduced relative risk associated with the lower eGFR is counteracted by the higher absolute risks for acute kidney injury, end-stage renal disease (ESRD), and death related to age. Of note, early diagnosing of CKD in elderly allows to focus on any other patient risks, leading to a better cardiovascular care. The evaluation of both the comorbid conditions and the trajectory of eGFR and urinary albumin together allows to better predict the outcomes; stable, slightly impaired renal function without other risk factors (i.e., eGFR 45–59 ml/min, no albuminuria) identifies a low-risk condition that usually can be followed without intensive cardiovascular care. In contrast, the presence of albuminuria, mainly above 300 mg albumin/g creatinine, identifies a true CKD irrespective of the eGFR level.

Likely to young peoples, the elderly with advanced CKD are at higher risk for myocardial infarction, kidney failure, stroke, and death as compared with age-/gender-matched individuals with normal or slightly reduced eGFR [7]. Though death is by far the most common hard outcome in elderly with advance CKD, older patients with severe CKD can benefit from timely renal care referral [8]. Even in the very old patients with advanced CKD, the appropriate intensive renal care may slow the kidney function decline rate; may improve the metabolic acidosis, the anemia, and the hyperparathyroidism; may lower the cardiovascular risk; and allows an aware choice of renal replacement strategies [9].

Nutritional Status and Evaluation in Elderly Patients with Renal Disease

Chronic kidney disease (CKD), especially in the advanced stages, can lead to the development of a compromised nutritional status or "a state of metabolic and nutritional derangements," termed protein energy wasting (PEW). This impacts negatively on hospitalizations and survival [10]. Older people with CKD are even more vulnerable to developing PEW which can affect physical and mental well-being [11]. The evaluation of nutritional status has added complexity in older people with CKD.

Several studies have demonstrated that as people on dialysis age, nutritional status worsens with the prevalence of PEW in older people ranging from 50% to 68% compared to 27–50% in younger people [12, 13]. As the dialysis population ages, nutritional status worsens [14, 15].

Aging leads to loss of muscle, strength, and dentition as well as cognitive ability, potentially culminating in sarcopenia and dementia. Emotional and social support networks can suddenly diminish with bereavements and changes in housing. Overlap this with ill health, such as CKD, and it is clear why older people experience greater nutritional issues.

Evaluating nutritional status/PEW therefore requires assessment of multiple systems to determine the outcome. A single system cannot reliably reflect overall nutritional status as indicated in Table 15.1. Composite nutritional assessment tools commonly used in evaluation of PEW in CKD are the subjective global assessment (SGA) and malnutrition inflammation score (MIS). SGA and MIS have several features in common such as weight loss, dietary intake, gastrointestinal symptoms, functional capacity, and fat and muscle wasting. MIS has additional features of comorbidity and time on dialysis, body mass index (BMI), and laboratory parameters. The Mini Nutritional Assessment (Short Form) was designed for older people and includes pertinent questions on chewing and swallowing problems, mobility, psychological stress, and neuropsychological problems. SGA, MIS, and MNA had hazard ratios of 2.63, 5.13, and 2.53, respectively, for mortality in participants identified with PEW compared to those who were well nourished [16] (Table 15.1 [17–24]).

Table 15.1 Assessment of nutritional status in elderly CKD patients

Systems	Indicators of poor nutritional status	Interpretation	Cutoffs for poor nutritional status and conclusions
Biochemical indices	Low serum albumin and prealbumin	Albumin reduces through loss of protein, e.g., through dialysis process	Low albumin = <38 g/L
		Albumin is a negative acute-phase protein so levels decrease with inflammation	Low albumin levels are not exclusively due to poor nutritional intake or poor nutritional status [17] so doubts as to whether this is an appropriate indicator for poor nutritional status [18]
		Levels dilute (i.e., decrease) if plasma volume increases as occurs in renal patients with fluid retention	
	Low total iron binding capacity (transferrin)	Levels reflect changes in nutritional status	Low total iron binding capacity = <250 mg/dL [18]
Whole body	Low body mass index (BMI)	Inappropriate method to determine obesity levels in older people (as body composition changes with age)	ESPEN consensus BMI <22 kg/m^2 in older people >70 years [18]
		Higher BMI needed in older people to capture cases of poor nutritional status	Protein energy wasting: BMI <23 kg/m^2 for adults [20]
		Weight must be edema free	
	Significant weight loss	Unintentional weight loss evaluated relative to body mass as a %	>5% over the last 3 months for acute illnesses
		Weight must be edema free	>10% of usual weight, independent of time for chronic condition [18]
Body composition	Decreased fat free mass	Fat free mass, in particular muscle, has important functions in relation to undertaking activities	Fat free mass index <15 kg/m^2 and <17 kg/m^2 for women and men [18] Skeletal muscle index for sarcopenia assessment ≤6.75 kg/m^2 in women and ≤10.75 kg/m^2 in men [23]
Physical function	Decreased muscle strength (by handgrip strength)	Used in diagnosis of sarcopenia and frailty as opposed to poor nutritional status	Mobility limitations <20 kg and <30 kg for women and men [24] Weakness <16 kg and <26 kg for men and women [22]
Dietary intake	Decreased energy intake	Significant contributor to a poor nutritional status	Unintentional low dietary energy intake <25 kcal/kg/day for at least 2 months [20]

Table 15.1 (continued)

Systems	Indicators of poor nutritional status	Interpretation	Cutoffs for poor nutritional status and conclusions
	Decreased protein intake	Significant contributor to a poor nutritional status	Unintentional low dietary protein intake <0.80 g/kg/day for at least 2 months for dialysis patients or <0.6 g/kg/day for patients with CKD stages 2–5
Symptoms	Anorexia/nausea/vomiting/diarrhea	Significant contributor to a poor nutritional status either through decreased dietary intake and/or through increased loss of nutrients	Daily for 2 weeks [21]

In summary, older people with renal disease are more at risk of PEW due to the additional risk factors that accompany aging and increased comorbidities. Evaluating these additional risk factors as part of the nutritional assessment would be expected to deliver a more accurate diagnosis of PEW; however, this has not been evidenced. Improving nutritional status in older people is likely to require a multifaceted approach by improving dietary intake, inflammation, and symptoms as well as support with managing shopping, cooking, cognitive dysfunction, depression, and social isolation.

Safe Approach for Nutritional Treatment in Elderly Non-dialysis Renal Patients

Global population is aging rapidly. The number of patients affected by chronic kidney disease (CKD) is growing, and this is mainly related to the increasing elderly patients, and more than half people reaching the end-stage renal disease (ESRD) are older than 65 years [25, 26]. The transition toward dialysis is critical in elderly patients. The functional capacity in the daily activities in older patients reduces before the start of dialysis, has a steep decline in few months and 1 year after dialysis start only 13% of patients maintain their non-dialysis functional status [27]. In older people, the functional status, that is the capacity to perform the common activities in the daily living, represents a priority according to the World Health Organization which promotes the health aging, that is, any strategies to preserve and maintain the individual functional ability in the older age in order to guarantee the well-being and a good quality of life [28]. Hence, the elderly CKD non-dialysis patients transiting toward dialysis need special healthcare.

A key question in elderly patients with advanced non-dialysis CKD is to start dialysis early with the risk to reduce the functional status or continue the conservative care as far as possible with the related risks. A cornerstone of the conservative treatment in CKD is the nutritional treatment based on the low-protein diet (LPD) which has advantages but also potential concerns [29]. The LPD may slow down the GFR progression rate, lower the uremic toxicity, and improve several renal and cardiovascular risk factors (i.e., proteinuria, hypertension, hyperparathyroidism, hyperphosphatemia, metabolic acidosis, insulin resistance), thus improving the outcome. In contrast, especially in the elderly the LPD may enable several conditions (low energy intake, negative nitrogen balance, impaired glucose homeostasis, etc.) which may cause protein-energy wasting (PEW) and the resulting worst clinical outcome [30]. Hence, the outcome advantages of the nutritional treatment in the elderly may be overcome by the PEW. Is this risk related to proteins or energy?

The minimum protein requirement to maintain a body neutral nitrogen balance in adult subjects is 0.46 g per kilo of body weight per day if essential amino acids are provided, otherwise the amount rise to 0.60 g/kg/day; it has been evidenced that also patients with advanced CKD can maintain a neutral nitrogen balance with such an amount of protein intake of 0.60 g/kg/day in absence of metabolic acidosis and catabolic illness [31]. Due to the individual variability the recommended dietary allowance for proteins to assure the metabolic requirements in 97.5% of the population has been fixed in 0.8 g/kg/day [32].

The protein intake progressively reduces with increasing age in all people [33]. In young people there is no difference between CKD at any stage and normal individual, but among elderly CKD patients the protein intake reduces along the renal disease and mainly in CKD stages 4–5 as compared to normal; nonetheless, the daily protein intake never falls below 1 g/kg/day, thus largely over the safe threshold [33]. In contrast, the mean actual energy intake in elderly CKD patients is around 25 kcal per kilo of body weight per day with a progressive reduction in advanced CKD; this reduction is related in part to the reduced protein intake but mostly to the spontaneous lowering of carbohydrates intake [34]. So, most elderly patients with advanced CKD have an adequate or even high intake of proteins but a low intake of energy. This is a critical condition since the suggested intake of energy to maintain the nitrogen balance in elderly is between 30 and 35 kcal/kg/day and, in presence of the minimum intake of proteins, a low energy intake make the body nitrogen balance negative [35].

In CKD elderly, indeed, a supervised low-protein and normal energy diet does not reduce the muscle mass as well as in young CKD patients [36]. In CKD stage V elderly patients, even a very low-protein diet, while was able to delay the start of dialysis, did not cause major adverse effect or death and had a lower morbidity [37]. Neither a negative impact on both nutrition and outcomes was observed also in the long-term during the dialysis period after the low-protein diet [38].

In CKD elderly patients a nutritional approach satisfying the nutrient needs, does not impact negatively on the nutritional status, may delay the start of dialysis and improve the morbidity, without a negative effect on survival. The practical recommendation for elderly, high-risk, frail patients with advanced CKD suggest to choose first the CKD conservative treatment, hence including the nutritional treatment, with the strong advice to preserve the nutritional status over any other nutritional intervention [39]. Consequently, the safe nutritional approach in elderly CKD patients is, first to provide high energy to preserve the nutritional status and, and second to introduce any other needed dietary restrictions, including the protein restriction [40].

Healthy Dietary Patterns in Elderly Patients with Chronic Renal Disease

Most specific nutritional recommendations for chronic kidney disease (CKD) are focused on the restriction of certain nutrients such as sodium, potassium, phosphates or animal proteins and this positioning leads to restrictive renal diets. In the elderly, the abrupt either modification of dietary habits or prescription of too restrictive diets could lead to a striking lowering of nutrients intake and, consequently, to a worsening of the nutritional status.

In either the general population [41] or the CKD patients, eating habits and lifestyle may impact on the both the onset and worsening of chronic diseases. For instance, the western diet rich in animal proteins, refined sugar and poor in fruits and vegetables is associated with chronic cardiovascular and kidney diseases. In opposite, diets rich in fruits and vegetables and poor in sodium and meat are now recommended as "healthy diets" for the general population and the elderly as well. In the dietary guidelines advisory board for US population, the global healthy diet such as healthy US pattern, Mediterranean diet or vegetarian diet had been recommended [42].

In the CKD patient a diet richer in fiber and less rich in salt, refined sugars and animal proteins is associated with a lower mortality as shown by a recent meta-analysis [43]. Likewise, in CKD the Mediterranean diet has been proposed as a diet of choice [44].

What about the elderly? Few data are available specifically in older adults but point towards a protective effect of healthy diets. Analysis of the NHANES study based on adherence scores to a DASH or Mediterranean diet shows that the association between healthy diet and chronic diseases is less evident in older age groups because of interaction with other factors such as physical activity [45]. These results are similar to those of Martins et al., which analyzes the multi-decade follow-up of the AHS-2 (Adventist Health Study). Age is associated with a reduction in protein intake and an increase in fruits and vegetables. Those who have kept the same healthy diet the longest, are the ones with the least metabolic complications [46]. In other words, it is preferable to propose a diet close to a Mediterranean diet for younger generations [42]. The results of maintaining a healthy diet over time is supported by the results of the NHANES study; the decline in renal function in 3121 women, mean age 67, who completed the nutritional questionnaires since 1984 was evaluated. A Western-type diet is associated with a faster decline in renal function and proteinuria while a DASH type regime is protective against the progression of CKD [47]. A Japanese study of 99,000 participants showed that the adoption of a healthy both diet and lifestyle is associated with a lower incidence of proteinuria even in the highest age groups including patients who have changed their diet a year ago [48].

Even if few studies report a specific effect of a healthy diet in elderly people with kidney failure, it has been shown that reducing the acid load slows the progression of kidney failure in this population. Two-hundred-seventeen elderly CKD patients (eGFR 23 ml/min, age 71 years) with normal serum bicarbonate were retrospectively studied; subjects with higher net endogenous acid production had a higher progression of CKD [49]. The same result was obtained in diabetic CKD from CRIC study [50]. Mediterranean diet and DASH diet are associated with lower dietary acid load and contribute to a lower CKD progression [51]. In the elderly, adherence to a Mediterranean diet is associated with a reduction in the risk of many comorbidities, such as the slightest risk of frailty [52], lower diabetes incidence [53], lower cognitive decline [54], and risk of osteoporosis [55].

In summary, in elderly people with CKD it may be advisable to maintain or adopt a healthy dietary pattern which is associated with better outcomes and possibly a lower kidney function decline.

Combination of Nutritional Treatment and Low-Frequency Dialysis

In CKD elderly subjects with extremely reduced renal function, the start of dialysis may prolong survival but reduces the quality of life, lowers the functional status making personal relationships and social life very poor [27]. In addition, in this conditions the nutritional status worsens due to anorexia, inflammation and metabolic derangements with consequent high risk of protein-energy wasting [56]. Moreover, the costs of the transition of elderly to dialysis are very high for the health system [57].

Delay the start of dialysis may be possible by mean of a strict comprehensive treatment associated with a rigorous control of the clinical complications related to the end-stage renal disease [29]. A dietary-nutritional treatment may target this aim, but in elderly, frail end-stage renal disease (ESRD) patients, it may also further expose the subjects to severe risks, and, therefore, this treatment alone cannot be always safe. A strategy which can help to solve this dilemma (i.e., conservative or dialysis treatment in elderly ESRD) may be the combination of both treatments, that is, a strict conservative/dietary treatment and a low-dose/low-frequency dialysis treatment, together.

The combination of a dietary treatment and a once-weekly hemodialysis session was tested in ESRD patients (residual renal function < 5 ml/min) with the aim to reduce the uremic toxins source and to attain a blood purification, with the final purpose to ensure an adequate metabolic control and to preserve the residual renal function [58]. This integrated program is based on a very low-protein diet (0.3–0.4 g proteins per kg/day) supplemented with a mixture of essential amino acids and keto acids for 6 days per week, a strict sodium and water restriction, one hemodialysis session per week, and unrestricted diet on the dialysis day [59].

A combined dietary/dialysis approach deserves a careful care and is demanding for patient itself, for his family and for the caretakers as well. Indeed, despite the promising clinical effects, some concerns can be related to diet adherence and nutritional status [60]. Thus, a close monitoring by physician, dietitian and caregivers is required to avoid complications in frail, elderly patients.

Recently, a more accurate combined dietary/dialysis program has been proposed with the aim to further improve the patient's adherence and reduce the nutritional risks [61]. The program was extended to patients with higher residual renal function (>5 ml/min), the dietary protein regimen was less severe (0.6 g of proteins per kg/day), and there was a more careful attention to phosphorus restriction and to high energy provision. As compared to patients on full dialysis regimen, the combined program showed better preservation of residual renal function and daily urine output, better metabolic control, lower drug need, reduced morbidity and hospitalization while deferring the start of full dialysis by almost 1 year [61].

In an integrated diet and dialysis strategy, the peritoneal dialysis (PD) is the ideal companion for the diet. The low-dose PD should be preferable to weekly HD for several reasons. Mainly, PD is an home-based, less invasive, and best tolerated treatment, and it is continuous with lower hemodynamic impact and less ischemic insult on the kidney. Therefore, PD may better preserve the patient functionality and the residual renal function. A preliminary report evidenced that in incident ESRD (GFR, >3 – <10 ml/min) patients over 60 years, a low-dose PD is safe and compared to standard PD has similar survival, lower hospitalization, and slower renal function decline [62].

Overall, in elderly ESRD patients the combined dietary/dialysis approach could be an actual bridge strategy in the transition toward full dialysis [63], allowing to preserve the functional status while not exposing the patients to high risks (Table 15.2). This strategy could be proposed to selected, motivated and supported patients in which may improve the quality of life and help the transition to end-of-life, even it is also cost-saving [64].

Table 15.2 Advantages and concerns of combined diet and dialysis in elderly ESRD patients

Advantages	Concerns
Improvement of metabolic control of uremia	Strict therapeutic regimen
Improvement of clinical symptoms	Low palatability diet
Maintenance of diuresis and RRF	Risk of malnutrition
Maintenance of physical function	Requirement of a renal dietician
Reduction of patient's hospital visits	Requirement of a multi-disciplinary approach
Favoring end-of-life dignity	Involvement of family or caregivers
Maintenance of direct and indirect costs	Requirement of close nutritional monitoring

Target Nutritional Needs in Elderly Dialysis Patients

Nutritional interventions must ensure that the nutritional needs for any individual dialysis patient are met. Most elderly dialysis patients have low, if not very low, spontaneous intakes, making this goal a challenge in order to maintain and/or improve their nutritional status. There are no specific clinical studies which exclusively investigated nutritional interventions in elderly dialysis patients. However, data from interventional studies in nonrenal geriatric patients and those in the overall dialysis population, which involve many elderly patients, provide useful information likely to be applied in elderly dialysis patients.

Nutritional interventions in elderly dialysis patients may be targeted to reach three aims:

(a) To tackle age-related causes of protein-energy wasting (PEW) such as reduced metabolic rate, loss of muscle mass and function, sedentary behavior, and anorexia
(b) To address psychosocial and medical issues related with advanced age such as loneliness, depression, dependency, poverty, dementia, early satiety, comorbidities, and polypharmacy
(c) To counteract dialysis-related causes including uremic toxicity, metabolic derangements, inflammation-related catabolism, dialysis-related acute, and chronic complications.

Interventions Tackling Age-Related Causes

Advanced age is associated with sarcopenia, progressive decline in skeletal muscle mass, strength, and function [65]. Sarcopenia, which is part of frailty, is prevalent in the elderly dialysis population and is associated with higher morbidity and mortality [66]. Several studies from nonrenal elderly patients investigated the use of oral nutritional supplements (ONS) to address sarcopenia. A recent non-blinded randomized study evaluated the addition of ONS, i.e., two daily cans of β-hydroxy-β-methylbutyrate (HMB) in patients aged 65 years and older with hip fractures admitted to rehabilitation facilities. The addition of HMB prevented the onset of sarcopenia, improved muscle mass, and was associated with functional improvement [67]. Another observer-blinded controlled randomized study in patients subjected to hip fracture surgery, aged 60 years and older, tested the addition of an ONS (18–24 g protein and 500 kcal per day) to the usual hospital diet. Both groups received rehabilitation therapy and calcium plus vitamin D supplements. Patients who received ONS, on top of standard diet, had a significantly shorter length of stay in the rehabilitation ward and a reduced number of infections [68]. Flakoll et al. evaluated the effects of a combination of arginine, lysine, and HMB dietary supplementation in 50 elderly female subjects (mean age of 76.7 years old) and observed an increase of 17% in the "get-up-and-go" test and an increased leg circumference and leg extensor and handgrip strengths in the experimental group, but not in the control group after 12 weeks [69]. Baier et al. showed an increase in lean body cell mass and lean mass after supplementation for 1 year with HMB, lysine, and arginine in elderly subjects aged 76 ± 1.6 years [70]. Similarly, de Luis et al. reported in an open-labeled study from elderly patients a beneficial effect of an enhanced enteral formula with HMB and vitamin D, on handgrip strength and some domains of quality of life [71]. Finally, Deutz et al. evaluated the effect of high-protein ONS containing HMB (two servings per day, with 1.5 g of HMB per serving) in malnourished hospitalized elderly patients. Mortality at 3 months was significantly lower and the nutritional status improved in the ONS group compared with the control group (placebo) [72]. Some studies evaluated the use of ONS in combination with exercise. A recent meta-analysis addressed this combination and showed that HMB supplementation in addition to resistance exercise resulted in better preservation of muscle mass versus resistance exercise alone [73]. Although most of studies reported an efficacy of ONS in maintaining or improving lean mass and increasing muscle strength in older adults suffering from nonrenal diseases, studies are warranted in renal elderly patients, in particular those undergoing dialysis.

Interventions Addressing Psychosocial and Medical Causes

A multicenter cross-sectional study on patterns of cognitive impairment in adult hemodialysis patients (median age of 70.9 years) showed that cognitive impairment was extremely common [74]. A longitudinal cohort study showed that hemodialysis patients had cognitive decline and older age was the only risk factor for steeper executive function decline [75]. Efforts should be made to identify modifiable risk factors for cognitive impairment in this population, of which nutritional and nutrient-dependent risk factors are of vital importance. Recently, raised plasma total homocysteine has been proposed as a modifiable risk factor for the development of cognitive decline and dementia in the older population [76]. Several interventional trials in elderly with cognitive impairment have indeed showed that homocysteine-lowering therapy with supplementation of B vitamins retarded cognitive decline [76]. However, studies exploring this issue are crucially needed in elderly dialysis patients. Finally, socialization at meal times can improve nutritional intake in older people. Locher et al. indeed showed that older people increased their intake during meals when eating in the presence of others [77].

Interventions Counteracting Dialysis-Related Causes

Eating during dialysis has been promoted by a recent consensus of the International Society of Renal Nutrition and Metabolism (ISRNM) [78]. It has been shown to reduce protein degradation [79]. In our dialysis center, snacks are routinely provided to hemodialysis patients with respect for eating habits, preferences, and cultural/religious interest. The nutrient content of typical snacks is shown in Table 15.3. The role of daily ONS to improve nutritional status has been demonstrated. An

Table 15.3 Nutritional content of common snacks during hemodialysis

	Kcal	Protein (g)	Glucose (g)	Phosphate (mg)	Potassium (mg)	Sodium (mg)
2 slices of bread	360	8.6	60	110	140	550
Ham sandwich	380	20	47	215	205	1175
Cheese sandwich	490	21	47	380	170	830
15 g protein powder + 2 slices bread	420	22	60	220	145	550
250 ml (2×) Renilon 7.5®	500	19	50	15	0.8	150
200 ml resource 2.0® fiber	400	18	44	180	320	120
200 ml Fortimel®	200	20	21	400	400	100

open-labeled randomized controlled trial in dialysis patients (mean age of 73 years old) with low nutritional intakes evaluated the effect of a renal-specific oral supplement (two daily packs of 125 ml Renilon 7.5® for 3 months) compared with standard care. ONS helped to meet energy and protein requirements, and nutritional status remained constant in the group supplemented, whereas nutritional parameters declined in the control group. In addition, quality of life improved in the supplemented group [80]. A randomized controlled trial in malnourished hemodialysis patients (mean age 68 years old) receiving ONS, with or without intradialytic parenteral nutrition (IDPN), reported improvements in nutritional parameters such as BMI, serum albumin, and prealbumin levels in both groups. An increase in prealbumin of >30 mg/L within 3 months was associated with a 54% decrease in mortality at 2 years [81]. Finally, a recent multicenter randomized controlled trial in hemodialysis patients with PEW (mean age of 73 years old) showed that the addition of IDPN three times weekly over 16 weeks to standardized nutritional counseling increased serum prealbumin compared to nutritional counseling alone [82].

In summary, although no studies have investigated nutritional interventions in elderly dialysis patients exclusively, nutritional interventions are effective in improving nutritional status and quality of life in randomized controlled trials including dialysis patients with an elevated mean age (68–73 years old). In nonrenal elderly patients, nutritional interventions have been shown to improve muscle strength, functional performances, and cognitive functions. In hospitalized elderly patients, some studies reported significant effects of nutritional supplementation on hard end points such as length of stay and mortality. These findings should convince nephrologists to integrate nutritional care in the overall management of elderly dialysis patients.

Conclusions

The majority of renal patients are old, more frail, and at high risk of impaired nutritional status; in these subjects, the nutritional intervention may have many benefits but also some harms and is a real challenge in the daily clinical practice. The older renal patients have to be regularly monitored for the nutritional status, the nutrient intakes, and the nutritional risk factors associated with aging and kidney disease by trained dietitians and physicians to early discover a nutritional impairment. In these people, the nutritional treatment requires a multifaceted approach not merely on dietary prescription but also on support with managing food preparation, cognitive dysfunction, depression, and social integration. A basically, safe dietary recommendation for elderly patients with advanced CKD is to first provide high energy and then introduce the other dietary restrictions. Elderly renal patients should be advisable to maintain or adopt a healthy dietary pattern (i.e., Mediterranean or DASH dietary regimens) and a healthy and active lifestyle which may reduce the risk of comorbidities, frailty, and cognitive decline also in these individuals. Also, the combination of nutritional treatment and low-frequency substitutive renal treatment could be a novel strategy to make more acceptable the transition of elderly patients to chronic dialysis. Overall, nephrologists should routinely integrate the nutritional care in the comprehensive management of elderly individuals in all the stages of renal disease in order to improve the nutritional status, the functional status, the quality of life, and the patient's outcomes.

Acknowledgments The European Renal Nutrition (ERN) Working Group is an initiative of and supported by the European Renal Association – European Dialysis Transplant Association (ERA-EDTA).

References

1. Gekle M. Kidney and aging – a narrative review. Exp Gerontol. 2017;87:153–5.
2. Musso CG, Jauregui JR. How to differentiate renal senescence from chronic kidney disease in clinical practice. Postgrad Med. 2016;128:716–21.
3. Coresh J, et al. Prevalence of chronic kidney disease in the United States. JAMA. 2007;298:2038–47.
4. Hommos MS, Glassock RJ, Rule AD. Structural and functional changes in human kidneys with healthy aging. J Am Soc Nephrol. 2017;28:2838–44.
5. Farrington K, et al. Clinical Practice Guideline Clinical Practice Guideline on management of older patients with chronic kidney disease stage 3b or higher (eGFR). Nephrol Dial Transpl. 2016;31:1–66.
6. Hallan SI, Gansevoort RT. Moderator's view: should we diagnose CKD using the 'one-size fits all' KDIGO 2012 guideline or do we need a more complex age-specific classification system? Nephrol Dial Transplant. 2014;29:780–2.
7. Hemmelgarn BR, et al. Relation between kidney function, proteinuria, and adverse outcomes. JAMA – J Am Med Assoc. 2010;303:423–9.
8. Tonelli M, Riella MC. Chronic kidney disease and the aging population. Kidney Int. 2014;85:487–91.
9. Stevens PE, Levin A, Kidney Disease: Improving Global Outcomes Chronic Kidney Disease Guideline Development Work Group, M. Evaluation and management of chronic kidney disease: synopsis of the kidney disease: improving global outcomes 2012 clinical practice guideline. Ann Intern Med. 2013;158:825–30.
10. Ikizler TA, et al. Prevention and treatment of protein energy wasting in chronic kidney disease patients: a consensus statement by the International Society of Renal Nutrition and Metabolism. Kidney Int. 2013;84:1096–107.

11. Johansson L, Hickson M, Brown EA. Influence of psychosocial factors on the energy and protein intake of older people on dialysis. J Ren Nutr. 2013;23:348–55.
12. Qureshi AR, et al. Factors predicting malnutrition in hemodialysis patients: a cross-sectional study. Kidney Int. 1998;53:773–82.
13. Cianciaruso B, et al. Nutritional status in the elderly patient with uraemia. Nephrol Dial Transplant. 1995;10(Suppl 6):65–8.
14. Rambod M, et al. Association of malnutrition-inflammation score with quality of life and mortality in hemodialysis patients: a 5-year prospective cohort study. Am J Kidney Dis. 2009;53:298–309.
15. de Mutsert R, et al. Subjective global assessment of nutritional status is strongly associated with mortality in chronic dialysis patients. Am J Clin Nutr. 2009;89:787–93.
16. de Santin FG, Bigogno FG, Dias Rodrigues JC, Cuppari L, Avesani CM. Concurrent and predictive validity of composite methods to assess nutritional status in older adults on hemodialysis. J Ren Nutr. 2016;26:18–25.
17. Don BR, Kaysen G. Serum albumin: relationship to inflammation and nutrition. Semin Dial. 2004;17:432–7.
18. Cederholm T, et al. Diagnostic criteria for malnutrition – an ESPEN consensus statement. Clin Nutr. 2015;34:335–40.
19. Kalantar-Zadeh K, Kopple JD, Block G, Humphreys MH. A malnutrition-inflammation score is correlated with morbidity and mortality in maintenance hemodialysis patients. Am J Kidney Dis. 2001;38:1251–63.
20. Fouque D, et al. A proposed nomenclature and diagnostic criteria for protein-energy wasting in acute and chronic kidney disease. Kidney Int. 2008;73:391–8.
21. Detsky AS, et al. What is subjective global assessment of nutritional status? JPEN J Parenter Enteral Nutr. 1987;11:8–13.
22. Studenski SA, et al. The FNIH sarcopenia project: rationale, study description, conference recommendations, and final estimates. J Gerontol – Ser A Biol Sci Med Sci. 2014;69A: 547–58.
23. Janssen I, Baumgartner RN, Ross R, Rosenberg IH, Roubenoff R. Skeletal muscle cutpoints associated with elevated physical disability risk in older men and women. Am J Epidemiol. 2004;159:413–21.
24. Lauretani F, et al. Age-associated changes in skeletal muscles and their effect on mobility: an operational diagnosis of sarcopenia. J Appl Physiol. 2003;95:1851–60.
25. United, U. S. R. D. S. U. 2011 A. D. R. A. of C. K. D. and E.-S. R. D. In the USRDS 2011 annual data report: Atlas of chronic kidney disease and end-stage renal disease in the United States. Bethesda, MD Natl. Institutes Heal. Natl. Inst. Diabetes Dig. Kidney Dis. Bethesda, MD 1–26. 2011.
26. Danfoss. Annual report 2013. 2013.
27. Kurella Tamura M, et al. Functional status of elderly adults before and after initiation of dialysis. N Engl J Med. 2009;361:1539–47.
28. World Health Organization. World report on ageing and health. 2015. Luxemb. Luxemb 1–260. 2015.
29. Bellizzi V, et al. Low-protein diets for chronic kidney disease patients: the Italian experience. BMC Nephrol. 2016;17:77.
30. Ko GJ, Obi Y, Tortorici AR, Kalantar-Zadeh K. Dietary protein intake and chronic kidney disease. Curr Opin Clin Nutr Metab Care. 2017;20(1):77–85. https://doi.org/10.1097/MCO.0000000000000342.
31. WHO/FAO/UNU Expert Consultation. Protein and amino acid requirements in human nutrition. World Health Organ. Tech. Rep. Ser. 1–265. 2007. ISBN 92 4 120935 6.
32. Young R. Special 1987 McCollum acid metabolism. 1987.
33. Moore LW, et al. The mean dietary protein intake at different stages of chronic kidney disease is higher than current guidelines. Kidney Int. 2013;83:724–32.
34. Luis D, et al. Renal function associates with energy intake in elderly community-dwelling men. Br J Nutr. 2014;111:2184–9.

35. Slomowitz LA, Monteon FJ, Grosvenor M, Laidlaw SA, Koppel JD. Effect of energy intake on nutritional status in maintenance hemodialysis patients. Kidney Int. 1989;35:704–11.
36. Hung KY, et al. Effects of diet intervention on body composition in the elderly with chronic kidney disease. Int J Med Sci. 2017;14:735–40.
37. Brunori G, et al. Efficacy and safety of a very-low-protein diet when postponing dialysis in the elderly: a prospective randomized multicenter controlled study. Am J Kidney Dis. 2007;49:569–80.
38. Bellizzi V, et al. Very low-protein diet plus ketoacids in chronic kidney disease and risk of death during end-stage renal disease: an historical, cohort, controlled study. Nephrol Dial Transplant. 2015;30(1):71–7.
39. Farrington K, et al. Clinical Practice Guideline on management of older patients with chronic kidney disease stage 3b or higher (eGFR<45 mL/min/1.73 m^2): a summary document from the European Renal Best Practice Group. Nephrol Dial Transpl. 2017;32:9–16.
40. Bellizzi V, et al. A Delphi consensus panel on nutritional therapy in chronic kidney disease. J Nephrol. 2016;29:593–602.
41. Eckel RH, et al. 2013 AHA/ACC guideline on lifestyle management to reduce cardiovascular risk: a report of the American college of cardiology/American heart association task force on practice guidelines. J Am Coll Cardiol. 2014;63:2960–84.
42. Millen BE, et al. The 2015 dietary guidelines advisory committee scientific report: development and major conclusions. Adv Nutr. 2016;7:438–44.
43. Kelly JT, et al. Healthy dietary patterns and risk of mortality and ESRD in CKD: a meta-analysis of cohort studies. Clin J Am Soc Nephrol. 2017;12:272–9.
44. Chauveau P, et al. Mediterranean diet as the diet of choice for patients with chronic kidney disease. Nephrol Dial Transplant. 2017. https://doi.org/10.1093/ndt/gfx085.
45. Park YMM, et al. Mediterranean diet, Dietary Approaches to Stop Hypertension (DASH) style diet, and metabolic health in U.S. adults. Clin Nutr. 2017;36(5):1301–9.
46. Martins MCT et al. A new approach to assess lifetime dietary patterns finds lower consumption of animal foods with aging in a longitudinal analysis of a health-oriented adventist population. Nutrients 2017;9.
47. Lin J, Curhan GC. Associations of sugar and artificially sweetened soda with albuminuria and kidney function decline in women. Clin J Am Soc Nephrol. 2011;6:160–6.
48. Wakasugi M, et al. Association between overall lifestyle changes and the incidence of proteinuria: a population-based, cohort study. Intern Med. 2017;56:1475–84.
49. Kanda E, Ai M, Kuriyama R, Yoshida M, Shiigai T. Dietary acid intake and kidney disease progression in the elderly. Am J Nephrol. 2014;39:145–52.
50. Scialla JJ, et al. Higher net acid excretion is associated with a lower risk of kidney disease progression in patients with diabetes. Kidney Int. 2017;91:204–15.
51. Banerjee T, Liu Y, Crews DC. Dietary patterns and CKD progression. Blood Purif. 2016;41:117–22.
52. Ntanasi E, et al. Adherence to Mediterranean diet and frailty. J Am Med Dir Assoc. 2017. https://doi.org/10.1016/j.jamda.2017.11.005.
53. Rossi M, et al. Mediterranean diet and glycaemic load in relation to incidence of type 2 diabetes: results from the Greek cohort of the population-based European Prospective Investigation into Cancer and Nutrition (EPIC). Diabetologia. 2013;56:2405–13.
54. Trichopoulou A, et al. Mediterranean diet and cognitive decline over time in an elderly Mediterranean population. Eur J Nutr. 2015;54:1311–21.
55. Savanelli MC, et al. Preliminary results demonstrating the impact of Mediterranean diet on bone health. J Transl Med. 2017;15:81.
56. Johansson L, et al. As we grow old: nutritional considerations for older patients on dialysis. Nephrol Dial Transplant. 2017;32:1127–36.
57. Vanholder R, Lameire N, Annemans L, Van Biesen W. Cost of renal replacement: how to help as many as possible while keeping expenses reasonable? Nephrol Dial Transplant. 2016;31:1251–61.

58. Mitch WE, Sapir DG. Evaluation of reduced dialysis frequency using nutritional therapy. Kidney Int. 1981;20:122–6.
59. Locatelli F, Andrulli S, Pontoriero G, Di Filippo S, Bigi MC. Supplemented low-protein diet and once-weekly hemodialysis. Am J Kidney Dis. 1994;24:192–204.
60. Locatelli F, Andrulli S, Pontoriero G, Di Filippo S, Bigi MC. Integrated diet and dialysis programme. Nephrol Dial Transplant. 1998;13:132–8.
61. Caria S, Cupisti A, Sau G, Bolasco P. The incremental treatment of ESRD: a low-protein diet combined with weekly hemodialysis may be beneficial for selected patients. BMC Nephrol. 2014;15:172.
62. Sandrini M, et al. Incremental peritoneal dialysis: a 10 year single-centre experience. J Nephrol. 2016;29:871–9.
63. Bolasco P, Cupisti A, Locatelli F, Caria S, Kalantar-Zadeh K. Dietary management of incremental transition to dialysis therapy: once-weekly hemodialysis combined with low-protein diet. J Ren Nutr. 2016;26:352–9.
64. Moss AH, Armistead NC. Improving end-of-life care for ESRD patients: an initiative for professionals. Nephrol News Issues. 2013;27:30–2.
65. Cruz-Jentoft AJ, et al. Sarcopenia: European consensus on definition and diagnosis: report of the European Working Group on Sarcopenia in Older People. Age Ageing. 2010;39:412–23.
66. Musso CG, Jauregui JR, Macías Núñez JF. Frailty phenotype and chronic kidney disease: a review of the literature. Int Urol Nephrol. 2015;47:1801–7.
67. Malafarina V, Uriz-Otano F, Malafarina C, Martinez JA, Zulet MA. Effectiveness of nutritional supplementation on sarcopenia and recovery in hip fracture patients. A multi-centre randomized trial. Maturitas. 2017;101:42–50.
68. Myint MWW, et al. Clinical benefits of oral nutritional supplementation for elderly hip fracture patients: a single blind randomised controlled trial. Age Ageing. 2013;42:39–45.
69. Flakoll P, et al. Effect of β-hydroxy-β-methylbutyrate, arginine, and lysine supplementation on strength, functionality, body composition, and protein metabolism in elderly women. Nutrition. 2004;20:445–51.
70. Baier S, et al. Year-long changes in protein metabolism in elderly men and women supplemented with a nutrition cocktail of β-hydroxy-β-methylbutyrate (HMB), L-arginine, and L-lysine. J Parenter Enter Nutr. 2009;33:71–82.
71. De Luis DA, Izaola O, Bachiller P, Perez Castrillon J. Effect on quality of life and handgrip strength by dynamometry of an enteral specific suplements with beta-hydroxy-beta-methylbutyrate and vitamin D in elderly patients. Nutr Hosp. 2015;32:202–7.
72. Deutz NE, et al. Readmission and mortality in malnourished, older, hospitalized adults treated with a specialized oral nutritional supplement: a randomized clinical trial. Clin Nutr. 2016;35:18–26.
73. Wu H, et al. Effect of beta-hydroxy-beta-methylbutyrate supplementation on muscle loss in older adults: a systematic review and meta-analysis. Arch Gerontol Geriatr. 2015;61:168–75.
74. van Zwieten A, et al. Prevalence and patterns of cognitive impairment in adult hemodialysis patients: the COGNITIVE-HD study. Nephrol Dial Transplant. 2017. https://doi.org/10.1093/ndt/gfx314.
75. Drew DA, et al. Cognitive decline and its risk factors in prevalent hemodialysis patients. Am J Kidney Dis. 2017;69:780–7.
76. Smith AD, et al. Homocysteine and dementia: an international consensus statement. J Alzheimers Dis. 2018;62:561–70.
77. Locher JL, Robinson CO, Roth DL, Ritchie CS, Burgio KL. The effect of the presence of others on caloric intake in homebound older adults. J Gerontol – Ser A Biol Sci Med Sci. 2005;60:1475–8.
78. Kistler BM, et al. Eating during hemodialysis treatment: a consensus statement from the International Society of Renal Nutrition and Metabolism. J Ren Nutr. 2018;28:4–12.
79. Veeneman JM, et al. Protein intake during hemodialysis maintains a positive whole body protein balance in chronic hemodialysis patients. Am J Physiol – Endocrinol Metab. 2003;284:E954–65.

80. Fouque D, et al. Use of a renal-specific oral supplement by haemodialysis patients with low protein intake does not increase the need for phosphate binders and may prevent a decline in nutritional status and quality of life. Nephrol Dial Transplant. 2008;23:2902–10.
81. Cano NJ, et al. Intradialytic parenteral nutrition does not improve survival in malnourished hemodialysis patients: a 2-year multicenter, prospective, randomized study. J Am Soc Nephrol. 2007;18:2583–91.
82. Marsen TA, Beer J, Mann H. Intradialytic parenteral nutrition in maintenance hemodialysis patients suffering from protein-energy wasting. Results of a multicenter, open, prospective, randomized trial. Clin Nutr. 2017;36:107–17.

Pharmacogeriatrics and the Kidney

16

Paula Scibona and Waldo H. Belloso

Introduction

Life expectancy is increasing in most parts of the world, probably in relation to improvements in health care and access to better treatment, but this trend toward longevity is associated with an increased demand on health services and health-care expenditure [1, 2].

Older people constitute a particular group regarding pharmacotherapeutics for many reasons. They are high consumers of prescription drugs (up to 30% of all commonly prescribed medications); the age-related pharmacokinetic and pharmacodynamic changes and high rate of comorbidities put them at an increased risk of drug interactions, adverse effects, and inadequate dosing. Furthermore, pharmacological studies and clinical trials in this age group are scant, especially in those with significant comorbidities, and so there is often inadequate information available to guide safe and effective use of drugs [3].

Pharmacological Considerations in Older Adults

Aging is associated with many changes that can affect pharmacokinetics and pharmacodynamics, even in the absence of specific disease [4]. Some of the changes relating to the aging are as follows: reduction in total body water determines a decrease in the volume of distribution (VD) for hydrophilic drugs, while increase in total body fat produces a 20–40% increase in VD for lipophilic drugs [5, 6].

P. Scibona (✉) · W. H. Belloso
Clinical Pharmacology Section, Internal Medicine Service, Hospital Italiano de Buenos Aires, Buenos Aires, Argentina
e-mail: waldo.belloso@hospitalitaliano.org.ar

C. G. Musso et al. (eds.), *Clinical Nephrogeriatrics*,
https://doi.org/10.1007/978-3-030-18711-8_16

VD increases with age partly due to a decrease in protein binding, and mainly due to a relative increase in fat mass [3, 16]. Nevertheless, the increase in free plasma fraction and the decrease in total clearance compensate for the aging effect on VD, and, with the exception of loading doses for some antimicrobials, dose increments are usually not necessary [17]. In contrast, when total clearance (Cl) of free-drug is reduced in older people due to end-organ disease, the need for dose reduction becomes increasingly apparent [16, 18]. Dose adjustments in older patients are especially required for drugs with a narrow therapeutic range [19, 20]. In this context, predictive tools for dose individualization and the availability of measuring plasma drug concentrations become highly desirable, since the net effect of age-related pharmacokinetic variations is particularly difficult to predict. Aging usually reduces gastrointestinal motility and blood flow, and gastric acid secretion is reduced, but the net effect of all these changes is difficult to predict, and variations in drug absorption in older patients are generally considered to be small [7, 8].

Age-related decrease in liver volume and blood flow determines a reduction in metabolic reactions, in particular those collectively known as Phase I, catalyzed by cytochrome P450 enzymes (CYP450), which in turn may reduce total and free-drug clearance [7, 9, 10].

Loss of renal parenchyma is another hallmark of increasing age, which in conjunction with a decrease in renal plasma flow determines a progressive decline in glomerular filtration rate (GFR) [11–13]. At least 0.4 mL/min of GFR is lost in individuals of Caucasian race per year [14], and this decline is also associated with an age-related prolongation in the half-life (T1/2) of different drugs that have first-order elimination. This is more evident when GFR is <30 mL/min, since the T1/2 rises in a hyperbolic manner in relation to renal function [4, 15].

Pharmacodynamics may also change in older people, mainly in relation to drug sensitivity [21]. This may, in turn, suggest the need for further dose adjustment for some drugs. The same pharmacokinetic concentration in biophase can produce reduced or, more frequently, increased effects (usually adverse effects) in older patients compared to those younger [22, 23]. The risk of fixed adjustment approaches is that the desirable effect could be missed due to the sigmoidicity of the relation between effect and concentration (known as Hill coefficient). In contrast, in some cases older patients show less sensitivity, such as with drugs affecting beta-adrenergic receptors [24]. The preferred therapeutic approach in older people has usually been to start with lower doses in order to avoid untoward effects, with the exception of antimicrobials; however, this poses a risk for potential suboptimal therapy [25–27].

The main pharmacokinetics aspects in the early people are those related to the renal excretion of the drugs. These renal physiological factors are GFR reduction; tubular back-filtration; sodium, calcium, and magnesium loss; potassium retention; altered dilution-concentration capability, tubular frailty, and genetics; internal milieu; body composition senile changes; and dysautonomy. Table 16.1 summarizes the major pharmacokinetic changes in older patients.

Table 16.1 Renal changes secondary to aging

Glomerulus	Reduced glomerular blood flow
	Glomerular degeneration
	Reduced glomerular filtration rate
Thick ascending limb of loop of Henle	Low free water clearance
	Low sodium, calcium and magnesium reabsorption
Renal medulla	Low tonicity
Collecting duct	Reduced sensitivity to antidiuretic hormone
	Reduced clearance of drugs and toxic
	Low water and sodium reabsorption
	Low potassium secretion

Glomerular Filtration Rate (GFR) Reduction According to Age

There is a physiologic trend toward a progressive GFR reduction secondary to senescence process. The GFR reduction secondary just to aging starts around age 30 and continues to decline at a rate of about 1 mL per year. It is worth noting that this GFR reduction typically runs with normal serum urea and creatinine levels [14] because serum creatinine does not reflect the real magnitude of a GFR reduction since muscle mass, which is the source of creatine (creatinine precursor), is reduced in this population [1] and the urea urinary excretion is increased [14]. Thus, a serum creatinine concentration of 1 mg/dL reflects a GFR of 120 mL/min in a 20-year-old person but 60 mL/min in an 80-year-old individual [12]. Similarly, the effective renal plasma flow (ERPF) is reduced by 50%; therefore it falls proportionally more than GFR during aging, and thus the fractional filtration (GFR/ERPF) is increased in the elderly [14]. Finally, regarding renal reserve, which is the kidney's ability to increase basal GFR by at least a 20% after an adequate stimulus (e.g., protein load), although it is preserved in healthy old and very old people, its magnitude decreases significantly with aging [13]. In elderly people, serum cystatin C was documented as a more reliable GFR marker with respect to serum creatinine [15–17].

As it has been mentioned above, there is a GFR reduction according to age, and this GFR decline is also associated with an age-related prolongation in the half-life (T1/2) of different non-lipophilic drugs which have predominant renal clearance [12, 14]. Since pharmacokinetics of these drugs (and their active by-products) which are excreted by GFR is affected by aging, their dose should be adjusted according to aging-related GFR reduction before their initial prescription [12, 18]. Thus, patient's GFR should be measured or calculated (GFR equations) in order to perform these required dose adjustments [12]. Several calculating GFR equations can be used for this purpose, such as calculated creatinine clearance obtained by Cockcroft-Gault formula or calculated GFR obtained by MDRD (creatinine-based), CKD-EPI (creatinine-based), BIS1 (creatinine-based), or BIS2 (creatinine and cystatin C-based) equations [11, 19–23]. The BIS2 equation is currently considered the most accurate equation to estimate GFR in persons aged 70 years or older with normal or mild to moderately reduced kidney function, but if cystatin C is not available, the BIS1 equation is an acceptable alternative [23].

Table 16.2 Aging physiologic changes and dose prescription

Aging body and renal changes	Recommendation
Dysautonomy	Beware of potential rapid deterioration of renal function in patients on ACE or ARA
GFR reduction	Measure or estimation of GFR should be performed before initiating any renal excreted drug in order to adjust their dose
Reduced tubular secretion	To adjust dose of drugs susceptible of renal secretion
Reduced sodium reabsorption	Beware of diuretics and cathartic drugs
Reduced potassium excretion	Beware of potassium-sparing drugs
Reduced free water clearance	Beware of hypotonic solution load
Hypotonic medulla	Beware of dehydrating drugs
Divalent ions renal handling	Beware of diuretics and cathartic drugs
Tubular frailty	Beware of nephrotoxic drugs
Low body water, fat and lean mass	Drug dose adjustment

ACE angiotensin converting enzyme inhibitors, *ARA* angiotensin II receptor antagonists, *GFR* glomerular filtration rate

Since this threshold represents a condition of advanced renal function decline irrespective of renal aging, the warning works also for young subjects. It should be noted that few drugs are to be avoided or even totally contraindicated when GFR is <60 mL/min such as methotrexate since it accumulates after 4–8 weeks of use and can cause long-lasting myelotoxicity, antidiabetics such as glibenclamide/glimepiride because of the risk of hypoglycemia, and enoxaparin because of the risk of hemorrhage.

Newer antiepileptic drugs present reduced clearance in older patients and therapeutic drug monitoring (TDM) might be helpful to guide changes in dosing. Similarly older patients may face a higher risk of concentration-dependent side effects of some antidepressants –particularly tricyclic compounds – and antipsychotics due to reduced clearance and an absolute increase in serum drug concentrations [23, 24].

Prevention and Recommendations Measure or estimation of creatinine clearance or GFR should be performed before initiating any renal excreted drug in the elderly (even in a setting of normal creatinine levels), and subsequent dose adjustments should follow changes in renal function (Tables 16.1 and 16.2).

Proximal Tubule Back-Filtration

It has been documented that creatinine secretion is reduced in healthy old persons, and it can even show a slightly reabsorption pattern: creatinine clearance/GFR = 0.9. It is possible that the senile tubular changes could make the aged tubules more susceptible to creatinine back-filtration, as it happens in newborns but in this case due to tubular immaturity [25, 26]. Since aging process reduces tubule secretion capability, this should be taken into account that pharmacokinetics of those drugs which are usually submitted to significant renal secretion can be affected, and consequently their retention promoted in the elderly [25].

Prevention and Recommendations Particularly for drugs that use the organic acid or basic transporters (such as penicillin, furosemide, indomethacin, amiloride, or dopamine), the possibility of higher plasma concentration due to back-filtration should be considered (Tables 16.1 and 16.2).

Reduced Sodium Reabsorption and Reduced Potassium Excretion

Sodium reabsorption is reduced in the thick ascending loop of Henle in the old and very old individuals, and consequently the amount of sodium loss is increased in this population [6, 27, 28]. Moreover, low serum aldosterone levels and reduced response to this hormone by collecting ducts can also explain the usually enhanced sodium loss in this aged group [12]. Finally, the elevated serum and urinary natriuretic peptide levels usually observed in the elderly may constitute another factor for the characteristic urinary sodium loss in this group [21] (Table 16.1). Because of the senile sodium loss, drugs which promote salt and water excretion (thiazides, loop diuretics, and cathartics) can induce hyponatremia, hypovolemia, and even acute renal failure, particularly in elderly patients who are on a low sodium diet, or their salt and water losses are in excess of sodium [12, 28].

Renal potassium excretion is significantly reduced in the elderly, and this phenomenon is justified by combined mechanisms: low aldosteronemia and aldosterone tubular resistance which induce a reduction in distal potassium secretion by principal cells and an increase potassium reabsorption by intercalated cells of the papillary ducts [6, 29, 30] (Table 16.1). It is worth to highlight, that despite the tendency to retain potassium usually observed in old people, they can also develop significant potassium depletion when they are submitted to an intense pharmacological therapy based on thiazides, loop diuretics or cathartics drugs in a context of an inadequate potassium supplementation. This phenomenon has been explained as a consequence of senile sarcopenia, since muscles are the potassium body reserve [21, 31] (Tables 16.1 and 16.2).

Due to the abovementioned potassium retention trend observed in the elderly, a group of drugs, such as ACEI, ARA, aliskiren, digoxin, potassium-sparing diuretics, nonsteroidal anti-inflammatory drugs (NSAIDs), and beta-blockers, can induce hyperkalemia even in elderly patients not suffering from any nephropathy [13, 21, 25, 31].

Prevention and Recommendations One should be aware of the use of cathartic drugs in oldest old patients since they can contribute to induce an excessive water and salt negative balance and consequently hypovolemia. Blood sodium levels, weight, and blood pressure should be closely monitored in patients of advanced age receiving major diuretic drugs (Tables 16.1 and 16.2).

Serum potassium levels should be monitored in older patients receiving NSAIDs, ACEI, ARA, beta-blockers, and potassium-sparing diuretics among other potentially hyperkalemia-inducing drugs.

Altered Calcium and Magnesium Renal Handling

Serum calcium and magnesium levels and their urinary fractional excretion are similar in the healthy young, old, and very old individuals [6, 32]. However, since elderly people usually have low vitamin D diet, reduced sun light exposure, decreased renal vitamin D hydroxylation (activation), poor calcium intestinal absorption and low serum levels of sexual hormones, then they have a tendency to develop calcium metabolism disorders [32, 33]. Even though magnesium renal reabsorption is preserved in old and very old people, magnesium urine excretion is significantly increased in volume expansion. Besides, elderly people often need magnesium supplements probably due to a combination of diminished spontaneous intake of magnesium, and poor intestinal absorption [6, 32, 33]. Because of the divalent cations handling characteristics in the elderly mentioned above, hypocalcemia can easily be induced by loop diuretics, and hypomagnesemia by loop diuretics, thiazides, cisplatin, amphotericin, aminoglycosides, and calcineurin inhibitors (cyclosporine and tacrolimus) in this population [31–34].

Prevention and Recommendations Serum magnesium levels should be regularly monitored in elder patients receiving diuretics, amphotericin B formulations, aminoglycosides, cisplatin, and calcineurin inhibitors (Tables 16.1 and 16.2).

Reduced Free Water Clearance

Urinary dilution capability is decreased in the healthy elderly. Thus, there is a minimum urine concentration of only 92 mOsmol/kg in the old people compared to 52 mOsmol/kg in the young. Maximum free water clearance is also reduced in the elderly from 16.2 to 5.9 mL/min in average. The functional impairment of the diluting segment of the thick ascending limb appears to account for the decrease in the capacity to dilute urine observed in the aged [6, 13, 21] (Table 16.1). Because of the senile reduction in urine dilution capability, drugs such as thiazides, thiazide-like diuretics, opioids, antiepileptic (carbamazepine), and psychotropic medications, increase their risk of inducing hyponatremia in this population [25, 31].

Prevention and Recommendations Free water overload should be avoided in this population, and the use of drugs with risk of inducing hyponatremia should be carefully monitored (Tables 16.1 and 16.2).

Hypotonic Medulla

Aging reduces the capacity of the kidney to concentrate the urine. The maximum urinary concentration capacity remains normal until about the third decade of life and then it falls by 30 mOsmol/kg per decade. This phenomenon can be explained by a relative increase of medulla blood flow (wash out), the defect in sodium reabsorption in the ascending limb of Henle's loop, and reduced distal urea reabsorption in the elderly. Another mechanism that contributes to the impairment of the urine concentration ability is the decreased responsiveness of tubular epithelium of the collecting tubules to antidiuretic hormone [6, 13, 28] (Table 16.1). Due to the reduced sense of thirst and reduced urine concentration capability observed in the elderly, all medications that may induce salt and water excretion in excess of water (loop diuretics and cathartics) or which can prevent an adequate water ingestion by consciousness impairment (e.g., benzodiazepines) may promote clinically significant dehydration in the elderly [12, 13, 21, 28].

Prevention and Recommendations Maintaining adequate water ingestion is paramount in this population particularly when receiving cathartics or diuretics (Table 16.2).

Tubular Frailty

It has extensively been documented that renal tubular cells are more vulnerable to any insult (ischemic or toxic), and also that they recover more slowly from acute tubular necrosis in the elderly [6]. Consequently, acute renal injury is a frequent complication in the elderly, and if the kidney does not recovered after approximately 3 months it remains as chronic kidney disease [6, 7]. On the other hand, polypharmacy, defined as the presence of five or more concomitant medications, makes old people more susceptible to develop severe acute renal injury, especially if they receive potential nephrotoxic substances such as NSAIDs, ACEI, statins, or radio-contrast, which for different reasons are frequently prescribed in this group [7, 13, 25].

Prevention and Recommendations One should be aware of potentially dangerous drug-drug interactions as inducers of severe acute renal injury in this population, particularly in the context of polypharmacy (Table 16.2).

Internal Milieu and Body Composition Changes in the Elderly

Total body water is diminished with age: it comprises only 54% of total body weight in older patients compared to 65% in the young [35, 36]. Since the reduction in aged-body water content takes place in the intracellular compartment, hypovolemia always represents a pathologic condition in the elderly [13, 35]. Total body potassium content is lower in this population and the correlation with age is linear. This phenomenon can be explained by the reduced muscle mass (senile sarcopenia), which constitutes the main body potassium store, and by poor potassium intake characteristic in the elderly [13, 35, 36]. Regarding body fat content, it is usually increased in healthy old people yet furtherly reduced in very old people. Conversely, despite the aforementioned exaggerated natriuresis in the elderly, total body sodium is not significantly decreased with age [13, 35]. Reduction in total body water determines a decrease in the VD for hydrophilic drugs, while increase in total body fat produces a 20–40% increase in VD for lipophilic drugs [36, 37]. VD increases with age partly due to a decrease in protein binding, and mainly due to a relative increase in body fat content [38, 39]. Nevertheless, the increase in free plasma fraction and the decrease in total clearance compensate for the aging effect on VD, and, with the exception of loading doses for some antimicrobials, dose increments are usually not necessary [40]. In contrast, when total clearance of free-drug is reduced in older people due to end-organ disease, the need for dose reduction becomes increasingly apparent [39, 41]. Dose adjustments in older patients are especially required for drugs with a narrow therapeutic range, such as some of the antiarrhythmic, antiepileptic, and anticoagulant drugs [42, 43]. In this context, predictive tools for dose individualization and the availability of measuring plasma drug concentrations become highly desirable, since the net effect of age-related pharmacokinetic variations is particularly difficult to predict. Modifications in VD must be taken into account when dosing a particular drug in older people. As such, loading dose for initial administration should be considered for some drugs – particularly antimicrobials – in order to obtain the target effect immediately [40]. Subsequent doses in repetitive administration should be adjusted as per the reductions in GFR [40, 41]. Different adjustment approaches can be used, based on reduction of individual maintenance doses, increase in administration interval, or a combination of both, depending on whether the area under the curve (frequency adjustment is preferred) or the peak concentration (dose adjustment is preferred) constitutes the main pharmacokinetic characteristic associated with efficacy and/or toxicity [44] (Table 16.2).

Atherosclerosis and Vascular Dysautonomy

Renal arteries suffer structural and functional changes in the elderly. These changes consist of a progressive atherosclerotic vascular stenosis, and a dysfunction of their autonomic vascular reflex, which usually protects renal parenchyma from blood flow alterations [6] (Table 16.1). Thus, all these vascular changes predispose elderly patients who are on vasodilator drugs to suffer from a decreased kidney perfusion, and consequently to develop an ischemic acute renal injury [7]. This phenomenon can particularly occur in those patients who are on angiotensin converting enzyme inhibitors (ACEI) and/or angiotensin II receptor antagonists (ARA) [8, 9]. Two clinical scenarios of acute renal injury associated to these drugs have been described: First, a reversible acute renal failure in patients with bilateral renal artery stenosis or unilateral renal artery stenosis in a solitary kidney, which improves after ACEI or

ARA withdrawal [8]. Second, a syndrome of unpredictable and rapid onset end-stage renal disease (SORO-ESRD) over a previously stable chronic kidney disease [9]. It seems that some aging renal changes, such as effective renal blood flow reduction and senile glomerulosclerosis, could represent risk factors for installing SORO-ESRD syndrome in situations of hemodynamic instability, particularly in the oldest old [9].

Prevention and Recommendations Evaluate renal artery flow (e.g., by renal Doppler ultrasound) in elder patients before prescribing ACEI or ARA [10, 11]. One should be aware of potential rapid deterioration of renal function in patients on ACE or ARA with stable kidney disease undergoing acute hemodynamic decompensation [10–12] (Tables 16.1 and 16.2).

Other Considerations

Pharmacogenetics and Therapeutic Drug Monitoring (TDM) in Older People

The pharmacological effects of most drugs depend on the result of a series of pharmacokinetic processes (including its renal handling), which determine the amount of a drug that reaches the biophase (target tissues), as well as on pharmacodynamics, involving the interaction between the drug and its site of action [25]. These processes occur at variable rate in different individuals and depend on many factors such as sex, age, diet, environmental factors, drug interactions, demographics, and clinical, but one of the major determinants of this variability is patient genetics [45]. The structure, function, and expression of most enzymes involved in drug transport and metabolism, as well as the specific drug receptors, may be affected by the presence of genetic variants, which may in turn modify the intended therapeutic effect or the appearance of adverse effects. In cases in which polymorphisms or mutations affect the structure or expression of these proteins, with corresponding implications for their function, genomic analyses can be applied prior to treatment to predict the patient's response. This concept represents the central aim of pharmacogenomics [24, 45]. However, importantly, pharmacogenomic knowledge does not explain all of the variability in drug responses. Consequently, the individualized therapy must combine genetic information and nongenetic factors. Given the consequences for the administration of drugs of the renal variations in the elderly, this population is a potential candidate for pharmacogenetic analysis, since both individual variability sources may overlap [25].

TDM refers to the individualization of drug dosing within a target range and involves measurement of plasma or serum concentrations of drugs in individual patients [46]. TDM may be useful as individual patients may respond differently to the same therapeutic dose regimen, based on changes and variability on drug absorption, distribution, and elimination, such as the pediatric population, the critically ill, and the elderly [44]. The aging process implies progressive loss in the functional capacities of organs and changes in kinetic performances [24, 48]. Furthermore, older patients present a higher susceptibility to toxic effects of medications. The unexpected or altered response to drugs in this group compared to younger individuals can thus be explained mainly by changes in pharmacokinetics, dynamic changes or polymedication interaction [24]. As such there are many different clinical scenarios (sepsis, cardiac arrhythmias, etc.) in older patients that may benefit from therapeutic drug monitoring [49–54].

Polypharmacy, Interactions, and Adverse Effects

It has been reported that older patients use up to 30% of all medications, although they account for only 12% of the total population [24]. Often, they receive a large number of medications prescribed by one or more different practitioners, and the risk of "polypharmacy" – the use of five or more concomitant medications usually being excessive or unnecessary – is greater when there is no primary health-care provider [28, 29]. Beyond the issue of unnecessary costs, polypharmacy runs the risk of inadequate dosing, increased adverse effects, and drug interactions [30, 31].

In elderly patients affected by multiple disorders, it is appropriate to set treatment priorities and always consider an initial non-pharmacological therapeutic approach (e.g., exercise and weight reduction). This helps to avoid polypharmacy, as well as to monitor and oversee the benefits and potential harms of the prescribed drugs in order to reduce their adverse effects. In addition, other strategies have been reported as effective for avoiding adverse drug events. These include adequate communication between health providers, particularly during transitions from hospital to outpatient care, the use of computer decision support systems, the use of low dose and slow titration, and the consideration of drug-drug and drug-disease interactions at the time of prescription [24, 32–35].

Adverse drug effects are responsible for 30% of ambulatory geriatric consultations and 10–17% of hospital admissions [24]. Adverse drug reaction should be suspected whenever an elderly patient has an unexpected change in function, for example, gait disorder, change in mental status or behavior, or urinary or fecal incontinence. Warfarin is implicated in about one third of these hospitalizations, while insulin, oral antiplatelet agents, and oral hypoglycemic agents accounted for about another third. Medications commonly designated as high risk or potentially inappropriate (according to widespread Beers Criteria) were rarely implicated [38, 39].

Dose Adjustments in Older Patients

This underscores the intrinsic difficulty of drug adjustments in older people based upon scant and insufficient data [42].

Different adjustment approaches can be used, based on reduction of individual maintenance doses, increase in administration interval, or a combination of both, depending on whether the area under the curve (AUC) or the peak concentration (C_{peak}), constitute the main pharmacokinetic characteristic associated with efficacy and/or toxicity [40].Modifications in VD must be taken into account when dosing a particular drug in older people. As such, a loading dose for initial administration should be considered for some drugs, in order to obtain the target effect immediately [17]. Subsequent doses in repetitive administration should be adjusted as per the reductions in GFR and total Cl. It should be noted that some drugs are to be avoided or even totally contraindicated when GFR is <60 mL/min: methotrexate since it accumulates after 4–8 weeks of use and can cause long-lasting myelotoxicity, antidiabetics such as glibenclamide/glimepiride because of the risk of hypoglycemia, and enoxaparin because of the risk of hemorrhage. When GFR is <30 mL/min, there is high prevalence of hyperkalemia with spironolactone/eplerenone and central nervous system toxicity with antibiotics such as cefepime [43]. A particular consideration involves regarded the use of antibiotics. Patients with renal insufficiency may need a higher starting dose, so beginning with the standard dose and then adjusting the maintenance dose to renal function depending on half-life should be the rule [4, 43].

Some drugs, regardless of their dosage, may be "inappropriate" for older people. For example, the use of long-acting benzodiazepines and psychotropics with anticholinergic properties has been clearly associated with an increased risk of falling in older people and with functional impairment [44, 45].

Successful dosing in older patients should also consider behavioral influences on compliance. Adherence rate is higher in acute rather than chronic conditions, and persistence among patients with chronic conditions is disappointingly low, dropping dramatically after 6 months. Organizing an easy medication schedule for older people therefore is paramount [46]. In a systematic review of the associations between dose regimens and drug compliance, Claxton et al. confirmed that the prescribed number of doses per day is inversely related to patient compliance. Drug compliance was significantly higher for once-daily versus three-times-daily ($P = 0.008$), once-daily versus four-times-daily ($P < 0.001$), and twice-daily versus four-times-daily regimens ($P = 0.001$) [47]. However, there were no significant differences between once-daily and twice-daily regimens, or between twice-daily and three-times-daily regimens. In multivariate, meta-regression analyses by Coleman et al., the adjusted, weighted-mean, percentage adherence rate for twice-daily, three-times-daily, and four-times-daily dosing regimens were all significantly lower compared with once-daily regimens [48]. Moreover, the risk of nonadherence is especially high in the presence of cognitive impairment, when the use of numerous medications for multiple chronic conditions is commonplace.

In a thorough review of pharmacokinetics and pharmacodynamics of the aging kidney, Aymanns et al. analyzed three major kinetic determinants of drugs ($T_{1/2}$, VD, Cl) from data published in PubMed. After recording approximately 90,000 values of 3000 drugs and metabolites, the data revealed an average 1.39-fold age-related prolongation of $T_{1/2}$ and, surprisingly, only modest changes in Cl and VD. This might mean that, from a kinetic point of view, only a few of the most commonly prescribed drugs may need significant dosage modifications [4].

Using a different approach, Denneboom et al. conducted a pharmacotherapy analysis by a multidisciplinary expert panel (including general practitioners and clinical pharmacists) of about 100 home-dwelling older patients on polypharmacy. In this study, the prescription of drugs in an inappropriate dosage was seen in 56% of cardiovascular drug users and in 40% of neurological drug users [41]. In addition, on a two-round modified Delphi survey, an expert panel of geriatric clinical pharmacists was convened to reach consensus for oral dosing in primarily renally cleared medications prescribed for older adults, based on the fact that approximately 25% of the population over 70 years old may have a Cl <60 mL/min. For ten of the reviewed medications (chlorpropamide, colchicine, cotrimoxazole, glyburide, meperidine, nitrofurantoin, probenecid, propoxyphene, spironolactone, and triamterene), a consensus was reached not to use when Cl <30 mL/min. For a group of eight medications (acyclovir, amantadine, ciprofloxacin, gabapentin, memantine, ranitidine, rimantadine, and valacyclovir), consensus was reached and a dosing reduction guideline was completed. Interestingly, there was no agreement on appropriate dosing for commonly prescribed drugs, such as metformin, allopurinol, atenolol, hydrochlorothiazide, and metoclopramide.

Despite significant methodological limitations, Zedler et al. systematically reviewed the available data from randomized controlled trials, concluding that calendar packaging, especially in combination with education and other reminder strategies, may be useful in improving adherence in long-term treatment [49].

Conclusions

Renal physiology changes secondary to aging, such as dysautonomy; glomerular filtration rate reduction; tubular back-filtration; sodium, calcium, and magnesium loss; potassium retention; altered dilution-concentration capability; tubular frailty; genetics; internal milieu; and body composition changes, can predispose elderly people to suffer from pharmacological adverse effects. Knowledge of these physiological modifications associated with aging and their impact over the pharmacology of particular drugs may help to optimize drug use and to avoid complications in this age group.

References

1. Waltman KWS. Preventing adverse drug reactions. Philadelphia: Hanley & Belfus; 2000.
2. Hajjar ER, Cafiero AC, Hanlon JT. Polypharmacy in elderly patients. Am J Geriatr Pharmacother. 2007;5(4):345–51.
3. Weiss BD, Lee JK. Aging: is your patient taking too many pills? J Fam Pract. 2012;61(11):652–61.
4. Bressler R, Bahl JJ. Principles of drug therapy for the elderly patient. Mayo Clin Proc. 2003;78(12):1564–77.
5. Willlams CM. Using medications appropriately in older adults. Am Fam Physician. 2002;66(10):1917–24.
6. Musso CG. Geriatric nephrology and the "nephrogeriatric giants". Int Urol Nephrol. 2002;34:255–6.
7. Musso CG. Acute renal failure in the elderly: pearls for its assessment and treatment. Electron J Biomed. 2005;1:1–93.

8. Renkke H, Denker B. Renal pathophysiology. Philadelphia: Lippincott Williams & Wilkins; 2007.
9. Onuigbo MA, Onuigbo NT. The Syndrome of Rapid Onset End-Stage Renal Disease (SOROESRD) – a new Mayo Clinic Dialysis services experience, January 2010–February 2011. In: Di Iorio B, Heidland A, Onuigbo M, Ronco C, editors. Hemodialysis: when, how, why, vol. 2012. New York: NOVA Publishers; 2012. p. 443–85.
10. Onuigbo M, Onuigbo N, Musso CG. Syndrome of rapid-onset end-stage renal disease in incident Mayo Clinic chronic hemodialysis patients. Indian J Nephrol. 2014;24:75–81.
11. Musso CG, Jauregui J. Renin-angiotensin-aldosterone system and the aging kidney. Endocrinol Metab. 2014;9(6):1–4.
12. Musso CG, Oreopoulos D. Renal changes in the elderly. In: Katlic M, editor. Cardiothoracic surgery in the elderly. Evidence-based practice. New York: Springer; 2011.
13. Musso CG, Macias Nunez JF, Oreopoulos DG. Physiological similarities and differences between renal aging and chronic renal disease. J Nephrol. 2007;20(5):586–7.
14. Musso CG, Oreopoulos DG. Aging and physiological changes of the kidneys including changes in glomerular filtration rate. Nephron Physiol. 2011;119(Suppl 1):1–5.
15. Hojs R, Bevc S, Antolinc B, Gorenjak M, Puklavec L. Serum cystatin C as an endogenous marker of renal function in the elderly. Int J Clin Pharmacol Res. 2004;24(2–3):49–54.
16. Törner A, Odar-Cederlöf I, Kallner A, Akner G. Renal function in community-dwelling frail elderly. Comparison between measured and predicted glomerular filtration rate in the elderly and proposal for a new cystatin C-based prediction equation. Aging Clin Exp Res. 2008;20(3):216–25.
17. Wei L, Ye X, Pei X, Wu J, Zhao W. Reference intervals for serum cystatin C and factors influencing cystatin C levels other than renal function in theelderly. PLoS One. 2014;9(1):e86066.
18. Keller F. Kidney function and age. Nephrol Dial Transplant. 1987;2(5):382.
19. Wetzels JF, Kiemeney LA, Swinkels DW, Willems HL, den Heijer M. Age- and gender-specific reference values of estimated GFR in Caucasians: the Nijmegen Biomedical Study. Kidney Int. 2007;72(5):632–7.
20. Aymanns C, Keller F, Maus S, Hartmann B, Czock D. Review on pharmacokinetics and pharmacodynamics and the aging kidney. Clin J Am Soc Nephrol. 2010;5(2):314–27.
21. Musso CG, Oreopoulos D. Geriatric nephrology. In: Pathy J, Sinclair A, Morley J, editors. Principles and practice of geriatric medicine. West Sussex: Wiley; 2012.
22. Schaeffner ES, Ebert N, Delanaye P, Frei U, Gaedeke J, Jakob O, Kuhlmann MK, Schuchardt M, Tölle M, Ziebig R, van der Giet M, Martus P. Two novel equations to estimate kidney function in persons aged 70 years or older. Ann Intern Med. 2012;157(7):471–8.
23. Alshaer IM, Kilbride HS, Stevens PE, Eaglestone G, Knight S, Carter JL, Delaney MP, Farmer CK, Irving J, O'Riordan SE, Dalton RN, Lamb EJ. External validation of the Berlin equations for estimation of GFR in the elderly. Am J Kidney Dis. 2014;63(5):862–5.
24. Denneboom W, Dautzenberg MG, Grol R, De Smet PA. Analysis of polypharmacy in older patients in primary care using a multidisciplinary expert panel. Br J Gen Pract. 2006;56(528):504–10.
25. Scibona P, Angriman F, Vazquez C, Ferreyro BL, Perelsztein AG, Simonovich VA, Jauregui JR, Musso CG, Belloso WH. Individualisation of drug therapy in older people. Rev Clin Gerontol. 2014;24:145–57.
26. Musso CG, Michelángelo H, Vilas M, Reynaldi J, Martinez B, Algranati L, Macías Núñez JF. Creatinine reabsorption by the aged kidney. Int Urol Nephrol. 2009;41(3):727–31.
27. Musso CG, Ghezzi L, Ferraris J. Renal physiology in newborns and old people: similar characteristics but different mechanisms. Int Urol Nephrol. 2004;36(2):273–6.
28. Musso CG, Macías-Núñez JF. Dysfunction of the thick loop of Henle and senescence: from molecular biology to clinical geriatrics. Int Urol Nephrol. 2011;43:249–52.
29. Musso CG, Rd M, Algranati L, Farias Edos R. Renal potassium excretion: comparison between chronic renal disease patients and old people. Int Urol Nephrol. 2005;37(1):167–70.
30. Musso C, Liakopoulos DMR, Imperiali N, Algranati L. Transtubular potassium concentration gradient: comparison between healthy old people and chronic renal failure patients. Int Urol Nephrol. 2006;38(2):387–90.
31. Lacy C, Armstrong L, Goldman M, Lance L. Drug information handbook. Philadelphia: Lexi-Comp; 2004. p. 646–8.

32. Musso CG, Juarez R, Vilas M, Navarro M, Rivera H, Jauregui R. Renal calcium, phosphorus, magnesium and uric acid handling: comparison between stage III- chronic kidney disease and healthy oldest old. Int Urol Nephrol. 2012;44(5):1559–62.
33. Musso CG, Alvarez Gregory J, Macías Núñez JF. Renal handling of uric acid, magnesium, phosphorus, calcium, and acid base in the elderly. In: Núñez M, Cameron S, Oreopoulos D, editors. Renal ageing: health and disease. New York: Springer; 2008. p. 155–71.
34. Musso CG. Magnesium metabolism in health and disease. Int Urol Nephrol. 2009;41:357–62.
35. Musso CG, Reynaldi J, Vilas M, De Miguel R, Imperiali N, Algranati L. Fractional excretion of K, Na and Cl following furosemide infusion in healthy, young and very old people. Int Urol Nephrol. 2010;42(1):273–7.
36. Musso CG, Macías Núñez JF. Renal handling of water and electrolytes in the old and old-old healthy aged. In: Núñez M, Cameron S, Oreopoulos D, editors. Renal ageing: health and disease. New York: Springer; 2008. p. 141–54.
37. Fulop T Jr, Worum I, Csongor J, Foris G, Leovey A. Body composition in elderly people. I. Determination of body composition by multiisotope method and the elimination kinetics of these isotopes in healthy elderly subjects. Gerontology. 1985;31(1):6–14.
38. Ginsberg G, Hattis D, Russ A, Sonawane B. Pharmacokinetic and pharmacodynamic factors that can affect sensitivity to neurotoxic sequelae in elderly individuals. Environ Health Perspect. 2005;113(9):1243–9.
39. McLean AJ, Le Couteur DG. Aging biology and geriatric clinical pharmacology. Pharmacol Rev. 2004;56(2):163–84.
40. Perucca E. Age-related changes in pharmacokinetics: predictability and assessment methods. Int Rev Neurobiol. 2007;81:183–99.
41. Noreddin AM, Haynes V. Use of pharmacodynamic principles to optimise dosage regimens for antibacterial agents in the elderly. Drugs Aging. 2007;24(4):275–92.
42. Butler JM, Begg EJ. Free drug metabolic clearance in elderly people. Clin Pharmacokinet. 2008;47(5):297–321.
43. Mallet L, Spinewine A, Huang A. The challenge of managing drug interactions in elderly people. Lancet. 2007;370(9582):185–91.
44. Wang L. Changes in pharmacokinetics in the elderly and therapeutic drug monitoring of anti-arrhythmic drugs. Life Sci J. 2007;4:1–7.
45. Dettli L. Drug dosage in renal disease. Clin Pharmacokinet. 1976;1(2):126–34.
46. Gardiner SJ, Begg EJ. Pharmacogenetics, drug-metabolizing enzymes, and clinical practice. Pharmacol Rev. 2006;58(3):521–90.
47. Ruiz JG, Array S, Lowenthal DT. Therapeutic drug monitoring in the elderly. Am J Ther. 1996;3(12):839–60.
48. Ghiculescu R. Therapeutic drug monitoring: which drugs, why, when and how to do it. Aust Prescr. 2008;31(2):42–4.
49. Klotz U. Pharmacokinetics and drug metabolism in the elderly. Drug Metab Rev. 2009;41(2):67–76.
50. Greenblatt DJ, Harmatz JS, Shader RI. Clinical pharmacokinetics of anxiolytics and hypnotics in the elderly. Therapeutic considerations (part II). Clin Pharmacokinet. 1991;21(4):262–73.
51. Lundmark J, Bengtsson F, Nordin C, Reis M, Walinder J. Therapeutic drug monitoring of selective serotonin reuptake inhibitors influences clinical dosing strategies and reduces drug costs in depressed elderly patients. Acta Psychiatr Scand. 2000;101(5):354–9.
52. Bonetti A, Franceschi T, Apostoli P, Cetto GL, Recaldin E, Molino A, et al. Cisplatin pharmacokinetics in elderly patients. Ther Drug Monit. 1994;16(5):477–82.
53. Greenblatt DJ, Abernethy DR, Shader RI. Pharmacokinetic aspects of drug therapy in the elderly. Ther Drug Monit. 1986;8(3):249–55.
54. Waade RB, Molden E, Refsum H, Hermann M. Serum concentrations of antidepressants in the elderly. Ther Drug Monit. 2012;34(1):25–30.

Conservative and Palliative Care in Old Age Individuals with End-Stage Renal Disease

17

Luis Miguel Gutiérrez Robledo and Ricardo Correa-Rotter

The phenomenon of population aging is inexorably accompanied by a rising numbers of deaths occurring among people at older age. A growing proportion of people will live into advanced age and, if current trends prevail, will die following a period of increasing dependency and disability associated with chronic illness and frailty. The World Health Organization (WHO) estimates that in high-income countries, seven in every ten deaths are among people aged 70 years and older. People predominantly die from chronic diseases: cardiovascular diseases, cancer, dementia, chronic kidney disease (CKD), diabetes, or a combination of them.

Epidemiology of Old Age End-Stage Renal Disease

The few population-based studies designed specifically to assess the prevalence of CKD in elderly population have shown great diversity, ranging from 23.4% to 58.5% [1, 2]. In developed countries, trends in adjusted end-stage renal disease (ESRD) incidence rate are displaying a rising trend, particularly in the older age group. For example, in the United States between 2009 and 2015, the annual number of incident cases of ESRD has increased by 7.5%, due to several factors, yet one of the most relevant ones is the aging of the population. Not surprisingly, hospitalization rates in older patients are greater than for younger age cohorts. In the advanced CKD group, those over 85 years of age had a 44.3% higher admission rate than those aged 66–69 years and, in 2015, Medicare spending for beneficiaries with

L. M. G. Robledo (✉)
National Institute of Geriatrics, Mexico City, Mexico
e-mail: lmgutierrez@inger.gob.mx

R. Correa-Rotter
Nephrology Department, National Institute of Medical Sciences "Salvador Zubiran", Mexico City, Mexico

C. G. Musso et al. (eds.), *Clinical Nephrogeriatrics*,
https://doi.org/10.1007/978-3-030-18711-8_17

CKD aged 65 and older exceeded $55 billion, representing 20% of all Medicare spending in this age group [3].

These trends pose major challenges to healthcare systems, given the greater healthcare utilization by and more comorbid conditions among elderly adults. Chronic kidney disease is a major concern for health systems, given the high and increasing prevalence of ESRD and of patients being treated with renal replacement treatments. With the rise in prevalence of obesity, diabetes, and hypertension in middle-aged adults, we will likely witness further increases. In countries where funding and universal health coverage is available, given the constant percentual increase of the aging population, a continued growth in the elderly dialysis population is also anticipated. In the United States and Europe, for example, the increase in the dialysis population is strongly driven by the increased incidence of octogenarians and nonagenarians starting dialysis. Their poor outcomes, in particular in elder individuals with multiple comorbidities, strongly suggest that alternative paths, such as decision for palliative care rather than initiation of dialysis, should be incorporated in discussions around chronic predialysis settings [4].

The changing demographics mandate a discussion of individual and societal goals and priorities. A recent study noted that elderly nursing home residents initiating dialysis in the United States experienced a marked decline in functional status during the period surrounding the initiation of dialysis and, by 1 year after the start of dialysis, only one of eight nursing home residents had functional capacity similar to the predialysis level [5].

It is now commonly agreed that the presence of advanced CKD (stages 4–5 of the Kidney Disease: Improving Global Outcomes (KDGIO) classification) identifies a higher risk state in older adults, with increased risk for multiple adverse outcomes, including cardiovascular disease, cognitive impairment, and death. Accordingly, ESRD in older adults is worthy of attention by both healthcare providers and patients, with the concomitant presence of frailty potentially informing therapeutic and diagnostic decisions for these individuals.

Characteristics and Outcomes of Old Age ESRD Patients

Major risk factors for progression of CKD to ESRD include hypertension and diabetes, both common in the elderly. Additionally, older persons are at high risk for development of acute kidney injury (AKI), which is also a major risk factor for progression in patients with some degree of CKD, for several reasons. First, a high prevalence of comorbid diseases, such as prostatic hypertrophy or congestive heart failure, both of which can directly induce and favor AKI development. Second, medications and medical interventions commonly used to treat comorbid conditions may either cause or predispose to the development of AKI (e.g., nonsteroidal anti-inflammatory drugs). And third, structural changes in the kidney that normally occur with aging may preclude successful compensation for acute decreases in glomerular filtration rate (GFR). Data from a large healthcare system demonstrate that on average patients developing AKI are approximately 10 years older than those who do not develop it [6] and elderly patients developing AKI are less likely to recover kidney function [7] and thus liable for rapid progression to ESRD.

Older patients with kidney disease face both a shortened life expectancy and a high symptom burden. They will benefit from early supportive care interventions. The goal of supportive care is to relieve suffering and to support the best possible quality of life for patients and their families, regardless of their stage of disease or the need for other therapies in accordance with their values and preferences. People affected by kidney failure usually have a difficult scenario ahead. They tend to be ill for many months or years with the possibility of sudden acute, severe relapsing episodes, and then remitting periods, but with an underlying downward trend in function. Usually relapsing episodes are associated with hospitalization and intensive treatment; possibly, every relapsing episode could be fatal. How to be accurate in predicting prognosis and time of death is very challenging in this context. In addition, there is a unique need for advanced care planning for these patients, most of whom have more than one life-limiting illness.

There is a growing recognition that skills in palliative and end-of-life supportive care are required for physicians, nurses, and others who treat patients with CKD and ESRD. The two principal reasons are as follows: they have a significantly shortened life expectancy; just over half of dialysis patients (52%) are still alive 3 years after the start of renal replacement therapy (RRT), and very often they have multiple comorbidities and a multiplicity of symptoms such as pain, fatigue, itching, and difficulty with sleep.

Palliative care will help with complex pain and symptom management and advance care planning, including shared decision-making about the goals of care. Collaboration with geriatrics departments and/or hospices, can help renal and dialysis units implement a palliative and supportive care program and appropriately treat or refer patients for palliative care at the end of life.

Person-Centered Care

Developing a patient-centered approach, with a patient-centered care plan, which includes conservative, nondialytic care, is increasingly recognized as an important issue when caring for advanced CKD patients, in particular those who are elder and with multiple comorbidities. In a patient-centered model, an attainable treatment goal for each patient is based upon the patient's medical condition and treatment options, the patient's preferences and expectations within his or her psychosocial context, and the patient's prognosis. Considering these variables, most of the time, one of the following three clinical pathways may follow for the treatment of ESRD:

- Dialysis as a bridging treatment
- Dialysis as a final destination treatment
- Active medical management without dialysis

Palliative or supportive care should be integral to each and every pathway within the view of patient-centered care.

The education of relevant healthcare providers regarding the importance of an integrated multidisciplinary renal palliative care approach in the overall care of patients with ESRD is then essential.

At all times, the patient is the focus of care, and he/she should be encouraged, together with his family to be actively involved in the decision-making process. In this vein, developing good and open two-way communication with patient, caregivers, and primary care practitioner regarding prognosis, expectations, and other issues which may arise is of upmost importance. It is necessary to be always aware and ready to recognize and manage debilitating symptoms in order to sustain and if possible improve continuously patient's functionality and quality of life.

Indeed, the management of the patient's symptoms should be based on the highest level of clinical evidence and the team must facilitate timely withdrawal from dialysis when indication arises. This will be easier if advanced healthcare directives are obtained early in the assessment process. In addition, this will facilitate, as well, the timely introduction of available palliative care support and services and may promote a smooth transition to end-of-life care by early decision-making and referral to community palliative care or hospice services to avoid unnecessary hospital admissions.

Advance Care Planning

Advanced care planning is the process by which patients, family members, and providers reflect upon the patient's goals and values to help inform current and future medical care plans, and this begins with the initial conversation of whether to elect or not conservative care. There should also be a meaningful discussion addressing the end-of-life trajectory with conservative care and outlining the patient's care preferences. Advanced care planning means also a continuous process of communication among patients, families, healthcare providers, and other important individuals about the follow-up of patient's preferences and the appropriate medical care. A significant proxy or tutor should be systematically considered if and when a patient is unable to make his or her own decisions.

The American Society of Nephrology and Renal Physicians Association have recommended that advance care planning for advanced CKD and ESRD patients should be considered, including a patient-specific estimate of prognosis and shared decision-making prior to dialysis initiation [8, 9]. Clinicians are responsible for advanced care planning, although aspects of this process can be shared with other health professionals. Advanced care planning is important for CKD KDIGO stages 4 and 5 patients as it can ensure that patients' wishes for end-of-life care are respected, that unwanted interventions are avoided, and that patients and their families are satisfied with the care provided. Although most clinicians are expected to possess primary palliative care skills, they are encouraged to consult geriatrics or palliative care physicians for more complex cases.

Treatment Decisions

Even though older adults facing ESRD will eventually consider the need of renal replacement therapy (RRT) and they may be offered hemodialysis (HD), peritoneal dialysis (PD), or kidney transplantation; increasingly, attention is driven to also consider the alternative of conservative treatment. All four options should generally be considered and unbiased information should be provided by the treating physician as there are no definitive age limits for any of the treatments.

Not every older adult with ESRD will accept RRT. During the last few years, conservative care for old ESRD patients has become a genuine alternative. There is a growing body of literature addressing issues of prognosis, quality of life, and symptom burden [10, 11]. The burden of transporting a frail elderly person, the effect of hypotension and fatigue related to ultrafiltration, and the feeling of dependence late in life all associated with performing HD make conservative management an appropriate option for many older ESRD patients, in particular for those with significant comorbidities.

A usual challenge faced by clinicians is to convey the necessary information to the patient and his family so that they will be able to make an informed decision about dialysis or conservative care, where the patient's perspective should be in the center of the decision process. A crucial element is that patient and family have a clear understanding of prognosis and of the fact that conservative management also means care. Even if it is difficult to estimate prognosis on an individual level, there is data that predicts carrying a poor prognosis such as comorbid conditions, particularly frailty, poor functional status, significant cardiovascular disease, diabetic nephropathy, and malnutrition [12, 13]. Quality of life is closely related to functional status. Older patients starting dialysis are likely to experience a decline in functional status [14, 15]. Thus, frailty, quality of life, and comorbid conditions should be incorporated into estimates of prognosis and outcomes for older ESRD adults and for informed decision-making about dialysis or conservative care. For certain patients a predefined period of time where dialysis treatment can be experienced may be helpful followed by a re-evaluation of decision. Survival in older adults with advanced CKD but low comorbidity and without frailty is generally better with dialysis treatment compared to conservative care. However, the benefit of living longer might be outweighed by a poorer quality of life in a significant percentage of elderly individuals undergoing dialysis.

Regarding prognosis, several illness trajectories have been used to conceptualize the life course of people dying for malignant and nonmalignant conditions. Beyond these trajectories a real challenge for physicians is to predict survival, communicate prognosis, and recognize the active process of dying in order to make appropriate choices regarding therapeutic decisions.

Patients who perceive themselves to be more ill will, every day that goes by, regularly question their physicians about whether they can be cured and if they will die of their current condition. It is essential to be prepared to answer to them and not to deny what could be a fact, and to evaluate the benefits, harms, and cost (social, economic, spiritual, and ethical) of medical decisions and interventions. That is why the ability to establish a prognosis should be a core skill in the practice of medicine, as it is the science of evaluating what is likely to happen in terms of health outcomes.

The success of scientific medicine carries the risk of the false assumption that science offers a cure for every illness and the indefinite postponement of death. Within this triumphant perspective, death has assumed a connotation of failure. The palliative care movement has contributed to reemphasize prognosis as a process of foreseeing. Thus, the abilities of estimating the likelihood of an illness to be life-threatening become crucial to balance the benefits of potential interventions. A physician in this clinical context should be confident in prognostication and recognition of dying for many reasons: Death is most common in elderly patients; frailty and dementia both common comorbidities are like a progressive illness which if you do not die with them, you will die from them. The use of prognostic tools to estimate life expectancy is necessary to move beyond arbitrary age-based cutoffs in clinical decision-making for older people. Prognostication will help to drive decision-making, balancing benefits and harms of tests and treatments, and identification of who is in need of palliative care and comfort measures. Recognition of active dying will allow the management of specific symptoms towards a dignified death.

Prognostication can be divided into two separate processes: on the one hand, the ability to formulate a prediction of survival, and on the other hand, the ability to communicate this prognosis to patients and families. These skills are learnable, and when appropriate, they play a central role in decision-making. The first task for a physician is to acknowledge uncertainty with an honest approach. Prognostic tools usually give a probabilistic prediction, and the vast majority have been developed and validated for cancer to assist clinicians in assessing short-term survival (e.g., ≤6 months). Nonetheless, in older adults, specific prognostic indicators have been developed with a much wider life span of several years.

In practical terms, the Charlson's comorbidity index [16], the patient's functional status, the presence of frailty [17], and the surprise question (would I be surprised if this patient died within the next year?) [12] are all useful in predicting prognosis, especially in older adults.

There is a need for accurate prognosis in order to shed light into decision-making. The challenge is to ameliorate current prognostic tools and develop innovative ones that are feasible, accurate in routine clinical use, and not just in research studies. However, current medical culture remains a significant challenge and educating healthcare professionals to consider the establishment of a prognosis as a learnable, core clinical competency is a priority. Recognition of dying and care during the last days/hours of life should also be a core competency of every physician.

Ethical Issues

When treating patients with ESRD, unavoidably ethical issues arise. Current clinical practice guidelines consider some of them but there is a lack of comprehensive information about the full range of relevant ethical issues in this condition.

Despite the wide possible range of ethical issues that can be present in healthcare decisions for patients with advanced CKD, major professional organizations mostly focus on the ethical issues of withdrawing dialysis. For example, the US Renal Physicians Association (RPA) and the American Society of Nephrology (ASN) issued a clinical practice guideline called "Shared Decision Making in the Appropriate Initiation of and Withdrawal from Dialysis" [18], while the Renal Association in the United Kingdom issued the guideline "Planning, Initiating and Withdrawal of Renal Replacement Therapy" [19].

Moral and technological imperatives to treat patients irrespective of age and prognosis, coupled with a push for earlier dialysis start, have the potential to disproportionately affect patients older than age 75 years. Clinicians should be aware of this and ensure that the patient's rights to be informed about the potential benefits and burdens of renal replacement therapy are respected, particularly because frailty, functional status, nutritional status, and comorbidities affect the net balance between benefits and burdens. Nephrologists in particular are called on to help patients make a decision, for which the patient's goals of care guide determination of potential benefit from dialysis in the elder population. There should be concern as well about potential overtreatment and eventual risk of under treatment of older adults with ESRD. Providers can ethically approach the question of initiation of renal replacement treatment in the older patient by including patient-specific estimates of prognosis, shared decision-making, and the use of specialist palliative care or geriatrics clinicians or ethics consultants for complex cases.

In order to approach the patient, the potential goals of care must be addressed: In this context, being cured is rarely possible, to live longer is usually an issue, but with increasing frailty. Improving or maintain function, quality of life, and independence and being comfortable become increasingly relevant. Within this perspective, achieving life goals and eventually the need to provide support for family or caregiver should also be considered in decision-making.

A compassionate and effective practical approach should:

- Assess the patient's goals of care and establish advance care planning.
- Assess the patient's risk profile and prognosis (assessment of frailty, functional and mental status, and comorbidities).
- Evaluate the patient's prognosis in the context of his/her goals of care.
- Communicate individualized treatment options and likely outcomes (best case/worst case).
- Engage both the patient and family in deliberation on treatment choice.
- Convene a meeting in order to make individualized treatment recommendations to fit the patient's goals of care if the patient prefers a physician-led decision-making process or if patients or surrogate decision struggle with their choices.
- Consider recommending against dialysis in patients with very poor prognosis, potential contraindications, or safety concerns.
- Consider a time-limited trial with predefined milestone measures of success/failure if there is significant ambivalence or lack of consensus.

- Consider involving a geriatrician and the ethics consult team or use other due process in challenging cases.
- Identify and treat burdensome symptoms and aim to minimize treatment burden. Involve specialist geriatric or palliative care physicians for complex cases.
- Periodically reassess the patient's willingness to continue dialysis as well as palliative care eligibility.
- Enable and support the patient to opt out of dialysis if continuation is no longer consistent with his/her goals of care.

Conservative and Supportive Care

A conservative approach to the management of CKD stages 4 and 5 may be appropriate for some patients who have opted not to receive RRT. Many renal specialists and organizations across the world are offering conservative management as a recognized treatment option [20]. In more recent data, an analysis of the Austrian Dialysis and Transplant Registry compared survival of 8622 individuals of >65 years old to 174 patients with eGFR <10 mL/min who were managed conservatively. In this study, while the hemodialysis group did demonstrate benefit in general survival, the comparative benefit of hemodialysis is lost after the first 2 months of follow-up; this is explained by early mortality among the conservative treatment group, which probably included very poor risk cases, some of which could have not been eligible for dialysis as well as a significant age difference, being those with conservative treatment 7 years older in average [21].

As those patients who are elder and have added comorbidities experience deterioration in their general health and increased frailty, the management focus should be shifted toward advanced care planning and planning for end-of-life care. Conservative care of ESRD means medical management without renal replacement therapy. Conservative care is appropriate for patients with coexisting advanced comorbidities who are not eligible for transplantation and who may not gain meaningful benefit from renal replacement therapy; or who prefer to avoid intensive medical therapies and instead want to receive care that focuses on quality of life. Conservative or palliative care in this context essentially means treatment of symptoms in the first place and the implementation of measures that delay the loss of the renal residual function that is present and that could be essential to prolong life as well as to reduce symptomatology, in particular the one related to fluid overload. Most common symptoms are fatigue which may be associated to anemia, which can be managed by proper iron store replenishment and erythropoiesis-stimulating agents, dyspnea treated with water restriction and diuretics in those patients with renal residual function, pain, pruritus, loss of appetite, nausea, and other concerns. Symptoms may resemble those of advanced cancer patients in the month before they die yet the renal patient is often resilient and may survive significantly longer periods [22]. The clinical relevance of these observations has prompted new practice guidelines addressing the issue of supportive care in advanced CKD and ESRD patients [23, 24]. Skills to communicate with patients and family members and to convey topics of existential content will have to be learned by specialized trainees. Thus, the ideal interdisciplinary setting is one which may include a nephrologist, a primary care physician ideally a geriatrician, a specialized nurse, a dietician, a palliative care specialist, a social worker, and/or psychologist.

The option for conservative care should be discussed with all patients who may not meaningfully benefit from dialysis or whose goals focus on quality over quantity of life. Conservative care is a reasonable treatment option alongside renal replacement options for those who are less likely to benefit from dialysis. In particular, frail and/or multi-morbid patients are candidates for conservative care since they tend to incur in more of the burdens and complications of dialysis rather than intended benefits. It is important to point out that conservative care should be offered only when all other options for renal replacement are discussed and the treatment plan must be reconsidered regularly, as shifts in the decision process are often present and could happen in either way.

The components of conservative care include medical management of kidney disease, symptom management, and advance care planning (ACP), including quality end-of-life care. All patients should have treatments designed to manage symptoms. The degree to which treatments to delay progression of kidney disease or prolong life are used is individualized for each patient and depends upon prognosis, quality of life, and patient desire to prolong life. The medical management is often essentially the same as that of advanced CKD patients who are awaiting the initiation of renal replacement therapies. Nevertheless, some considerations are specific to patients undergoing conservative care: While renin-angiotensin system (RAS) inhibitors may be used, there should be a low threshold to discontinue them in the setting of hyperkalemia or hypotension. Erythropoiesis-stimulating agents (ESAs) and iron administration are used to treat anemia which often is the cause of symptoms of fatigue and weakness. Doses of ESAs may exceed standard guidelines to achieve improvement in symptoms, but it is clear we should not target hemoglobin (Hb) levels >12.5 g/dL, as this has been demonstrated to be deleterious and of cardiovascular risk. Phosphorous-binding agents and vitamin D analogs should be used to treat hyperphosphatemia and hyperparathyroidism only in order to avoid accompanying symptoms such as pruritus and renal-related bone disease but would then allow higher parathyroid hormone (PTH) and phosphorus concentrations than commonly recommended, given the difficulty of achieving standard target PTH and phosphorus goals in advanced kidney disease in the absence of dialysis. Hyperkalemia that persists in the absence of RAS inhibitors should be treated with cation exchange resins such as sodium polystyrene sulfonate (Kayexalate), other more modern hyperkalemia treating agents as patiromer and in cases with residual renal function, diuretics may be of use. We should always remember that attention should prioritize symptom relief as a critical component of conservative care. Symptoms should be evaluated at each visit and assessment tools or surveys can be useful for a systematic approach [25]. Symptoms are more effectively managed in conjunction with a geriatric or palliative care team.

Symptom management can occur concurrently with medical management or as the primary treatment goal, yet symptom treatment alone can be more appropriate for patients who have a predictable poor prognosis, and for those whose prognosis is uncertain but whose goals are focused on comfort. Medications that do not address comfort or whose benefits will not be reached because of a limited survival should be stopped.

The most common and disturbing symptoms usually are: fatigue, anorexia and nausea, pain, dyspnea, pruritus and psychological symptoms; mainly depression, anxiety, and delirium.

Conservative management should also incorporate community and palliative support services to maximize quality of life until the terminal phase of life is reached. At this point, specialized supportive care should be provided with particular attention directed to bereavement care for the family following the patient's death.

Palliative Care

The World Health Organization (WHO) defines palliative care as "an approach that improves the quality of life of patients and their families facing the problem associated with life-threatening illness, through the prevention and relief of suffering by means of early identification and impeccable assessment and treatment of pain and other problems, including those of physical, psychosocial and spiritual natures" [26].

Palliative care provides relief from pain and other distressing symptoms, affirms life and regards dying as a normal process intends neither to hasten nor to postpone death. It integrates the psychological and spiritual aspects of patient care offering a support system to help patients live as actively as possible until death and helping the family cope during the patient's illness and in their own bereavement.

Palliative care uses a team approach to address the needs of patients and their families, including bereavement counseling, if indicated and focuses on enhancing the quality of life, and whenever possible, positively influence the course of illness. For best results, it should be introduced early in the course of illness, in conjunction with other therapies intended to prolong life, such as chemotherapy or renal conservative therapies and includes those investigations needed to better understand and manage distressing symptoms and clinical complications.

Palliative care is sometimes referred to as supportive care; its goal is always to achieve the best possible quality of life by controlling symptoms, relieving pain, and restoring functional capacity while respecting the patients personal, cultural, and spiritual beliefs and practices. The traditional belief that palliative care is associated with only end-of-life care tends to remain firm in the general community. But there is an increasing awareness among physicians that palliative care is not just end-of-life management but rather a supportive care pathway leading over time to a dignified end of life for an individual patient.

Providing palliative care to patients with advanced CKD begins at diagnosis and continues throughout the patient's life. Palliative care assumes increasing importance with time and leads to "good deaths" as the disease progresses. The concept of a renal palliative care approach within renal units, to provide supportive care to patients, their family, and primary caregivers in addition to their usual renal care, is not new. However, the actual delivery around the world is inconsistent as there is no systematic and formalized pathway model yet, with some exceptions as is the case for Australia [27].

Palliative care addresses as well the physical, psychological, social, spiritual, and existential needs of patients within the context of family and community. The goal of palliative care is to achieve the best possible quality of life by relieving suffering, controlling symptoms, and restoring functional capacity, while maintaining sensitivity to personal, cultural, and spiritual beliefs and practices. Palliative care in patients with ESRD incorporates all members of the interdisciplinary team (physicians, nurses, social workers, peers, and families). Important aspects of palliative care include assessment of quality of life and prognosis and the development of appropriate advance directives through an advance care planning process. The advance care planning process should include options for conservative care versus dialysis, symptom control after dialysis discontinuation, and bereavement care for family and community. Dialysis patients have symptoms (pain, fatigue, and pruritus, among other) that are commonly undertreated. Hospice is underutilized in those with ESRD and should be considered in any patient refusing or withdrawing from dialysis.

Specific elements to be considered within its scope comprise [23]:

- Pain and symptom assessment/management
- Shared decision-making for informed consent
- Patient-specific estimates of prognosis using the surprise question
- Timely discussions prompted by prognosis
- Inclusion of family/legal agent in discussions
- Completion of advance directives
- Completion of physician orders for life-sustaining treatment paradigm form as appropriate
- Immediately actionable medical orders
- Transferrable throughout healthcare setting specifications, and referral to hospice when indicated.

Consider for eligibility the following groups as suitable candidates for palliative care service:

- Patients with advanced CKD who have opted for conservative management
- Patients with advanced ESRD who are considering withdrawal from RRT
- Patients with advanced CKD with unresolved symptoms affecting quality of life
- Patients under dialysis who have exhausted all options for on-going dialysis access, for example, peritoneal dialysis catheter or arteriovenous fistula methods in hemodialysis

- Patients with declining transplant graft function who have opted not to return to dialysis therapy
- Patients with advanced CKD who have other life-limiting comorbidities resulting in physical and functional decline. For example: malignancy, end-stage cardiac and/or respiratory disease, Alzheimer's disease, or other forms of dementia

Palliative Care Needs in Low- and Middle-Income Countries

Improving access to affordable palliative care is an important priority in response to the challenges posed by the global rise in ESRD. This need is not reflected at present in the emerging body of literature related to the global response to CKD [28]. Palliative care needs of patients with ESRD not treated with renal replacement treatment in low- and middle-income countries (LAMIC) settings concur with what has been described in high resource settings where patients express concerns about symptom burden limiting their functional ability. Other areas identified reflect some of the contextual realities of a low-resource environment. The diagnosis and consequent treatment of ESRD poses extreme financial challenges and in many LAMIC nations, universal health coverage is not provided. This therefore impacts on the quality of medical care, including routine visits to hospital and purchase of essential medication. In many instances, roles within the family, as caregiver, sexual partner, and breadwinner constitute losses of great importance. Nevertheless, in some instances, spiritual and cultural beliefs are a source of hope as well as framing understanding and acceptance of the disease itself [29]. A growing number of patients with ESRD managed without renal replacement treatment will require care in this context in the coming years. For the majority of patients who are diagnosed and reviewed by renal services without access to renal replacement therapy or formal palliative care provision, clinicians and nurses should adopt some simple tools, using a symptom-based approach. By asking the patient about his main concerns, patient-centered priorities can be identified and supported to optimize the quality of life up to and beyond the time of death.

Research Priorities

Older adults with advanced CKD often have frailty, functional impairment, multiple comorbid conditions, a high symptom burden, and limited life expectancy. There is growing concern that the intensive patterns of care that many of these patients tend to receive at the end of their lives are often not aligned with their values and preferences. This has been underlined in a recent report by WHO, where the geriatric community recognizes that person-centered care is often not considered and besides that there are significant unmet needs in this population [30]. Also, there are several areas of knowledge deficit where more evidence is needed to support the best possible care for this population: knowledge about intrinsic capacity and frailty and the role they play in advanced CKD evolution and therapeutic needs; knowledge about person-centered care and what matters most to older adults with advanced CKD and their caregivers near the end of life; better knowledge about how can we best support older adults with advanced CKD to prepare timely advanced directives so that they can navigate complex treatment decisions throughout their illness; and evidence to support the adaptation of the healthcare system in order to serve the best interest particularly of frail older adults with advanced CKD and ESRD. Research priorities should include identifying opportunities for improving the end-of-life experience of older adults with CKD and their caregivers and developing and testing clinical pathways before and during dialysis and communication strategies to ensure that treatment decisions reflect patients' preferences. Besides, more evidence is needed on assessing the effectiveness of palliative care in improving quality of life for patients and caregivers, satisfaction with care, and aligning treatment decisions with patient goals and preferences particularly in low resource settings.

Conclusion

Palliative and supportive care must be considered as alternatives from the outset when dealing with ESRD in frail patients. A patient-centered approach and early definition of advance care planning are essential to fulfil patient's expectations.

References

1. Zhang Q-L, Rothenbacher D. Prevalence of chronic kidney disease in population-based studies: systematic review. BMC Public Health. 2008;8:117.
2. Abdulkader RCRM, Burdmann EA, Lebrão ML, Duarte YAO, Zanetta DMT. Aging and decreased glomerular filtration rate: an elderly population-based study. PLoS One. 2017;12(12):e0189935.
3. 2017 USRDS annual data report.
4. Thakar CV, Quate-Operacz M, Leonard AC, Eckman MH. Outcomes of hemodialysis patients in a long-term care hospital setting: a single-center study. Am J Kidney Dis. 2010;55(2):300–6.
5. Kurella Tamura M, et al. Functional status of elderly adults before and after initiation of dialysis. N Engl J Med. 2009;361(16):1539–47.
6. Hsu CY, et al. The risk of acute renal failure in patients with chronic kidney disease. Kidney Int. 2008;74:101–7. AKI. [PubMed: 18385668].
7. Schmitt R, et al. Recovery of kidney function after acute kidney injury in the elderly: a systematic review and meta-analysis. Am J Kidney Dis. 2008;52(2):262–71.
8. Renal Physicians Association. Shared decision-making in the appropriate initiation of and withdrawal from dialysis. 2nd ed. Rockville: Renal Physicians Association; 2010.
9. Williams AW, Dwyer AC, Eddy AA, Fink JC, Jaber BL, Linas SL, Michael B, O'Hare AM, Schaefer HM, Shaffer RN, Trachtman H, Weiner DE, Falk AR, American Society of Nephrology Quality, Patient Safety Task Force. Critical and honest conversations: the evidence behind the "Choosing Wisely" campaign recommendations by the American Society of Nephrology. Clin J Am Soc Nephrol. 2012;7:1664–72.
10. Chandna SM, Da Silva-Gane M, Marshall C, Warwicker P, Greenwood RN, Farrington K. Survival of elderly patients with stage 5 CKD: comparison of conservative management and renal replacement therapy. Nephrol Dial Transpl. 2011;26:1608–14.

11. Morton RL, Turner RM, Howard K, Snelling P, Webster AC. Patients who plan for conservative care rather than dialysis: a national observational study in Australia. Am J Kidney Dis. 2012;59:419–27.
12. Cohen LM, Ruthazer R, Moss AH, Germain MJ. Predicting six-month mortality for patients who are on maintenance hemodialysis. Clin J Am Soc Nephrol. 2010;5(1):72–9.
13. Chowdhury R, Peel NM, Krosch M, Hubbard RE. Frailty and chronic kidney disease: a systematic review. Arch Gerontol Geriatr. 2017;68:135–42.
14. Kurella Tamura M, Covinsky KE, Chertow GM, et al. Functional status of elderly adults before and after initiation of dialysis. N Engl J Med. 2009;361:1539–47.
15. Jassal SV, Chiu E, Hladunewich M. Loss of independence in patients starting dialysis at 80 years of age or older. N Engl J Med. 2009;361:1612–3.
16. Gomez AT, Kiberd BA, Royston JP, Alfaadhel T, Soroka SD, Hemmelgarn BR, Tennankore KK. Comorbidity burden at dialysis initiation and mortality: a cohort study. Can J Kidney Health Dis. 2015;2:34. https://doi.org/10.1186/s40697-015-0068-3. eCollection 2015.
17. Pugh J, Aggett J, Goodland A, et al. Frailty and comorbidity are independent predictors of outcome in patients referred for pre-dialysis education. Clin Kidney J. 2016;9(2):324–9.
18. RPA. Shared decision-making in the appropriate initiation of withdrawal from dialysis. Rockville: Renal Physicians Association (RPA); 2010.
19. Warwick G, Mooney A, Russon L, Hardy R. Planning, initiating and withdrawal of renal replacement therapy UK Renal Association 2014.
20. Burns A, Davenport A. Maximum conservative management for patients with chronic kidney disease stage 5. Hemodial Int Int Symp Home Hemodial. 2010;14(Suppl 1):S32–7.
21. Reindl-Schwaighofer R, Kainz A, Kammer M, Dumfarth A, Oberbauer R. Survival analysis of conservative vs. dialysis treatment of elderly patients with CKD stage 5. PLoS One. 2017;12(7):e0181345. https://doi.org/10.1371/journal.pone.0181345.
22. Murtagh FE, Addington-Hall J, Edmonds P, et al. Symptoms in the month before death for stage 5 chronic kidney disease patients managed without dialysis. J Pain Symptom Manag. 2010;40:342–52.
23. Douglas C, Murtagh FE, Chambers EJ, Howse M, Ellershaw J. Symptom management for the adult patient dying with advanced chronic kidney disease: a review of the literature and development of evidence-based guidelines by a United Kingdom Expert Consensus Group. Palliat Med. 2009;23:103–10. https://doi.org/10.1177/0269216308100247.
24. Levin A, Hemmelgarn B, Culleton B, et al. Guidelines for the management of chronic kidney disease. CMAJ. 2008;179:1154–62.
25. Brown SA, Tyrer FC, Clarke AL, et al. Symptom burden in patients with chronic kidney disease not requiring renal replacement therapy. Clin Kidney J. 2017;10(6):788–96.
26. http://www.who.int/cancer/palliative/definition/en/.
27. Department of Health, Western Australia. Pathway for renal palliative care services in Western Australia. Perth: Health Networks Branch, Department of Health, Western Australia; 2012.
28. The Lancet Global Health. End-stage kidney disease in LMICs: rising to the challenge. Lancet Glob Health. 2017;5(4):e370.
29. Bates MJ, Chitani A, Dreyer G. Palliative care needs of patients living with end-stage kidney disease not treated with renal replacement therapy: an exploratory qualitative study from Blantyre, Malawi. Afr J Prim Health Care Fam Med. 2017;9(1):e1–6.
30. WHO world report on ageing and health 2015. http://apps.who.int/iris/bitstream/10665/186463/1/9789240694811_eng.pdf.

Index

C. G. Musso et al. (eds.), *Clinical Nephrogeriatrics*,
https://doi.org/10.1007/978-3-030-18711-8

D

E

The manufacturer's authorised representative in the EU is Springer Nature Customer Service Centre GmbH, Europaplatz 3, 69115 Heidelberg, Germany. If you have any concerns regarding our products, please contact ProductSafety@springernature.com

Printed and bound by CPI Group (UK) Ltd, Croydon, CR0 4YY
30/07/2026
02181710-0002